Impairment Rating *and* Disability Evaluation

Impairment Rating *and* Disability Evaluation

ROBERT D. RONDINELLI, MD, PhD
Professor and Chairman
Department of Rehabilitation Medicine
University of Kansas Medical Center
Kansas City, Kansas

RICHARD T. KATZ, MD
Associate Clinical Professor of Internal Medicine and Orthopedics
St. Louis University School of Medicine
St. Louis, Missouri

W.B. SAUNDERS COMPANY
A Division of Harcourt Brace and Company
Philadelphia, London, Sydney, Toronto

W.B. SAUNDERS COMPANY
A Division of Harcourt Brace & Company

The Curtis Center
Independence Square West
Philadelphia, Pennsylvania 19106

Library of Congress Cataloging-in-Publication Data

Impairment rating and disability evaluation / [edited by] Robert D. Rondinelli. Richard T. Katz.

p. cm.

ISBN 0-7216-7772-X

1. Disability evaluation. I. Rondinelli, Robert D. II. Katz, Richard T.
[DNLM: 1. Disability Evaluation—Canada. 2. Disability Evaluation—United States. 3. Social Security—Canada. 4. Social Security—United States. 5. Workers' Compensation—Canada. 6. Workers' Compensation—United States. W 925 R7711 2000]

RC963.4.I48 2000
362.4′042—dc21

DNLM/DLC 99-26872

Cover art from Dürer A: Hierin sind begriffen vier Bücher von menschlicher Proportion, Nürenberg, 1528. (Courtesy of the Clendening History of Medicine Library, University of Kansas Medical Center, Kansas City, Kansas.)

IMPAIRMENT RATING AND DISABILITY EVALUATION ISBN 0-7216-7772-X

Printed in the United States of America

Last digit is the print number: 9 8 7 6 5 4 3 2 1

Contributors

Richard P. Bonfiglio, MD
Medical Director,
HealthSouth Harmarville Rehabilitation Hospital;
Chairman,
Department of Physical Medicine and Rehabilitation;
Medical Director, Rehabilitation Services,
Suburban General Hospital;
Division Chief, Physical Medicine and Rehabilitation,
The Western Pennsylvania Hospital,
Pittsburgh, Pennsylvania

Mikel Cook, RPT, MPA
Director of Rehabilitation Services,
Employer Health Services and Baptist Medical Center,
Health Midwest,
Kansas City, Missouri

Glenn Dabatos, RPT
Progressive Physical Therapy,
Santa Clarita, California

Pamela W. Duncan, PT, PhD
Professor, Health Policy and Management,
University of Kansas Medical Center,
Kansas City, Kansas

Richard Z. Freemann, Jr., BS, JD
Attorney at Law,
Philadelphia, Pennsylvania

Steve R. Geiringer, MD
Professor,
Department of Physical Medicine and Rehabilitation,
Wayne State University,
Detroit, Michigan

Andrew J. Haig, MD
Assistant Professor,
Departments of Physical Medicine and Rehabilitation and Surgery;
Medical Director,
Spine Program and WorkWise Program,
University of Michigan Spine Program,
University of Michigan,
Ann Arbor, Michigan

Steven R. Hinderer, MD, MS, PT
Assistant Professor,
Department of Physical Medicine and Rehabilitation,
Wayne State University School of Medicine;
Medical Director of Research and the Clinical Rehabilitation Research Unit,
Rehabilitation Institute of Michigan,
Detroit, Michigan

Richard T. Katz, MD
Associate Clinical Professor of Internal Medicine and Orthopedics,
St. Louis University School of Medicine,
St. Louis, Missouri

Michel Lacerte, MDCM, MSc
Associate Professor,
University of Western Ontario,
Faculty of Medicine and Dentistry,
Department of Physical Medicine and Rehabilitation,
London, Ontario, Canada

Alan K. Novick, MD
Medical Director of the Interdisciplinary Programs,
Park Place Therapeutic Center,
Plantation, Florida

Steven Oboler, MD
Associate Clinical Professor of Medicine,
University of Colorado Health Sciences Center;
Clinical Director, Compensation and Pension Unit,
Veterans Affairs Medical Center,
Denver, Colorado

Atul T. Patel, MD
Associate Professor,
Department of Rehabilitation Medicine,
University of Kansas Medical Center,
Kansas City, Kansas

Mohammed I. Ranavaya, MD, MS, FACPM
Associate Professor, Occupational Medicine,
West Virginia University School of Medicine;
Medical Director,
Appalachian Institute of Occupational and Environmental Medicine,
Morgantown, West Virginia

James P. Robinson, MD, PhD
Clinical Assistant Professor,
Department of Rehabilitation Medicine,
University of Washington,
Seattle, Washington

Robert D. Rondinelli, MD, PhD
Professor and Chairman,
Department of Rehabilitation Medicine,
University of Kansas Medical Center,
Kansas City, Kansas

Steven J. Scheer, MD
Voluntary Professor,
Department of Physical Medicine and Rehabilitation,
University of Cincinnati Medical Center,
Cincinnati, Ohio

William Stiers, PhD
Clinical Associate Professor,
Chief, Rehabilitation Psychology and Neuropsychology,
University of Kansas Medical Center,
Kansas City, Kansas

Raymond C. Tait, PhD
Professor,
Department of Psychiatry,
St. Louis University School of Medicine,
St. Louis, Missouri

Claire V. Wolfe, MD
Clinical Assistant Professor,
Physical Medicine and Rehabilitation,
Ohio State University College of Medicine;
Active Staff,
Department of Medicine,
Mt. Carmel Medical Center,
Columbus, Ohio

To our parents, who guided us to be productive; to our wives and children for their patience, love, and dedicated understanding; and to our students and teachers who make this all worthwhile.

Preface

It may be as humane to save one who is disabled from years of dependency, as to save his life.

Frank H. Krusen

Our purpose in writing this textbook is to provide, under single cover, an overview of the concepts and models of disablement and the major U.S. and Canadian disability systems. Particular attention has been paid to the definitions and terminologies inherent to each system and to the evaluating and reporting requirements each system poses to the disability examiner.

The impetus to develop this textbook has been spurred on, in part, by the realization that a majority of medical residents in training receive little or no formal didactic teaching about disability evaluation during their residencies. This includes residents in neurology, neurosurgery, occupational medicine, orthopedic surgery, plastic surgery, physical medicine and rehabilitation (PM&R), psychiatry, and rheumatology, to mention a few. Furthermore, the past decade has witnessed a rapid growth of interest within the field of medicine concerning disability evaluation. The educational demands thus created have fostered the emergence of the American Academy of Disability Evaluating Physicians (AADEP), the introduction of the American Board of Independent Medical Examiners (ABIME) certification exam, and the development of several formal didactic courses offered by organizations such as the American College of Occupational and Environmental Medicine (ACOEM), AADEP, and the American Academy of PM&R. Although such courses typically offer a printed syllabus, there has been no general reference textbook beyond the American Medical Association's *Guides to the Evaluation of Permanent Impairment* (AMA *Guides*) to assist in tackling the broader aspects of this topic.

Impairment and disability are the conceptual linchpins for the specialty of PM&R and provide the major focus for virtually all of rehabilitative problem solving. As physiatrists (PM&R specialists), we have developed clinical practices that emphasize the evaluation, treatment, rating, and reporting of impairment and disability. Our collective expertise draws largely from self-taught procedures and insights we have gathered through a cumulative 32 years of clinical experience. We have had opportunity to train our colleagues and students—initially through informal lectures and invited presentations—and subsequently as organizing faculty for the American Academy of PM&R Disability Evaluation Certificate Course. Along the way, we were disappointed with the limited quantity and quality of contemporary references available and applicable to our teaching efforts. Furthermore, the most notable and accessible references had been authored by specialists primarily outside the field of PM&R. This includes the AMA *Guides*. Historically, PM&R representation on the list of contributing authors to the AMA *Guides* has been disproportionately low, and particularly so for a profession that claims a clinical expertise encompassing nonoperative musculoskeletal medicine. Indeed, less than 5% of PM&R physician consultants contributed to the most recent (fourth) edition of the AMA *Guides,* whereas at least 40% of the content remains devoted to discussing the musculoskeletal system alone. We feel that this topic is most deserving of our professional attention, and that physiatrists should be at the forefront of contributions to current clinical thinking about evaluation of impairment and disability.

The book comprises four sections. The first is intended to provide a historical overview of disability systems as a form of social justice, to explore concepts and terminology inherent to disability evaluation, and to examine practical and theoretical limitations to measurement of impairment and disability, with applications to the AMA *Guides*.

In the second section, we review clinical assessment tools available with applications toward measurement of physical and psychological impairment and disability, examine the therapist's role in evaluating disability through functional capacity evaluation, and examine the physician's role in work disability management.

In the third section we examine each of the major U.S. disability systems including Workers' Compensation, Social Security, and compensation and pensioning within the Veterans Administration. We also provide a comparative overview of the Canadian disability system.

In our final section, we discuss key medicolegal and practical aspects of a physician disability practice including the Independent Medical Evaluation (IME), managing the "difficult patient," life care planning, and medicolegal aspects of disability-related documentation and testimony.

This textbook is in no way intended to be a critique of the AMA *Guides*. As clinicians and educators, we continue to find the AMA *Guides* to be a highly useful reference that provides a current, widely-accepted, standard framework for evaluating and reporting impairment and disability. In addressing shortcomings of the AMA *Guides*, we are implicating the field, and our hope is to call attention to the much-needed scientific scrutiny of practices inherent to this field.

We are hopeful that our textbook will prove useful to a variety of disability evaluating clinicians—including primary care physicians, specialty physicians, and chiropractic specialists alike—who may be practicing disability evaluations within one or more of the U.S. and Canadian disability systems. It will hopefully prove useful to allied health professionals, including physical, occupational, and speech therapists; rehabilitation psychologists; exercise physiologists; vocational rehabilitation counselors; nurse practitioners; and physician extenders dealing with medical impairment and disability. It is also intended to address the needs of insurance case managers for Workers Compensation, Social Security, personal injury claims, and for enlightened attorneys dealing with disability claims litigation.

Robert D. Rondinelli
Richard T. Katz

Acknowledgements

In addition to our contributing authors, we would like to acknowledge the following individuals, whose time, effort, and input helped make this project possible:

Randall Braddom, MD, Past President of the American Academy of PM&R, for his foresight in organizing the Academy Disability Evaluation Course and for showcasing us as course developers and faculty.

The University of Kansas Rehabilitation Association provided direct and indirect support and encouragement during all phases of this project.

Tamara Tipton provided tireless clerical and secretarial support.

The following individuals provided helpful ideas, suggestions, encouragement, criticism, and/or feedback at various stages of this project, and their assistance is gratefully acknowledged: Thomas Beller, MD; Susan Blaney, Esq.; David Cifu, MD; Linda Cocchiarella, MD; David Frayer, PhD; Ernest Johnson, MD; Robert Jurmain, PhD; Robert King, RPT; Robert Martensen, MD, PhD; Robert Meier III, MD; Jerry Misiw, MD; and Gale Whitekeck, PhD.

Any shortcomings, oversights, or errors are, of course, regrettable and remain our sole responsibility.

Robert D. Rondinelli

Richard T. Katz

Contents

Impairment Rating *and* Disability Evaluation

SECTION I

Conceptual Overview

CHAPTER 1

The Major U.S. Disability and Compensation Systems: Origins and Historical Overview

Mohammed I. Ranavaya MD, MS   *Robert D. Rondinelli MD, PhD*

It is written in the Bible that "if any would not work, neither should he eat."[35] Hence there has been a long-standing expectation among individuals within society that members must contribute individually to benefit and share collectively. It appears equally true that individual members who cannot contribute because of disability may be exempt from such expectation and yet still enjoy benefits to which other group members are entitled. It is also possible for an individual to exploit society through unfair and exaggerated claims of disability, which becomes an issue of social justice. Although social justice systems compensate in some way for bodily illness or injury, they must also afford protection against benefits being paid to those who choose not to be productive and fake or exaggerate their disability. Disability and compensation systems provide rules defining disability and entitlement as well as procedures for determining who qualifies as disabled. These rules are intended to provide fair and equitable distribution of limited system resources to those whose needs are greatest and whose disabilities are most compelling.

Within the United States, various disability and compensation systems have arisen to ensure that members of society with a medically determinable impairment that may lead to disability have recourse to compensation from various avenues, including state and federal workers' compensation laws, veterans benefits, and social welfare programs where appropriate. These systems have diverse historical origins and statutory requirements; consequently, there remains considerable variability between them with respect to definitions of disability, entitlement, benefits, claims application procedures, adjudication, and the role and relative weight given to medical versus administrative deliberations. In most cases, a medical determination of physical or psychological impairment is necessary, and in some cases the physician is empowered to render an opinion regarding the nature and extent of medically determined impairment resulting in disability. It is imperative that physicians be familiar with precise meanings and definitions of the terms *impairment* and *disability,* as well as the fundamental requirements, nuances, and jurisdictional variations of the particular disability system within which they are working.

This overview examines the historical origins of the major U.S. disability systems and highlights the fundamental similarities and contrasts between them.

EVIDENCE FROM PRIMITIVE AND PREHISTORIC SOCIETIES

Tolerance of and care for the disabled may be elemental components of our social fabric rooted in the very origins of human society. From the outset, our earliest ancestors may have been afforded communal benefits in terms of improved odds of survival of hereditary and acquired physical impairments that might otherwise prove fatal to the individual.

Evidence exists within contemporary species of nonhuman social primates to suggest that this is so. For example, individual society members frequently suffer incapacitating injuries and disfigurement during their lifetime, yet survive into adulthood and thrive within their group. To illustrate, Schultz [29, 30] describes advanced crippling arthritic changes in 55% of skeletons from mature and aged specimens of wild-shot gibbons, who are traditionally socially monogamous. Furthermore, diseases affecting dentition (including severe caries, alveolar abscesses, and maxillary sinus infections) and those that produce pathological and disfiguring changes in the skull are commonly seen among free-ranging chimpanzees and gorillas. Many arboreal primates are prone to life-threatening falls and, if not killed outright, can frequently survive joint dislocations, single and multiple fractures of limb bones, and even cranial fractures. Such fractures may heal to a serviceable degree, or with nonunion, lead to pseudarthrosis and foreshortening of limbs in some cases (Fig. 1–1).[17, 30] The relationship between observed patterns of social behavior within higher primate species and the incidence, prevalence, morbidity, and mortality associated with such disabilities remains incompletely understood, but a facilitative and supportive role is suggested.

Among the earliest evidence of survival and recovery from major trauma among prehuman hominid species is a fossil specimen of *Australopithecus* (KNM ER 738) from Kenya that is believed to be between 1 and 2 million years old.[21] The remains include the neck and proximal shaft portion of a left femur

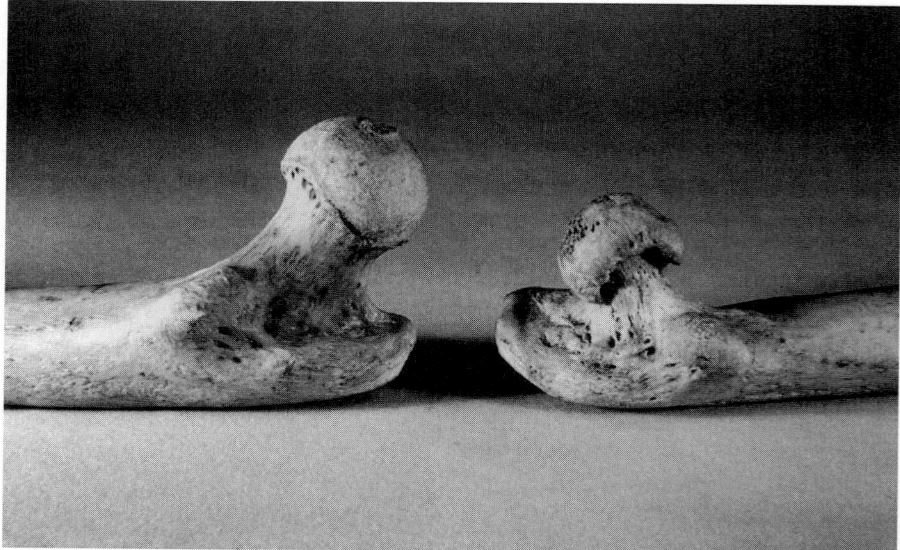

FIGURE 1–1
Right and left femora of an adult female gorilla, Powell-Cotton collection. The left femur head and neck are severely remodeled after fracture and dislocation. (Courtesy Robert Jurmain, PhD.)

that reveal signs of a healed fracture callus distal to the lesser trochanter, suggesting that the original owner once survived a catastrophic and potentially disabling injury.

Other evidence from the fossil record suggests that severe trauma was indeed prevalent among Pleistocene human populations and that survival was clearly possible after catastrophic injury. Perhaps the best example of this can be seen among skeletons excavated at Shanidar Cave in northeastern Iraq, dating to approximately 60,000 years ago. Partial skeletons of nine Neanderthals from the site have been described.[33] Four of the six reasonably complete adult skeletons show some form of trauma-related abnormality, and at least two were severely incapacitated by their injuries. The best known of these, Shanidar 1, was an adult male who died between 35 and 50 years of age after surviving a crushing blow to the left orbit, frontal, and zygomatic portion of the skull during his lifetime (Fig. 1–2). As a result of this injury, he was presumably blind and severely disfigured from enucleation of his left eye, and apparently suffered right arm and leg paralysis and associated long-bone atrophy/hypotrophy and joint deformity. Ultimately, he suffered an amputation of the right elbow, and was later killed when a ceiling collapsed on him. In another well-known Croatian Neanderthal site at Krapina, the remains of an amputated and healed proximal half of a right ulna have been found.[25] These findings reflect a remarkably high incidence of traumatic injury and recovery coupled with a level of societal development in which the disabled were somehow well cared for by other members of the group.[33]

Excavations from an Upper Paleolithic (11,000 years old) site in southern Italy yield evidence of dwarfism in a hunter-gatherer society. An adolescent individual has been described with characteristic deformities reflecting severe growth deficiency and restrictions in elbow mobility. These physical impairments undoubtedly interfered with the individual's participation in subsistence activities and may have been a substantial handicap for such a nomadic hunter-gatherer. Yet there is no evidence of nutritional stress according to skeletal and dental indicators (i.e., dental hypoplasia). Furthermore, the individual received a funeral, as evidenced by his burial in an important cave—a privilege typically reserved for those of special social status among the group at that time. Consequently, the capacity for group acceptance and support, despite severe nontraumatic handicaps that would limit the ability to contribute to group subsistence, was already evident among the stone-age populations of Europe.[14]

These examples are but a brief account of the widespread acceptance of the physically disabled in prehistoric societies, as evidenced by the fossil record.

HISTORICAL EVIDENCE

Historical evidence suggests that social justice and systems of compensation have existed and been linked since ancient times. Records exist from ancient Persian societies detailing compensation for injuries suffered in relation to the social order of that time. As far back as 4000 years ago, Babylon compensated for loss of life or limb while in service of the state. For example, the Code of Hammurabi (1750 BC) was an ancient Babylonian legal code, written in cuneiform, and containing laws purportedly given to King Hammurabi by Shamash, the Babylonian god of justice.[12] The code represents an advanced attempt to legislate justice in moral, social, and economic spheres[18] with

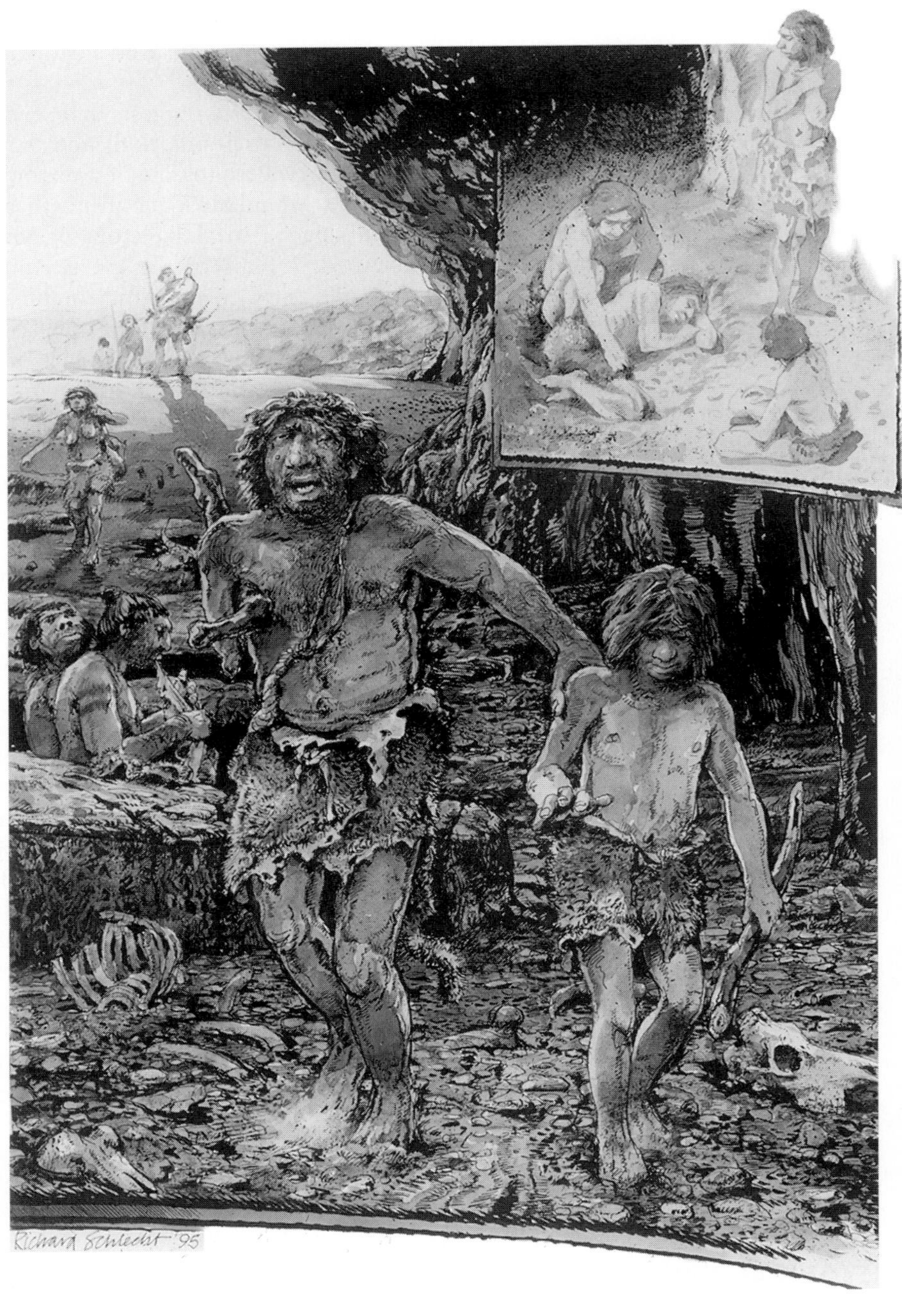

FIGURE 1–2
Neanderthal man. (With permission from Schlecht R: Neanderthals. National Geographic 189(1): 20, 1996.)

provisions that decreed punitive action to be taken against a person causing bodily injury, and it bears a striking resemblance to the Mosaic laws.[34] Among these was the principle of Lex Talonis, the "law of retaliation" or "principle of equivalence," which existed to compensate for wrongful bodily injury but dictated that societal retribution should be the same in kind as the offense, as in an "eye for and eye and a tooth for a tooth."[13]

The Laws of Eshnunna were a more enlightened yet contemporary approach, as evidenced from the cuneiform text of the Old Babylonian kingdom of Eshnunna. The laws were a compilation of rules and ordinances recommending monetary compensation for bodily harm, as the writing attests: "If a man bit and severed the nose of a man, 1 mina silver he shall weigh out. An eye, 1 mina; a tooth, ½ mina; an ear, ½ mina. A slap in the face, 10 shekels silver he shall weigh out."[38]

Among the ancient Egyptians, similar laws provided compensation for wrongful acts resulting in injury. Punitive actions, often severe, could be taken against physicians for acts of malpractice, such as amputating a physician's hands for causing blindness to a patient after removal of cataracts.[24]

Evidence of social compensation exists for other Western societies, including the ancient Greeks, who provided compensation for injured parties. The soldiers or survivors of Alexander the Great's army were compensated for losses of life and limb incurred during the course of military service. In Roman society, compensation was available for both free men and slaves, yet social status dictated that slaves received less compensation than free men.[16] Furthermore, Roman masters were obligated to care for their injured slaves. The concept of Respondeat Superior was also introduced, which created the legal obligation of a master to answer for the wrongful doings of his servants. This concept still exists in common law and in military doctrine in which subordinate members who are bound to obey their superiors in turn derive legal protection and immunity for actions taken and consequences of following orders.[6]

Around the birth of Christ the Germanic and Nordic tribes (Lombards) were establishing themselves on the western edge of the Roman empire as civilized members of the empire. Consequently, the blood feud, formerly used as a means of securing justice, was formally prohibited and the state assumed the role of administering justice between the injured and the accused. The compensation for injuries was based on a "whole person" concept. Each tribesman was considered to have an intrinsic monetary value—his wergild or "man value"—which varied according to social status and was typically worth 200 Roman solidi. This was the value of his life, or 100% whole-body impairment. There was a schedule for all sorts of injuries, from as trivial as injury to a toe to loss of limbs, eyes, and life itself. An even greater compensation was awarded for cosmetic loss; thus if one knocked out one's molar tooth, the compensation was eight solidi (4% of the wergild), but loss of a tooth that showed on a smile was equal to 16 solidi (8% of the wergild).[8] The impairment values are extraordinarily similar to those used today.

State-sponsored care for the poor and disabled without a responsible party (the concept of social security) has a tradition in history as well. The first state-sponsored social security system was established by Muslims in 640 AD during the reign of the second Caliph Omar. The state treasury provided monthly benefits to those afflicted with blindness, and to widows and orphans.

During the Middle Ages a paternalistic system existed in which feudal lords were obligated to care for subjects within their serfdom who became ill or injured. Various craft guilds were formed and developed an early form of disability insurance whereby healthy members of the guild contributed regularly to a fund that was made available to members in the event of injury or illness.[26]

Social compensation systems were not unique to civil society.[22] During the sixteenth and seventeenth centuries the buccaneers of America were engaged in acts of maritime piracy against vessels of trade between Europe and the colonies. Their system of laws was embodied in the ship's "articles of association" and was agreed to by signature of each crew member at the outset of any voyage. The articles specified sums of salary to be paid to the captain and various crew members, the source being the common stock of illegally acquired goods from that particular expedition. Furthermore, they contained an early form of workers' compensation agreement to recompense crew members for serious bodily harm suffered during the voyage. An example follows:

> ". . . they order for the loss of a right arm 600 pieces of eight or 6 slaves; for the loss of a left arm 500 pieces of eight or 5 slaves; for a right leg 500 pieces of eight or 5 slaves; for a left leg 400 pieces of eight or 4 slaves; for an eye 100 pieces of eight or 1 slave; for a finger of the hand the same reward as for the eye."[9]

CHANGES OF INDUSTRIALIZED SOCIETY

During the nineteenth century, London society regarded the working class and poor in terms of three categories—those who would work, those who could not work, and those who would not work. "Poor laws" were devised to determine those destitute but worthy of charity versus those deserving punishment. Sums of money were set aside under the auspices of local parishes and able-bodied members of the parish regularly contributed to the fund. Such funds were to be used to aid the lame, blind, elderly, and otherwise disabled poor. A board of commissioners was appointed to manage these funds by overseeing their disbursement. An able-bodied person who refused to work risked imprisonment or other punishment and faced "life on the street" unless he could successfully plead his case before such a commissioner.[23]

Among the changes brought about as nineteenth-century society became increasingly industrialized was the increase in the proportion of society members working for low wages. Fear of injury or death in the workplace was a significant concern. Local governments became increasingly concerned with strategies for provision of medical service to the poor and destitute, the systematic and equitable spreading of costs of indigent care, and compensating for lost wages among the working and middle class.[1]

Medical care was often provided by low-paid or unpaid doctors in training at hospitals maintained through charity and public subsidy. Medical insurance policies, per se, did not exist, and workers often went into debt or failed to pay medical bills altogether.[15] Workers fearing loss of income because of injury or illness resorted to the purchase of disability insurance to provide "sick pay" or "death benefits" to cover funeral costs.[1]

COMMON LAW AND THE RISE OF TORT CLAIMS

The United States inherited most of its common law from England, which has its roots dating back to the twelfth century in the reign of King Henry II when he delegated his judicial powers to various magistrates and judges. The country was divided into six circuits, and the king appointed three judges for each circuit who were charged with deciding civil cases based on precedent (prior decisions and the common customs of society), hence the term *common law.* This is based on the legal doctrine of *stari decicis,* which means "let the decision stand." The idea is to have a certain predictability in the law for those cases with circumstances similar to cases from the past. The aspect of common law most applicable to the practice of disability medicine involves tort liability. A tort is defined as a "breach of duty that gives rise to an action for damages"[28] and implies civil wrongdoing. Typically, there are four elements of a tort claim that must be proved before an adjudicating authority: (1) a legal duty existed, (2) a breach of legal duty occurred, (3) this breach of duty was the proximate or direct cause of harm or injury, and (4) harm or damage occurred as a result.

Liability under common law was often the only recourse whereby an injured worker could obtain compensation after injury in the workplace. It was burdensome to the plaintiff in terms of time and expense, and exceedingly difficult to prove employer negligence in a court of law because of three powerful defense strategies available to the employer that were often referred to as the "unholy trinity"[31] or the three "Wicked Sisters." The first defense was contributory negligence. If claimants could be shown to have contributed to their injuries through their own negligent actions, this would preclude their ability to recover damages against the employer, regardless of the extent of employer negligence. A second defense involved assumption of risk. If it could be shown that an injury was related to the inherent risks of the job, of which the worker knew or should have had prior knowledge, the injured worker could not recover damages by virtue of having accepted the job and thereby assumed its hazardous risks. A third defense was the "fellow servant doctrine." An employee could not recover damages if it could be shown that the injury resulted from a fellow worker's negligent actions. With these three defense strategies, it was unlikely that an injured employee could collect for damages under common law, where less than one in five tort claims were settled in favor of the plaintiff.[20]

At present, tort claims may arise out of a personal injury caused by motor vehicle accidents, toxic exposure, medical malpractice, or defective products. Criteria for recovery for damages may vary depending on jurisdiction.

WORKERS' COMPENSATION

Because of inadequacies of recovery from claims under common law, various workers' compensation statutes were enacted around the turn of the century. A Workmen's Accident Insurance Law was passed in 1884 as part of a comprehensive social insurance system in Germany. In England the Employers' Liability Act of 1880 and the Workers' Compensation Act of 1887 were passed to afford disability insurance protection to injured workers. In 1907 at St. Petersburg, Russia a disability indemnification schedule was introduced for regional bodily injury according to the concept of the "whole person."

In the United States the first Workers' Compensation Act was enacted in 1908 as a Federal Employers Liability Act, which was designed to provide for injured railroad workers. Wisconsin became the first state to sign Workers' Compensation into law on May 3, 1911[32] and New Jersey followed suit in 1912.[27] The California Industrial Accident Act of 1914 created a schedule of indemnification according to claimant's age, occupation, and physical impairment. By 1949 all states had enacted a Workers' Compensation Law, which is now mandatory in most employment in almost all states.

Under Workers' Compensation, a "no fault" system was adopted to resolve the dilemmas of the tort claims process by providing automatic coverage to employees whose claims of injury arise "out of and in the course of employment." In exchange, covered employees forego the right to sue the employer in most instances, except in cases of wanton neglect.

Further developments concerning the U.S. Workers' Compensation system are discussed in detail in Chapter 8.

SOCIAL SECURITY

A loosely structured welfare system existed within the United States as far back as colonial times.[37] Initial programs were informal, voluntary, and operated at the community level. By the early 1900s social and state-funded programs were in place. The Social Security Act of 1935 was the first federally mandated program and was implemented during the administration of Franklin D. Roosevelt as an attempt to create a federal social welfare system after the Great Depression. Initially, the program was intended to address the needs of individuals disadvantaged by means of old age, unemployment, disability, or death of a spouse. Under Title II of the act, an Old Age Insurance pension was established for workers when they reached age 65.

The Social Security Administration (SSA) is the largest disability program in the United States, assisting between 33% and 50% of all persons qualified as disabled.[7] It includes two separate disability benefits programs. The first is Social Security Disability Insurance (SSDI), a program established in 1956 to create a separate fund for workers over age 50 who were totally and permanently disabled. SSDI is federally administered through the SSA and funded through a payroll tax that combines deductions for old age and disability (OASDI). The application process is initiated at the state level with the Bureau of Disability Determination. To be eligible, an individual must have worked in a job covered by SSDI for a minimum period (in general, 5 of the 10 years preceding the onset of disability). Pension benefits are provided to disabled individuals who have contributed through payroll taxes (FICA) during the requisite period, and whose disability involves total incapacitation.

Supplemental Security Income (SSI) is a second disability benefits program within the SSA, which operates as a federal-state partnership. SSI provides benefits to disabled individuals whose income and assets meet minimum criteria according to a "means test." It is funded through general revenue (i.e., income tax revenues) and does not require work history for eligibility. For further detailed discussions of SSA, SSDI, and SSI, see Chapter 9.

FEDERAL EMPLOYERS LIABILITY ACT

The Federal Employers Liability Act (FELA) was enacted in 1908 to provide disability benefits to employees of the interstate railroad industry for job-related injuries. At that time railroads were the largest employer and rail work was exceptionally hazardous. Before passage of the act, injured employees would seek redress under tort claims as previously described. FELA limited employer defenses to only contributory negligence (and now modified to comparative negligence for which an award is apportioned according to percentage of employer versus employee culpability) and increased employers' awareness for liability and incentive for prevention of workplace injuries.

FELA remains a potentially adversarial system in which the injured employee may negotiate an out of court settlement. Alternatively, a claimant may file suit for personal losses against the railroad in either a state civil court or federal court. Under FELA, a claimant must prove negligence on the part of the railroad. In turn, the railroad may assert a defense of comparative negligence, whereby recovery for damages can be proportionately reduced. FELA enables a claimant to recover economic damages as well as compensation for pain and suffering. Additional benefits might include retirement and sickness and disability annuities.[10]

JONES ACT (MERCHANT MARINE ACT)

The Jones Act (Merchant Marine Act) of 1920 is similar to FELA but covers civilian sailors for permanent injury suffered while in the service of a ship in navigable water. To collect, the claimant must bring suit against the master or owner of the ship. Cases are typically settled out of court because seamen are regarded as wards of the states and thereby enjoy liberal treatment by the court system in general.

FEDERAL WORKERS' COMPENSATION PROGRAMS

Federal Employees Compensation Act

The Federal Employees Compensation Act (FECA) was enacted to provide compensation benefits to civilian employees of the federal government for work-related disability. Presently, it covers more than 3 million civilian employees of the U.S. Government, Postal Service, and Peace Corps, as well as such nonfederal employees as state and local law enforcement personnel and employees of the Civil Air Patrol. FECA is a no-fault system and, consequently, a federal employee cannot sue the federal government or recover damages under any other statute for work-related injuries. Changes in the law in 1974, whereby continued pay was offered to workers injured on the job, resulted in a dramatic increase in the incidence of claims.[19] There is no time limit on wage loss or medical benefits and no cap on medical benefits. FECA is federally administered under the Office of Workers' Compensation Program (OWCP) in Washington, D.C.[11]

Longshore and Harbor Workers' Compensation Act

The Longshore and Harbor Workers' Compensation Act (LHWCA) was enacted in 1927 to provide compensation benefits to shoreside maritime employees for occupational disabilities received while engaged in longshore work, ship building and repair, and other maritime activity. It is a no-fault system federally administered under the U.S. Department of Labor.[11]

Federal Black Lung Program

The Federal Black Lung Program was created by the Federal Mine Safety & Health Act of 1977 to provide coverage for coal miners engaged in surface or underground activity. The act provides monthly pension and medical benefits for total disability caused by pneumoconiosis (black lung) arising from employment in and around coal mines.[16] It is administered through the U.S. Department of Labor.

The diagnosis of pneumoconiosis under the act may be ascertained through findings on a chest x-ray according to the International Lave Office (ILO)

Classification system. Chest x-rays of claimants are read by "B-readers," who are medical specialists with certification by the National Institute of Occupational Health and Safety (NIOSH) to read chest x-rays of dust-exposed individuals according to the ILO classification. The miner must also show total disability from pulmonary causes as documented by pulmonary function testing. The U.S. Department of Labor has published predetermined disability standards for spirometric values and arterial blood gas values against which a disability claim is referenced.[27] It is estimated that the average cost per miner found eligible for disability benefits under the program is from $350,000 to $500,000 over their remaining life span.

Physicians desiring to serve as evaluators for claims arising within FECA, LHWCA, and the Federal Black Lung Program should contact the Office of Workers' Compensation Programs (OWCP), 200 Constitution Avenue, Room 53522, Washington, DC 20210.

DEPARTMENT OF VETERANS AFFAIRS

The Department of Veterans Affairs (VA) was established in 1930 as the Veterans Administration to "consolidate and coordinate" government activities affecting American veterans of war. The Veterans Benefits Administration (VBA) was originally established as the Department of Veterans Benefits within the VA in 1953 to administer the GI Bill and VA compensation and pension programs. Presently, the Compensation and Pension Service rests within the VBA.

Eligibility for compensation and pensioning within the VA is extended to all veterans who receive honorable or general discharge from active military service.[3] Entitlement decisions are administratively handled by the Adjudication Division of the Compensation and Pension Service. Service-connected entitlement refers to conditions determined by adjudication to be related to injury or disease incurred or aggravated while on active duty, whereas non–service-connected entitlement refers to conditions determined to be unrelated to active duty.[4] VA benefits include disability pensions in the form of monthly monetary support to the veteran because of service-connected disability, or to a spouse, child, or parent of the veteran in the event of service-connected death.[5] Additional benefits include hospitalization and medical care, orthotic and prosthetic devices, durable medical equipment, and allowances for adaptive modifications to the veteran's home and/or motor vehicle where necessary.

Title 38 of the Code of Federal Regulations contains both the VA's Schedule for Rating Disabilities (Part 4) and other VA regulations pertaining to compensation and pension (Part 3). Volume I of Title 38 contains Parts 0 to 17. Ten of the 16 body systems in the rating schedule have been recently revised. The 1997 edition does not contain the current versions of rating systems for muscle injuries and cardiovascular system, which were published in the Federal Register on June 3, 1997 and December 11, 1997, respectively. Each went into effect 30 days after the date of publication. They are available online through the Library of Congress website at *lcweb.loc.gov.*

The process of compensation requires a veteran to apply for compensation for a particular condition. The claim must be well-grounded, which means certain legal requirements must be met. If they are, the rater in a regional office may grant the benefit if the medical evidence of record is sufficient on which to rate (e.g., the service medical records may suffice in a recently discharged veteran), and the regulatory and statutory requirements for service connection are met. Some conditions may only be service connected directly; that is, there must be evidence that the condition began while the veteran was in the service. Many chronic conditions may be service connected if they began within a 1-year period after service was completed; some may be service connected much later if linked to service (e.g., because of herbicide or radiation exposure while in service). If a medical examination is needed, the rater will request one from a VA medical facility through a computerized request process. Some of the examinations may be contracted out if, for example, the required specialist is not available at a particular VA facility.

The VA examiner will receive a computer-generated set of worksheets for guidance as to the requirements of the particular examinations requested. If the examination, and any requested opinions about relationships, etc., are sufficient for rating purposes, the rater will apply the medical information to the rating schedule and assign a rating. Rating decisions require either one or two signatures. A physician need not sign any rating. Physicians make diagnoses only and give medical opinions or interpretations.

There is a local appellate process for veterans who have been denied benefits. Beyond that, there is the Board of Veterans Appeals in Washington, D.C., and, finally, there is the U.S. Court of Veterans Appeals. Rarely, cases may go to the Federal District Court and have the potential to go the Supreme Court. In the almost 10 years since the Court of Veterans Appeals began, a large body of case law has developed. Private medical evidence is considered as valid as VA medical evidence if it is sufficient for rating purposes, and veterans may apply for benefits with only private medical evidence. Examination guideline worksheets are available online in the benefits section of the VA's website at *www.va.gov.*

A detailed discussion of the VBA and the role of the physician in VA disability evaluation is provided in Chapter 10.

AMERICANS WITH DISABILITIES ACT

The Americans with Disabilities Act (ADA) was enacted in 1992 to guarantee equal rights for disabled individuals to employment opportunities, public transportation, and public access. The ADA broadly defines disability as ". . . a physical or mental impairment that substantially limits one or more of the major life activities of the individual; or a record of such an impairment; or being regarded as having such an impairment."[2] Discrimination against the disabled in the workplace is prevented under Title 1 (Employment), which applies to businesses in the private sector with 25 or more employees. Title 1 compels the employer to afford equal employment opportunities to an "otherwise qualified" individual with a disability, who meets the "essential functions" of an employment position with or without "reasonable accommodation." "Such accommodation can include structural modifications at the work site to improve access, availability of modified duty, adaptive equipment and devices." Accommodation is reasonable if it does not pose an "undue hardship" (logistically or financially) on the employer, or pose a "direct threat" to the health and safety of disabled individuals and their co-workers. The Equal Employment Opportunity Commission (EEOC) oversees compliance with the law and has an excellent technical manual for those who wish to further educate themselves on the topic.

FAMILY MEDICAL LEAVE ACT

The Family Medical Leave Act (FMLA) was enacted in 1994 to provide up to 12 weeks of unpaid leave under circumstances of medical necessity. The law applies to employers of 50 or more persons, and employees become eligible after having worked for the employer for 12 months or at least 1250 hours during the period before the requested leave. Leave may be granted to either gender and for purposes of the birth or adoption of a child, care of immediate family members, or an employee's own illness. It provides for unpaid leave and continued hospitalization and life insurance protection to an employee during the period of absence.

PRIVATE DISABILITY SYSTEMS

It is estimated that 40 million Americans have private, long-term disability insurance, usually through the workplace. Private insurance plans lack statutory provisions in favor of contractual language that stipulates the criteria for disability and entitlement as well as the benefits of coverage under the policy.[36] Employees who become disabled are initially covered by short-term disability for a period typically of 90 days. If the period of disablement must be extended, a long-term disability policy takes effect after 90 days.

Long-term disability policies may be individual or group policies. Group policies are typically sold to companies and are more affordable than individual policies. Group policies provide coverage to disabled employees who are unable to perform the requirements of their usual and customary job over a finite and specified period, typically 2 years; subsequently, the disabled will continue to receive benefits only if they are unable to perform the functions of "any occupation" as provisionally defined by the policy. Individual policies are available at higher premiums but may afford greater duration of protection to the individual who ultimately cannot perform his or her particular job over an extended, and perhaps indefinite, period.

Private disability generally pays up to 60% of the individual's wages, to a maximum allowable cap, and may have built-in cost-of-living allowances with adjustments for future inflation.

SUMMARY

Systems of social justice exist to ensure equitable compensation and societal care for the disabled. It is quite probable that caring and concern for the disabled has been an integral part of human society from its earliest inception. Rules governing societal compensation for losses suffered are common throughout antiquity and remain with us to date.

Disability systems in the United States have diverse historical origins, and a considerable diversity remains in respect to the definitions of disability, means of entitlement, benefits, provisions for application, and the role of and weight given to medical disability examinations. This historical overview is intended to acquaint physician disability examiners with the fundamental requirements and variations among the disability systems within which they may choose to work.

ACKNOWLEDGEMENTS

The authors are indebted to David Frayer, PhD, of the Department of Anthropology at the University of Kansas, Lawrence, Kansas. Dr. Frayer gave helpful and detailed technical advice concerning evidence of disablement in prehistoric and primate societies and provided assistance with illustrative materials for this manuscript.

Dr. James Robinson of the University of Washington Hospital in Seattle helped with historical information concerning the Social Security Administration.

REFERENCES

1. Bynum WF, Porter R (eds): Companion Encyclopedia of the History of Medicine, Vol 2. London, G. Routledge & Sons, 1993, pp 1210–1211.
2. 29 Code of Federal Regulations. Part 1630. Americans With Disabilities Act (ADA): equal employment opportunity for individuals with disabilities. Federal Register, 1991, pp 35726–35753.
3. 38 Code of Federal Regulations. 3.1–3.100: Pension, compensation and dependency and indemnity compensation. Washington, DC, U.S. Government Printing Office, 1997.
4. 38 Code of Federal Regulations. 3.358: Determinations for disability or death from hospitalization, medical or surgical treatment, examinations or vocational rehabilitation training. Washington, DC, U.S. Government Printing Office, 1997.
5. 38 Code of Federal Regulations. 4.1–4.150: Schedule for rating disabilities. Washington, DC, U.S. Government Printing Office, 1997.
6. Dinstein Y: The Defense of "Obedience to Superior Orders" in International Law. Leyden, A.W. Stijthoff, 1965.
7. Disability Evaluation Under Social Security. U.S. Department of Health and Human Services. Social Security Administration, SSA Publication No. 64-039, ICN No. 468600, 1994.
8. Drew Fischer K: The Lombard Laws. Philadelphia, University of Pennsylvania Press, 1973, p 62.
9. Esquemeling J: The Buccaneers of America, 1684–5. In: Stallybrass W (ed): Broadway Translations. London, G. Routledge & Sons, 1924, p 60.
10. Federal Employers' Liability Act. Issues associated with changing how railroad work-related injuries are compensated. GAO/RCED-96-199, August, 1996, pp 12–13.
11. Op. cit, pp 15–16.
12. Ferm V: An Encyclopedia of Religion. New York, The Philosophical Library, 1945, p 320.
13. Op. cit, p 442.
14. Frayer DW, Horton WA, Macchiarelli R, Mussi M: Dwarfism in an adolescent from the Italian late Upper Paleolithic. Nature 330(6143):60–62, 1987.
15. Hadler NM: The disabling backache: an international perspective. Spine 20(6): 640–649, 1995.
16. Johns RE: Compensation and impairment rating in the United States. J Disability 1(4):188–213, 1990.
17. Jurmain R: Skeletal evidence of trauma in African apes, with special reference to the Gombe chimpanzees. Primates 38(1):1–14, 1997.
18. Kauffman DT: The Dictionary of Religious Terms. Westwood, New Jersey, FH Revell Company, 1967, p 223.
19. LaDou J, Whyte AA: Workers compensation: the Federal experience. J Occup Med 23(12):823–828, 1981.

20. Larson A: The Law of Workmen's Compensation. New York, Matthew Bender & Co., 1985.
21. Leakey REF, Mungai JM, Walker AC: New Australopithecines from East Rudolf, Kenya (II). Am J Phys Anthrop 36:235–252, 1972.
22. Luck J, Florence D: A brief history and comparative analysis of disability systems and impairment rating guides. Orthop Clin North Am 19:839–844, 1988.
23. Mayhew H, Rosenberg JD: London Labour and the London Poor, Vol IV. New York, Dover Publications, Inc., 1968, pp 394–395.
24. Papyrus Archives, Cairo Museum, Egypt.
25. Radovcic J, Smith FH, Trinkhaus E, Wolpoff MH: The Krapina Hominids: An Illustrated Catalog of the Skeletal Collection. Zagreb, Mladost and the Croatian Natural History Museum, 1988, p 90.
26. Raffle PAB, Lee WR, McCallum RI, Murray R (eds): Hunter's Diseases of Occupations, 3rd ed. Boston, Little, Brown & Company, 1987, p 24.
27. Ranavaya MI: Impairment, disability and compensation in the United States: an overview. Disability 5:1–20, 1996.
28. Sanbar SS, Gibofsky A, Firestone MH, LeBlang TR: Legal Medicine, 3rd ed. American College of Legal Medicine, St. Louis, Mosby, 1995, p 129.
29. Schultz AH: Notes on diseases and healed fractures of wild apes. In: Brothwell DR, Sandison AT (eds): Diseases in Antiquity. Springfield, Illinois, Charles C Thomas, Publisher, 1967, pp 47–55.
30. Schultz AH: The Life of Primates. New York, Universe Books, 1969, pp 187–199.
31. Somers HM, Somers AR: Workmen's Compensation: Prevention, Insurance, and Rehabilitation of Occupational Disability. New York, John Wiley and Sons, 1954, p 18.
32. Op. cit, p 32.
33. Trinkaus E, Zimmerman MR: Trauma among the Shanidar Neanderthals. Am J Phys Anthrop 57:61–76, 1982.
34. Tyndale W: New Testament, English King James Version: Exodus 21:23–25.
35. Op. cit, 2 Thessalonians 3:10.
36. U.S. Department of Labor: Employee Benefits in Small Private Establishments. Washington, DC, U.S. Department of Labor, 1994, pp 20–34.
37. Weaver CL: The Crisis in Social Security. Durham, North Carolina, Duke Press Policy Studies, 1982.
38. Yaron R: The Laws of Eshnunna, Section 42. Jerusalem-Leiden, The Magnes Press, The Hebrew University, 1988, p 69.

CHAPTER 2

The Concepts of Impairment and Disability

Robert D. Rondinelli, MD, PhD *Pamela W. Duncan, PT, PhD*

The practices of impairment rating and disability determination have traditionally been the purview of the physician examiner. However, the conceptual underpinnings and practical issues that these processes address are not solely medical, but rather are largely socioeconomic, political, and legal in nature. The physician disability examiner is typically expected to diagnose and treat a medical impairment and to determine its disabling effect on a variety of physical, social, and vocational functions. Physician disability determinations have varying connotations and applications ranging from indemnity compensation and pensioning to return-to-work assessments and permanent work restrictions. Physicians must have a working knowledge of and be able to apply concepts and definitions of the terms *impairment* and *disability* according to criteria and guidelines of the various federal, state, and jurisdictional systems within which they are working. However, there is no clear consensus about definitions of impairment and disability among these systems. Conceptual models of the process of disablement are ever changing and, in the past, have been dominated by issues of medical management rather than social and political concerns.

One might ask, how does a conceptual understanding of the process of disablement help? The answer becomes clear with each attempt to determine the significance (or lack thereof) of physical impairment toward disablement in any given case. Physicians and other health care providers, and perhaps society in general, have come to regard impairment as disabling when, in fact, an enabling outlook (i.e., what tasks can the injured worker still perform?) is often needed. Furthermore, the lack of any coherent synthesis of concepts regarding disablement and the process of evaluating and treating impairment and disability across systems has contributed to the sense of chaos that the disability examiner must face. A synthesis of existing models is needed to help generate an approach that is less confusing, internally consistent, yet generally applicable to the various disability systems currently in place.

Conceptual models of the process of disablement have been developed to help evaluate the societal impact of disability, to develop appropriate rehabilitation programs and interventions, and to measure outcomes of such programs and interventions. Traditionally, such models have been designated as medical or social. In the medical model, disablement is viewed as a problem with the individual, who is afflicted with a disease or trauma that causes *observable* impairment and gives rise to disability. In this model, medical impairment is the primary focus of evaluation and treatment (e.g., the American Medical Association's *Guides to the Evaluation of Permanent Impairment* or AMA *Guides*[2]) and presumably determines the level of disability. The primary intervention is medical care, in which the goals are to cure or minimize the disease or trauma, thereby reducing impairment and any ensuing disability. Alternatively, the social model views disablement as a complex and interactive condition of the individual and his or her environment, and not solely the result of the impairment. Environmental modifications and other social accommodations are the focus of treatment within the social model.

Imbedded within these models are the fundamental concepts of impairment and disability—separate entities whose distinction is readily apparent, yet whose defining features are frequently confused and whose complex interrelationships remain poorly understood. Proper evaluation and management of impairment and disability demands that the physician or other health care provider be thoroughly familiar with these concepts, including their definitions, conceptual underpinnings, practical applications, and potential misapplications. Effective management of disablement at a societal level may require social-political actions to effect attitudes that are enabling and environmental changes that are accommodating to those with disabilities. A more coherent characterization of impairment and disability appears desirable and requires a reexamination and synthesis of existing models at this time.

The purpose of this chapter is to review old versus new conceptual models of disablement, with particular attention to the concepts of impairment and disability and the relationship between them. Special attention will be given to practical applications of these concepts to the area of Workers' Compensation and the associated rating practice of the physician disability examiner.

EVOLUTION OF MODELS OF DISABILITY

World Health Organization Model (1980)

The most commonly used and internationally accepted conceptual model of disablement is the World Health Organization (WHO) International Classification of Impairments, Disabilities, and Handicaps (Fig. 2–1).[30] The WHO model provides a conceptual framework that focuses on the individual and extends from pathology to handicap. The four levels of disablement of the WHO model are pathology, impairment, disability, and handicap.

Pathology is a disease or trauma that causes changes in the structure or function of the body or of a specific tissue or organ.

Impairment occurs at the organ level and is defined as "any loss or abnormality of psychological, physiological, or anatomical structure or function."[30, 31] Impairments are observable and can be objectively defined and measured in most cases. Examples of impairment include joint ankylosis, amputation of a limb, disfigurement of a body part, loss of joint motion (flexibility), loss of strength (manual muscle test), or loss of endurance (cardiopulmonary).

Disability occurs at the personal level and is defined as "any restriction or lack (resulting from impairment) of ability to perform an activity in the manner or within the range considered normal for a human being."[30, 31] Disability is most commonly defined in terms of dependent functioning within one's personal sphere. Activity domains may include mobility (i.e., transfers and ambulation), or activities of daily living (ADL) and self care such as feeding, personal hygiene, bathing, toileting, grooming, and dressing. For example, in the field of rehabilitation, the Functional Independence Measure (FIM)[13] has been developed to measure disability across a range of impairments. The FIM includes 18 tasks that are graded on a 7-point scale to characterize the level of dependence on task performance.

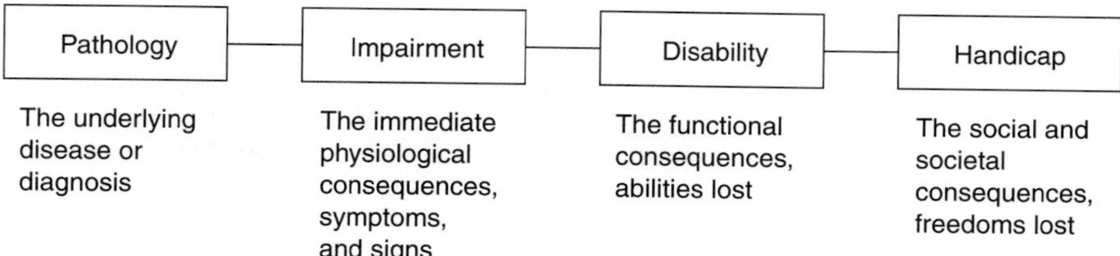

FIGURE 2–1
World Health Organization's international classification of illness. (Reproduced with permission from the World Health Organization.)

Handicap, at the societal level, is defined as "a disadvantage for a given individual that limits or prevents the fulfillment of a role that is normal (depending upon age, sex, social and cultural factors) for that individual."[30, 31] Handicaps may affect expected roles such as employee, family member, and community member. Examples of handicap may include lack of access to a public facility because of wheelchair confinement, loss of a telemarketing job because of Broca's aphasia, and inability to resume a scuba-diving hobby after severe decompression sickness.

The WHO model assumes unidirectional causality. For example, impairments cause disability that cause handicap. Medical rehabilitation practice has often focused on minimizing impairments to minimize disability. For instance, a therapist may try to improve muscle strength (impairment), which will theoretically decrease disability (impaired ability to climb stairs) and improve the ability to ambulate in the community. Or, perhaps an injured laborer undergoes work hardening to recapture sufficient material-handling ability to resume his occupation and thereby reduce or eliminate handicap.

Nagi Model (1969)

Saad Nagi[20] developed a conceptual model of disablement in the 1960s that has similarities to the WHO model. In the Nagi model, the term *disability* is replaced with *functional limitation* and the term *handicap* is replaced with *disability.* The Nagi model also differentiates disability at three levels: organ level, person level, and societal level. Nagi recognized that the correlations between impairments, functional limitations, and disability were poor, and he suggested that environmental factors may modify the relationships between impairments, functional limitations, and disability. Even though Nagi considered the environmental factors, his model still emphasizes the characteristics of the medical conditions and impairments and characterizes the relationship between impairments, functional limitations, and disability as unidirectional.

Institute of Medicine (1991)

In 1991 the Institute of Medicine (IOM) suggested another model of the disablement process adapted directly from the Nagi model. The IOM model defines disability as "a function of the interaction of the person with the environment."[22] The IOM model identified a subset of factors that could modify the relationships between impairments, functional limitations, and disability. These factors include biology, environment (physical, social, and psychological), lifestyle, and behavior (Fig. 2–2). In the IOM model, these

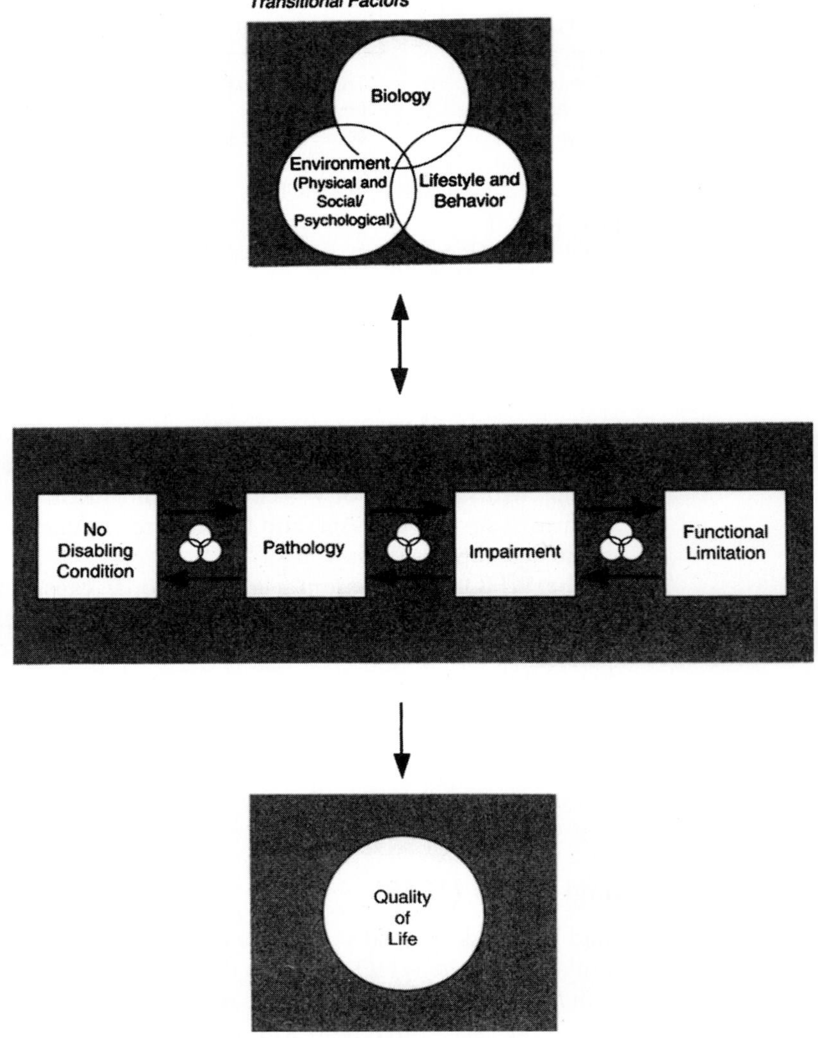

FIGURE 2–2
The enabling-disabling process. (Reproduced with permission from the National Academy Press.)

factors are independent variables that can modify all levels of the disablement process and affect quality of life.

The National Center for Medical Rehabilitation Research (1993)

In an attempt to link rehabilitation to the disability classification systems, the advisory board of the National Center for Medical Rehabilitation Research (NCMRR) developed yet another conceptual model of classifying the dimensions of disability.[21] The advisory board expanded the original IOM model to include societal limitations as a major aspect of disability. They also recognized that the relationships between pathology, impairment, functional limitations, disability, and societal limitations are not sequential or unidirectional. The

NCMRR terminology includes *pathophysiology, impairment, functional limitation, disability,* and *societal limitations*. The definitions are as follows:

- **Pathophysiology:** Interruption of or interference with normal physiological and developmental processes or structures
- **Impairment:** Loss or abnormality of cognitive, emotional, physiological, or anatomical structure or function, including all losses or abnormalities, not just those attributable to the initial pathophysiology
- **Functional limitation:** Restriction or lack of ability to perform an action in the manner or within the range consistent with the purpose of an organ or organ system
- **Disability:** Inability or limitation in performing tasks, activities, and roles to levels expected within physical and social contexts
- **Societal limitation:** Restriction attributable to social policy or barriers (structural or attitudinal), which limits fulfillment of roles or denies access to services and opportunities that are associated with full participation in society

With this broader classification of the disablement process, the NCMRR advisory board expanded the scope of rehabilitation sciences from the level of the individual to consideration of societal interactions This classification moved rehabilitation from simply a medical model to a medical-social model.[21]

RECONSIDERATION OF DISABLEMENT MODELS

The multiple models of disability have produced confusion. They limit our ability to define disability (as required by Workers' Compensation) and to develop coherent and effective rehabilitation programs. Additionally, there are major criticisms of the existing models. First, they have overemphasized the medical model. The AMA's *Guides to the Evaluation of Permanent Impairment, 4th ed*, in particular, has put forward the notion that physical impairment is a medical issue to be addressed and rated by physicians, whereas disability is an "administrative" issue to be addressed by nonmedical means and according to local jurisdictional guidelines and procedures.[2] Development of successful rehabilitation programs to minimize work disability must consider the multiple interacting environmental factors (e.g., work satisfaction, work environment, work tasks, local economy). Additionally, any comprehensive disability assessment must consider the cognitive, emotional, and motivational factors of affected individuals. A second major criticism of the existing models is that the models have assumed causal relationships between the different levels.[32] For example, in some models disability is directly caused by the observed impairments, whereas in reality, impairments may explain 25% or less of the variance in disability or handicap.[11, 12, 25] A third criticism of the existing models is that a unidirectional relationship exists between the levels. This unidirectional representation does not allow for reverse effects. For example, handicap (role limitations) may cause less mobility (disability), and less mobility causes declines in strength and endurance (impairments). Most importantly, the unidirectional representation implies that disability is not reversible. Lastly, the models are expressed in negative dimensions (handicap) rather than positive (enabling) terms (i.e., residual abilities). Given these limitations, two initiatives in 1997 put forth additional models to characterize disability.

Modified IOM Model (1997)

The new IOM model clearly defines disability as the interaction of the person with the environment and includes a bidirectional dimension (possibility of improvement) (Fig. 2–3). Disability has been moved from being a part of the process to being a product of the interaction of the individual with the environment. In the new model, enabling factors are identified rather than risk factors,[4] which are associated with increased likelihood of disability. Enabling factors are associated with an increase in likelihood of fewer limitations. The environment is represented in a multidimensional model and is portrayed as having two characteristics: social and physical. With less supportive environments, a person will experience more disability (Fig. 2–4). Individuals with disability must cope with impairments and functional limitations, but the true impact of these on their lives is more a function of the environment. For example, research on disability in the work setting indicates that the economic status of the overall labor market has a far greater impact on the employment status of people with disabling conditions than the willingness of individual employers to provide accommodation.[35]

New World Health Organization Model (1997)

The WHO has recently modified the 1980 model of the disablement classification.[33] In the June 1997, beta-1 draft for the second International Classification of Impairments, Disabilities, and Handicaps (ICIDH-2) manual for dimensions of disablement and functioning, the WHO has changed terminology from

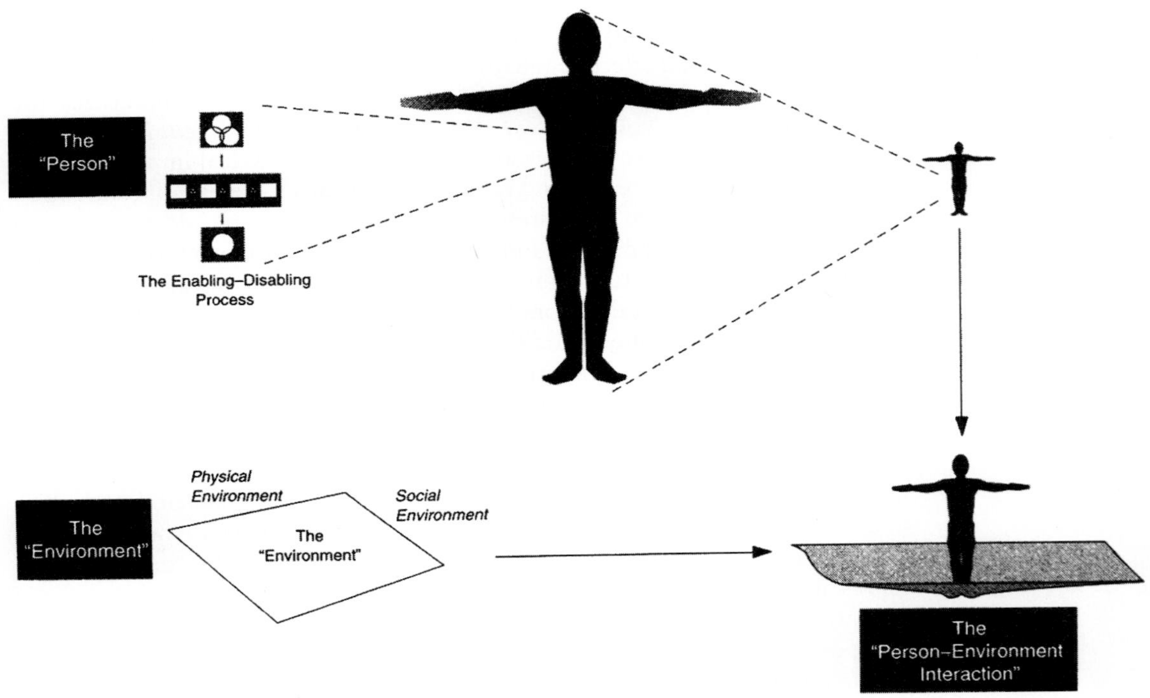

FIGURE 2–3
The person-environment interaction. (Reproduced with permission from the National Academy Press.)

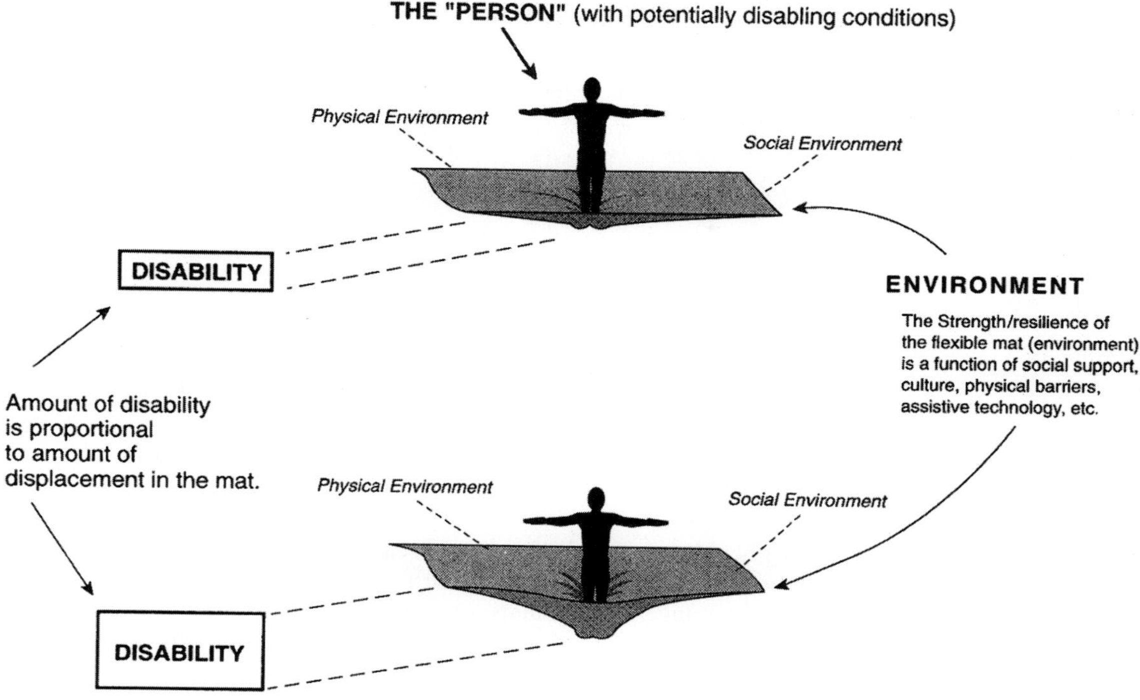

FIGURE 2–4
Disability is a function of the interaction between the person and the environment. (Reproduced with permission from the National Academy Press.)

impairments, disability, and handicap to *impairments, activities, and participation.* The purpose of the ICIDH-2 classification is to provide a unified and standard language that characterizes the consequences of health conditions. The ICIDH-2 classification is being tested internationally and is being developed for many users, including individuals with disabilities, and social-political sectors such as social security, insurance, education, and legislation. The principal aims of the ICIDH-2 include the following:

- Provide a scientific basis to understand and study the consequences of health conditions
- Establish a common language for describing consequences of health conditions to improve communications between health care workers, other sectors, and disabled people/people with disabilities
- Provide a basis to understand the impact of disablement phenomena on the lives of individuals and their participation in society
- Define consequences of health conditions to provide better care and services to improve the participation in society of people with health conditions

In the proposed ICIDH-2 model (Fig. 2–5), the consequences of health conditions are viewed as multidimensional phenomena that are interactive and evolutionary by nature. In this new model, the following operational definitions are suggested.[33]

- **Health condition:** An alteration or attribute of the health status of an individual that may lead to distress, interference with daily activities, or con-

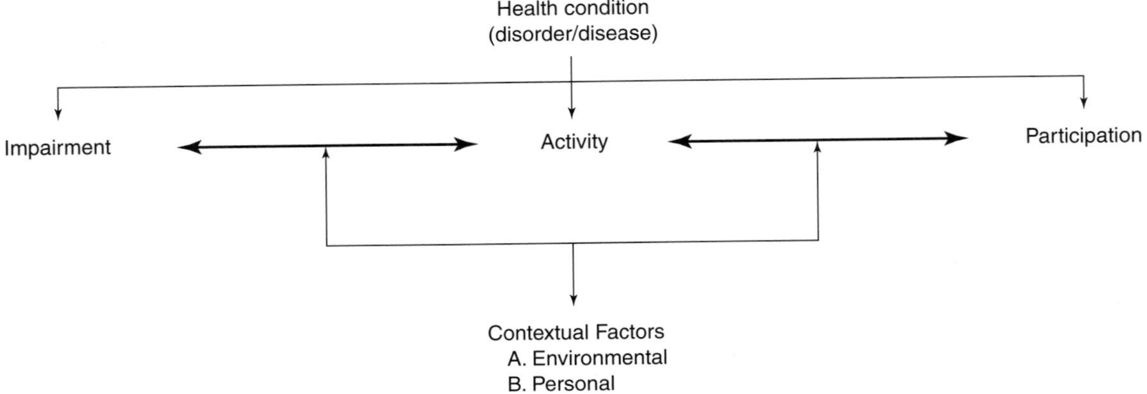

FIGURE 2–5
Health condition (disorder/disease). (Reproduced with permission from the World Health Organization.)

tact with health services. It may be a disease (acute or chronic), disorder, injury, or trauma, or reflect other health-related states such as pregnancy, aging, stress, congenital anomaly, or genetic predisposition.

- **Impairment:** A loss or abnormality of body structure or a physiological or psychological function.
- **Activity:** The nature and extent of functioning at the level of the person. Activities may be limited in nature, duration, and quality.
- **Participation:** The nature and extent of a person's involvement in life situations in relationship to impairment, activities, and contextual factors. Participation may be restricted in nature, duration, and quality.
- **Contextual factors:** The factors that interact with the person with disability to determine the level and extent of the person's participation in his or her surroundings. These factors include environmental and personal factors. Environmental factors are extrinsic to the individual (e.g., attitudes of the society, architectural characteristics, legal system). Personal factors have an impact on how the disablement is experienced (e.g., age, gender, other health conditions, fitness, lifestyle, coping style, social and educational background, individual psychological assets).

At this time, the new ICIDH-2 classification appears to be the best model for conceptualizing impairment and disability. It acknowledges the complex and dynamic interactions between a given health condition, the environment, and personal factors. The relationships between impairment, activity limitations, and participation are not assumed to be unidirectional. For example, one may have impairments without activity limitations (disability) or limitations in participation (handicap), or one could have activity limitations (disability) without limitations in participation (handicap). On the other hand, one could have limitations in activities or participation without documented impairments (e.g., pain). The new ICIDH-2 model also recognizes that limitations in participation may secondarily produce limitations in activities, which may also produce impairments. For example, inability to participate in fitness programs may cause poor performance in daily activities, which can produce impairments (decreased cardiovascular endurance and diminished muscle strength).

PRACTICAL APPLICATIONS FOR THE DISABILITY EVALUATING SPECIALIST

Current disability systems should integrate the emerging models of disablement into practice. For example, in Workers' Compensation it may no longer be considered optimal nor sufficient to base a disability rating solely on impairments derived according to the AMA *Guides*. Attention must be given to premorbid (baseline) functioning, psychosocial and vocational background, and feasability of contextual adaptations available to the impaired individual before weighing the purported functional impact of the impairment itself. To illustrate the current dilemmas and proposed solutions, we will examine and attempt to integrate the concepts of impairment and disability under the ADA and Workers' Compensation according to the AMA *Guides*.

ADA Model for Work Disability

Title 1 (Employment) of the ADA was signed into law in 1992 and applies to private-sector employers of 15 or more persons.[7] The ADA defines *disability* as "a physical or mental impairment" that "substantially limits" one or more of the "major life activities" of the individual, or "a record of such impairment," or being "regarded as having such an impairment."[7] This is a broad definition similar to the concept of impairment put forth by the AMA *Guides*. However, *employment* is considered a major life activity for which provisions regarding disability can become job specific. A *job description* is the formal description of an employment position by title and according to a list of *essential functions* and associated physical task demands that comprise that specific job. (A job description is typically available from the employer on request.) The essential functions are those fundamental duties of the job that, if removed, would change the nature of the job itself. Failure of the employee to perform the essential functions of his or her job could result in termination for cause. *Accommodation* refers to modification of a job or workplace to enable the disabled employee to meet the essential functions of his or her job. *Reasonable accommodation* is accommodation that can be carried out without imposing *undue hardship* (whether financial or economic) on the employer or posing a *direct threat* to the health and safety of the disabled employee or his or her co-workers. It is possible to conceptualize work disability under Title 1 as job specific and relative to the essential functions. Important variables include the nature and severity of impairment, job category and associated essential functions, and the need for and availability of accommodation in each case. Although impairment may be fixed at a particular level, the associated work disability and handicap may be minimized or eliminated altogether by availability and feasibility of reasonable accommodation. In essence, the disability or handicap may vary inversely with ability to accommodate.

To illustrate, consider the following example of a specific impairment (e.g., partial hand amputation affecting the metacarpophalangeal region of the thumb on the dominant hand) (Table 2–1). If the affected individual is a construction worker whose job requires successful operation of heavy equipment, it appears likely that the essential functions can be successfully performed without accommodation, and hence work disability and/or handicap are not present. If the affected individual is a peace officer whose job demands proficient use of a handgun for self-defense, and if said proficiency is lost, accommodation would be necessary. A potential reasonable accommodation might be to

TABLE 2–1 Examples of Medical Impairment and Work Disability Relative to Reasonable Accommodation and the ADA

Impairment	Job category	Sample essential functions	Essential functions performed	Accommodation needed	Reasonable accommodation afforded	Work disability present	Handicap present
Partial hand amputee (dominant)	Construction worker	Operates heavy equipment	+	–	Not applicable	–	–
	Policeman	Proficiency with handgun	–	+++	+ (reassign as dispatcher)	–	+/– if resulting loss in earning power
	Concert musician	Live concert appearances	+/–	+++	+ (provide synthesizer for studio performance)	+/–	+/– if resulting loss in work availability and earning power
	Surgeon	Operates on chest	–	+++	– (physician extender not feasible)	+	+

Modified and reproduced with permission after Delisa JA: Rehabilitation Medicine: Principles and Practice, 3rd ed. Philadelphia, JB Lippincott Co, 1998, Table 10–4.

reassign the individual to a dispatch role, thereby eliminating the need for handgun proficiency as well as the work disability. If the individual is a concert pianist whose ability to perform is significantly compromised, significant work disability and handicap would likely result. Accommodation in such a case might necessitate use of a synthesizer to enable composition and studio-level performance to continue. Some level of work disability and handicap would likely remain. If the affected individual were a surgeon whose job performance demanded the highest level of manual dexterity, accommodation may no longer suffice or be feasible, and work disability and handicap would be severe.

The example considered in Table 2–1 can be further expanded to consider amputation levels of varying severity (i.e., partial hand versus transradial versus shoulder disarticulation). For each level, accommodation needs may vary according to severity of impairment, and in more severe cases will likely include the need for and provision of a prosthesis. The construction worker with a transradial amputation and a below-elbow, body-powered prosthesis could, in all likelihood, operate heavy equipment and perform heavy manual labor to a degree comparable to before the amputation occurred. Accommodation would include the prosthesis, training in prosthetic use, and equipment maintenance. If the level was a shoulder disarticulation, heavy bimanual labor might not be possible even with a prosthesis, and accommodations to operate heavy equipment might not be possible. In that case, work disability and associated handicap would be expected to occur in inverse relationship to ability to accommodate. As the above examples illustrate, work disability and handicap under ADA are situationally specific, may vary with type and severity of impairment, and are inversely related to availability of reasonable accommodation.

Whereas work disability caused by impairments of the musculoskeletal system may be minimized or eliminated by environmental modifications, disabilities related to central neurological, cognitive, and behavioral impairments are more complex, hence less likely to be minimized and more challenging to accommodate. The individual who is severely impaired as a result of traumatic spinal-cord injury must contend with limitations to physical independence that require attendant physical care, limitations to access and transportation that require special equipment and transportation arrangements, and limitations to social interaction and economic self-sufficiency.[29] Collectively, such limitations may transcend obstacles and barriers of an occupational nature and require broader social accommodations before employment becomes feasible. An individual who has suffered severe traumatic brain injury may experience deficits in arousal level, impulse control, communication, and/or higher cognitive functioning that may require additional caregiver support and supervision for cognitive reasons and pose further obstacles toward reasonable and feasible accommodation in the workplace.

American Medical Association Model: Measuring Impairment and Disability (1958–1970)

The AMA *Guides* was developed out of a series of 13 separate publications in the *Journal of the American Medical Association (JAMA)* from 1958 to 1970. It has undergone multiple revisions from inception. The purpose of the AMA *Guides* is to provide a standard framework for physician evaluating and reporting about medical impairments of any organ or system. The AMA *Guides* is the preferred medical reference on impairment for Workers' Compensation being mandated or recommended by law in a majority of jurisdictions.[2] In its present form there are a number of theoretical shortcomings and practical pitfalls and limitations.[3, 5, 6, 9, 10, 23, 25, 26] Pursuant to this discussion, major concerns include the following:

- Definitions and terminology employed by the AMA *Guides* is fraught with inconsistency and ambiguity.[3, 5, 6, 9, 10] The distinctions between impairment, disability, and handicap are operationally blurred.
- Content validity of impairment ratings is not well established (see Chapter 3 for a detailed discussion of measurement validity and its significance to the AMA *Guides*). Functional losses continue to be inferred from medical impairment ratings linked to compensible injuries. Impairment ratings put forth by the AMA *Guides* represent a validation by consensus that is unsupported by rigorously collected, empirical, behaviorally based data. A sound scientific foundation is consequently lacking at this time.[25]
- Predictive validity is also not well established. For example, prediction of neurological outcome after traumatic spinal-cord injury in terms of sensory and motor impairment and corresponding functional ability can be done with precision and sensitivity.[17] However, prediction of extent of work disability according to these same criteria is not possible without added knowledge of other dimensions of handicap, including cognitive independence, occupation, social integration, and economic self-sufficiency of the individual involved.[28] Moreover, severity of impairment after traumatic brain injury, however measured, remains controversial as a predictor of postrecovery global functioning and return-to-work ability.[8]
- Reliability of specific measures of impairment (i.e., loss of spinal flexibility as measured by surface inclinometry) remains open to debate. For example, significant measurement error and unacceptably low reliability estimates have been shown by intraclass correlation for several common techniques of surface inclinometry, even when applied by experienced observers to healthy and cooperative subjects.[26]
- Subjectivity and bias on the part of claimant and examiner, as well as performance effort and consistency, may affect the ratings obtained. Exaggeration of presentation (symptom magnification) is a frequent occurrence.[16] When properly accounted for, exaggeration and inconsistency of presentation should not produce inflated ratings nor should it inappropriately penalize the claimant guilty of such displays. The AMA *Guides* fails to adequately proscribe ratings in the face of symptom magnification, leaving this most arduous task to the whims of the physician disability examiner.

Historically, impairment ratings of the spine and extremities have been identified according to an "anatomical model." Rating criteria include amputation, ankylosis, or loss of motion.[1, 14, 15, 18, 24, 27] More recently, a "diagnosis-based" system has been put forward in an attempt to minimize or eliminate the conceptual and methodological flaws inherent to the anatomical model as listed above.[2] The AMA *Guides* is subject to periodic revision in an ongoing attempt to correct its shortcomings. Under a revised impairment rating system, we believe that the following suggestions and considerations should be taken into account:

- The concept of "diagnosis-related estimates (DREs)" recently put forward in the AMA *Guides* has several desirable features and advantages over earlier models that hopefully can be carried forward and expanded on. The

DRE approach uses nominal-ordinal rather than interval-ratio data and descriptors that can be easily and consistently identified (hence "rater friendly"), and can thus be expected to show high inter-rater reliability (see Chapter 3). The DRE system is relatively simple to learn and to apply. Since physicians are inherently good diagnosticians, the applicability of a diagnosis-based approach to physician impairment ratings appears self-evident.

- We suggest that the AMA *Guides* abandon attempts to separate the issues of impairment and disability as medical and nonmedical, respectively. Alternatively, we recommend that physicians address medical impairment in diagnostic terms and the associated medical disability in terms of functionally based criteria.
- A diagnostic taxonomy and classification of impairment can be based on existing *International Classification of Diseases, 9th Revision (ICD-9)/ Diagnostic and Statistical Manual of Mental Disorders, 4th Edition (DSM IV)* criteria that physicians can recognize and apply with regularity. In systems where "causality" is at issue, and the condition may or may not be the direct result of injury, a modifier for "associated with or aggravating to" can be applied within a degree of medical certainty. The impairment rating per se would then be a nominal-ordinal (i.e., qualitative) diagnostic measure.
- In cases in which medical impairment is diagnosed, a matrix approach can aid the physician in rendering an opinion on associated disability within each of four possible domains: mobility (transfers and ambulation), self care (feeding, personal hygiene, bathing, toileting, grooming, dressing), and vocational and avocational pursuits. ADL assessments can be carried out in addition to self-report assessments of functional independence in each domain. Level of disability for each domain can be categorized in ordinal fashion to one of four possible levels: independent, independent with accommodation and/or adaptive equipment, helper required, or cannot perform. Consequently, a 4 × 4 "disability" grid can be established (Table 2–2) with a row for each functional domain and a column for each level of independence. If the columns are weighted from 1 to 4 points for "independent" to "cannot perform," respectively, it becomes possible to summarize

TABLE 2–2 Disability Matrix

	Functional status			
	1 Independent	2 Independent with accommodation/ adaptive equipment	3 Helper needed	4 Cannot do
I Mobility (ADL)				
II Self-care (ADL)				
III Vocational (Job specific)				
IV Avocational				

Ordinal disability score: 1–4: Mild; 5–8: moderate; 9–12: severe; 13–16: total.

an individual's row scores across functional domains to get a total (ordinal) score for disability. The magnitude of disability is functionally based and devoid of any impairment "weighting." Furthermore, the resulting disability score can be collapsed and simplified into four descriptive categories of mild (1 to 4 points), moderate (5 to 8 points), severe (9 to 12 points), and total (13 to 16 points) disability for any medical impairment in question. Such an approach can be expected to be sensitive to functional losses associated with catastrophic injury or illness, and yet remain robust in the face of the "symptom magnifier" who may tend to over-report symptoms but cannot demonstrate corresponding functional losses of a global nature. (The authors note that ordinal data, when treated as having interval properties, can be the subject of misinference,[19, 34] and that an ordinal disability scale such as we have illustrated does not imply comparable magnitude of disability between categories. The reader is referred to Chapter 3 for a more detailed discussion of this issue.)

To illustrate, an individual with high cervical tetraplegia (complete) who works part time as a switchboard operator via sip-and-puff technology, and whose hobby is painting by mouth-brush technique, may require the following: a power wheelchair with sip-and-puff control, a wheelchair accessable dwelling and workstation, a specially adapted van for transportation, and a full-time personal-care attendant. Ostensibly, such an individual would score 4 points each on ADL mobility and self-care scales and 3 points each on vocational and avocational scales, for an overall disability score of 14 points, and would be considered "totally" disabled. By contrast, an individual with lumbar degenerative disc disease and chronic low back pain claims inability to work because of severe back pain. A careful functional history reveals that all mobility and self-care activities can be carried out unassisted and without adaptive aids, although the individual infrequently resorts to help if available. A functional capacity evaluation suggests that the individual is capable of at least sedentary activity, and modified sedentary activity is available but being refused. Avocational pursuits are also possible but have largely been abandoned because of lack of interest and in favor of sedentary activity. Ostensibly, this individual would score 1 point each for ADL mobility and self-care scales, 2 points for vocational, and possibly 2 points for modification of avocational pursuits, for an overall disability score of 6 points, and would be considered only "moderately" disabled.

- Many states/jurisdictions allow application of physician impairment ratings for purposes of indemnity payments or compensation and pensioning. Such determinations can be more equitably accomplished by examining loss of earning power and/or loss of task performance in the workplace, and would appear to have greater validity if based on the functionally weighted physician assessment of disability, in preference of or in addition to medical impairment ratings.
- During treatment and at Maximum Medical Improvement (MMI) after work-related injury or personal injury claims, the treating physician (or ultimately the disability-evaluating physician) must make recommendations with respect to limited versus full duty, work restrictions and duration, and issues of accommodation. The AMA *Guides* does not address this aspect of disability determination; however, a conceptual blueprint for ADA-compatible return-to-work determinations is outlined below.

Integration of the ADA and AMA Models for Work Disability

It is possible to integrate concepts of work disability according to the ADA, Workers' Compensation, and the AMA as follows: At present, the ADA concepts and mandates[7] have not been fully integrated into Workers' Compensation law but represent a separate and parallel system. The physician may render an ADA-compatible return-to-work determination for an injured worker by addressing fitness to perform the essential functions of a specific job, if available, and the need/willingness/ability of the employer to accommodate in a given case.

In determining "fitness for duty" after work-related injury, a job-worker profile can be developed with input from a vocational analyst and physical or occupational therapist, and based on a functional capacities evaluation specific to the job and worker in question (see Chapters 5 and 7). A sample profile can be developed, as outlined in Chapter 5, that lists a menu of essential functions and physical task requirements of the job and the worker's associated functional capacities according to the U.S. Department of Labor criteria and guidelines. The need for accommodation arises when the worker's performance fails to meet or exceed task demands for any essential function listed in the job description. In a situation in which the physician disability specialist is asked to render a return-to-work statement, a valid functional capacity evaluation and job analysis may be helpful. Opinions should be based, with medical probability, on the patient's demonstrated ability to safely meet or exceed the physical task demands of each essential function listed, with or without accommodation. If an invalid performance effort is given on the part of the patient, the physician may ultimately qualify his or her opinion in terms of medical probability, and may opt for a more conservative estimate of task performance ability in that particular case.

SUMMARY

The community of health care providers devoted to the evaluation and management of medical disability requires a more coherent and internally consistent conceptual and methodological infrastructure, both for diagnosing and treating medical impairment and determining its disabling effects or consequences. The physician disability examiner is empowered to make such determinations and is expected to transcend the conceptual limitations and procedural restrictions of each system in which he or she operates, including Workers' Compensation, Social Security, Compensation and Pensioning within the Veteran's Administration, and others. A synthesis of concepts, definitions, and analytical approaches with common applications to all systems is needed and will be invaluable to physicians who rise to accept the challenges of impairment rating and disability determination.

Conceptual models are available to assist with our fundamental understanding of the complex relationship between impairment and disability. The emerging consensus from these models is a view that there is no direct causal link between these phenomena, that impairment and disability are bidirectionally interactive, and that attention must be paid to contextual and environmental factors as determinants of disablement for any given individual with a medical impairment.

Impairment ratings in and of themselves have little relevance, apart from being a standard means whereby medical disability determinations are made and legitimized. If coupled with functionally based assessments of the impact of impairment on the individual, the resulting disability determinations become more relevant by providing an objective and valid means for the brokerage of social justice according to medical losses suffered.

Medical impairment rating is, in essence, a diagnostic exercise, which plays to the physician's strength as diagnostician. As the process becomes more "diagnosis based," as opposed to anatomically based, physician-rater reliability and feasibility is expected to be enhanced. Medical disability determination is inherently more complex and requires physicians to broaden their scope of inquiry beyond the medical domain and to investigate environmental and personal modifiers of the process of disablement. Furthermore, physicians will be called on to exercise principles and approaches to functional assessment to derive determinations that are more functionally relevant and inherently valid than has traditionally been the case. A matrix approach based on ADL assessment of function in the presence of medical impairment is offered here as one possible solution.

Finally, the ADA offers several useful and relevant concepts applicable to physician disability determinations under Workers' Compensation and elsewhere. These include the notion that disability can best be approached and understood in terms of major life activities, such as employment. Components of such activity (e.g., essential functions of the job) become measurement criteria in and of themselves, for which disability is weighed according to need for, availability, and feasability of accommodation.

REFERENCES

1. American Academy of Orthopedic Surgeons: Manual for Orthopedic Surgeons in Evaluating Permanent Physical Impairment. Chicago, American Academy of Orthopedic Surgeons, 1975.
2. American Medical Association: Guides to the Evaluation of Permanent Impairment, 4th ed. Chicago, American Medical Association, 1993.
3. Brand RA, Lehmann TR: Low-back impairment rating practices of orthopedic surgeons. Spine 8:75–78, 1983.
4. Brandt EN, Pope AM: Models of Disability and Rehabilitation. In: Brandt EN PA (ed): Enabling America: Assessing the Role of Rehabilitation Science and Engineering. Washington DC, National Academy Press, 1997, pp 62–80.
5. Burd JG: The educated guess: doctors and permanent partial disability percentage. J Tenn Med Assoc 73:441, 1980.
6. Carey TS, Hadler NM: The role of the primary physician in disability determination for Social Security Insurance and Workers' Compensation. Ann Intern Med 104:706–710, 1986.
7. 29 Code of Federal Regulations. Part 1630. Americans with Disabilities Act (ADA). Equal employment opportunity for individuals with disabilities. Federal Register 56(144):35726–35753, 1991.
8. Cifu DX, Keyser-Marcus L, Lopez E, et al: Acute predictors of return to work one year after traumatic brain injury: a multicenter analysis. Arch Phys Med Rehabil 78:125–131, 1997.
9. Clark WL, Haldeman S: The development of guideline factors for the evaluation of disability in neck and back injuries. Spine 18:1736–1745, 1993.
10. Clark WL, Haldeman S, Johnson P, et al: Back impairment and disability detertmination: another attempt at objective, reliable rating. Spine 13:332–341, 1988.
11. DeHaan R, Horn J, Limburg M: A Comparison of Five Stroke Scales With Measures of Disability, Handicap and Quality of Life. Stroke 24:1178–1181, 1993.

12. Gloss DS, Wardle MG: Reliability and validity of American Medical Association's Guide to ratings of permanent impairment. JAMA 248:2292–2296, 1982.
13. State University of New York at Buffalo: Guide for the Uniform Data Set for Medical Rehabilitation (Adult FIM). Version 4.0 ed, Buffalo, New York, 1993.
14. Kessler HH: Disability: Determination and Evaluation. Philadelphia, Lea & Febiger, 1970.
15. Luck J, Florence D: A brief history and comparative analysis of disability systems and impairment rating guides. Orthop Clin North Am 19:839–844, 1988.
16. Matheson LN: Symptom magnification syndrome structured interview: rationale and procedure. J Occup Rehabil 1:43–56, 1991.
17. Maynard FM et al: International standards for the neurological and functional classification of spinal cord injury. Chicago, ASIA, 1996.
18. McBride ED: Disability Evaluation and Principles of Treatment of Compensible Injuries, 6th ed. Philadelphia, JB Lippincott Co, 1963.
19. Merbitz C, Morris J, Grip JC: Ordinal scales and foundations of misinference. Arch Phys Med Rehabil 70:308–312, 1989.
20. Nagi S: Disability and Rehabilitation: Legal, Clinical, and Self-Concepts and Measurement. Columbus, Ohio, Ohio State Univeristy Press, 1969.
21. National Institutes of Health: Research Plan for the National Center for Medical Rehabilitation Research. Washington DC, U.S. Department of Health and Human Services, 1993.
22. Pope AM, Tarlov AR: Disability in America: Toward a National Agenda for Prevention. Washington DC, National Academy Press, 1991.
23. Pryor ES: Flawed promises: A critical evaluation of the American Medical Association Guides to the Evaluation of Permanent Impairment. Harvard Law Rev 103: 964–976, 1990.
24. Rice CO: Calculation of Industrial Disability of the Extremities and the Back, 2nd ed. Springfield, Illinois, Charles C Thomas, Publisher, 1968.
25. Rondinelli RD, Dunn W, Hassanein KM, et al: A simulation of hand impairments: effects on upper extremity function and implications toward medical impairment rating and disability determination. Arch Phys Med Rehabil 78:1358–1363, 1997.
26. Rondinelli RD, Murphy J, Esler A, et al: Estimation of normal lumbar flexion with surface inclinometry: a comparison of three methods. Am J Phys Med Rehabil 71:219–224, 1992.
27. Smith WC: Principles of Disability Evaluation. Philadelphia, JB Lippincott Co, 1959.
28. Whiteneck GG: Evaluating outcome after spinal cord injury: what determines success? J Spinal Cord Med 20(2):179–185, 1997.
29. Whiteneck GG, Charlifue SW, Gerhart KA, et al: Quantifying handicap: a new measure of long-term rehabilitation outcomes. Arch Phys Med Rehabil 73:519–526, 1992.
30. WHO: International Classification of Impairments, Disabilities and Handicaps: A Manual of Classification Relating to the Consequences of Disease. Geneva, Switzerland, World Health Organization, 1980.
31. WHO: International Classification of Impairments, Disabilities and Handicaps: A Manual of Classification Relating to the Consequences of Disease. Geneva, Switzerland, World Health Organization, 1993.
32. WHO: International Classification of Impairments, Disabilities and Handicaps: A Manual of Classification Relating to the Consequences of Disease. Geneva, Switzerland, World Health Organization, 1997.
33. WHO: ICIDH-2 International Classification of Impairments, Activities and Participation: A Manual of Dimensions of Disablement and Functioning Beta-1 Draft for Field Trials. Geneva, Switzerland, World Health Organization, 1997.
34. Wright BD, Linacre JM: Observations are always ordinal; measurements, however must be interval. Arch Phys Med Rehabil 70:857–860, 1989.
35. Yein E: Disability and the Displaced Worker. New Brunswick, New Jersey, Rutgers University Press, 1992.

CHAPTER 3

Measurement Issues in Impairment Rating and Disability Evaluation

Steven R. Hinderer, MD, MS, PT *Robert D. Rondinelli, MD, PhD* *Richard T. Katz, MD*

When you cannot measure it, when you cannot express it in numbers, you have scarcely, in your own thoughts advanced to the stage of science, whatever the matter may be.

Lord Kelvin

Within the field of impairment rating and disability determination, the physician examiner is asked to describe the nature and extent of physical impairment as objectively as possible. The AMA *Guides* is intended to provide a uniform, standardized, and objective approach to impairment ratings and requires the examiner to follow standard measurement procedures. In so doing, the examiner can document impairment in conformance with a set of measurement parameters for which normative data exists and abnormal departures can be gauged. Commonly accepted measurement tools for the assessment of physical, psychological, and functional impairment and disability are described in detail in subsequent sections of this textbook (see Chapters 4 to 6, respectively). Before further discussion, it is worthwhile to consider the acceptability of the measurement tools themselves, according to criteria of adequacy.

It is important to understand the principles of measurement and the characteristics of good measures to be an effective and responsible user of measurement tools. Methods to evaluate measurement adequacy have been developed primarily in the psychology literature, but are equally applicable to those tests and measures used in impairment rating and disability determination. Standards for implementation of tests and measures have already been established within physical therapy[4, 44, 45] psychology,[1] and medical rehabilitation[26] to address quality guidelines and ethical expectations concerning the application of such clinical measures.

The purpose of this chapter is to briefly review basic criteria of measurement adequacy to better acquaint the reader with the rationale for selecting particular measures of impairment and disability and to critically assess the applications and interpretations drawn from their general use. The items of interest to this discussion include examination of the four possible levels of measurement (to define what is to be measured) and criteria of adequacy (reliability, validity, precision, range, feasibility, and practicality), as well as the relevance of measurement to the issues under study or questions being addressed. Applications to current impairment rating practice guidelines[3] are discussed in the final section of this chapter, to which the casual or quantitatively disinclined reader is directly referred.

LEVELS OF MEASUREMENT

The process of impairment rating is a diagnostic one. The criteria whereby an impairment determination is made may be discrete (i.e., amputation) or continuous (i.e., loss of range of motion, or ROM). The severity of the impairment can vary according to discrete (i.e., the level of amputation) or continuous (i.e., percentage of loss of ROM) criteria as well. Disability determination according to payments for economic losses associated with disability may also be discrete (i.e., permanent total disability cap in dollar amount) or continuous (i.e., percentage of permanent partial disability to the "whole person").

There are four levels of measurement that determine how test results should be analyzed and interpreted: nominal, ordinal, interval, and ratio.[29] Nominal and ordinal scales are used to classify discrete measures because the scores produced fall into mutually exclusive categories. Interval and ratio scales are used to classify continuous measures because the scores produced can fall anywhere along a continuum within the range of possible scores.

A *nominal* scale is used to categorize objects into different, internally equivalent groups based on a specific property when there is no rank ordering or difference of magnitude involved in the classification. An example of nominal groups may be dichotomous (i.e., only two possibilities, such as male-female, black-white) or nondichotomous (i.e., more than two possibilities, such as red-yellow-blue). Most medical diagnoses can be considered as nominal categories.

Ordinal scales are used to categorize objects into mutually exclusive, internally equivalent groups arranged in a hierarchy based on order of magnitude. The intervals between each category are not assumed to be equal, and the order of magnitude may differ between different groups. Ordinal scales are the most commonly used level of measurement in clinical practice. Common examples of ordinal scales are the 5-point manual muscle test scale[23, 25, 28] and the Functional Independence Measure.[19]

Interval scales are continuous and rank ordered according to uniform and sequential increments. Interval data are often generated from quantitative instrumentation as opposed to clinical observation. An example of an interval scale measure is ROM scores reported in degrees.

A *ratio* scale is an interval scale in which the zero point on the scale represents a total absence of the quantity being measured. An example of a ratio scale measure is grip pressure generated with a Jamar dynamometer.

Nominal and ordinal scales are generally less sophisticated and complex than interval and ratio scales and, perhaps, owe their appeal to the ease with which they are created. However, their analysis requires special considerations given to avoid misinference from test results.[38, 55] The major controversies surrounding the use of these scales concern problems of unidimensionality and whether scores of items and subtests can be summed and averaged to provide an overall score. Continuous-scale measures have a higher sensitivity and allow more rigorous statistical analyses to be performed than is possible with discrete measures.

CRITERIA FOR MEASUREMENT ADEQUACY

Reliability and Agreement

Unless measurements can be shown to be valid and reliable, they tend to generate numbers or categories that give a false impression of being meaningful.[44] A general definition of *reliability* is the extent to which a measurement provides consistent information. Another way to state this is that the data provided by the outcome measure are free from random error. Reliability may be thought of as the extent to which the data obtained contain information with a high "signal-to-noise ratio" versus "irrelevant static confusion."[20] A simple way to conceptualize reliability is to think of a measurement instrument as a gun, and the measurements as shots fired at a target. If the shots tend to cluster tightly, the gun is shooting with high reliability, regardless of where the shots cluster on the target (Fig. 3–1, *A* and *B*). If the shots fail to cluster, the reliability of the gun is poor. In contrast, agreement is defined as the extent to which identical measurements can be made with a given measure or instrument. For example, if there is strong agreement between shooters operating the gun, the shots fired will cluster to a similar degree. If there is poor agreement, the degree to which the shots cluster will vary among shooters (Fig. 3–2, *A–D*). The level of reliability and agreement required of a measure may differ, and they are estimated using different statistical techniques.[32] Unfortunately, these concepts and their respective statistics are often treated interchangeably in the literature.

The level of reliability may not parallel the level of agreement. For example, measurement scores may consistently cluster toward the same end of the scale, resulting in high reliability coefficients, and yet these scores may not be equivalent. High reliability does not indicate whether the raters absolutely agree. It can occur concurrently with low agreement when each rater scores subjects differently but the relative differences in the scores are consistent for all subjects rated. To illustrate, consider two therapists who independently rate the performance of a group of clients on a specific task. One therapist may consistently rate more strictly than the other and, consequently, tends to score the group lower in an overall sense (i.e., there is not precise agreement between

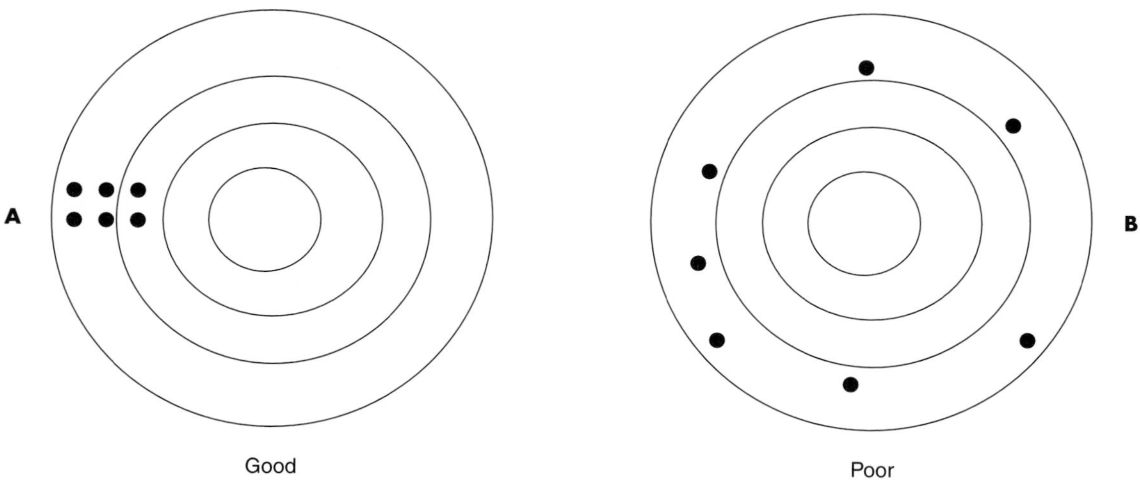

FIGURE 3–1
Reliability conceptualized as shots on a target. A tight cluster indicates high reliability (**A**). Failure to cluster indicates poor reliability (**B**).

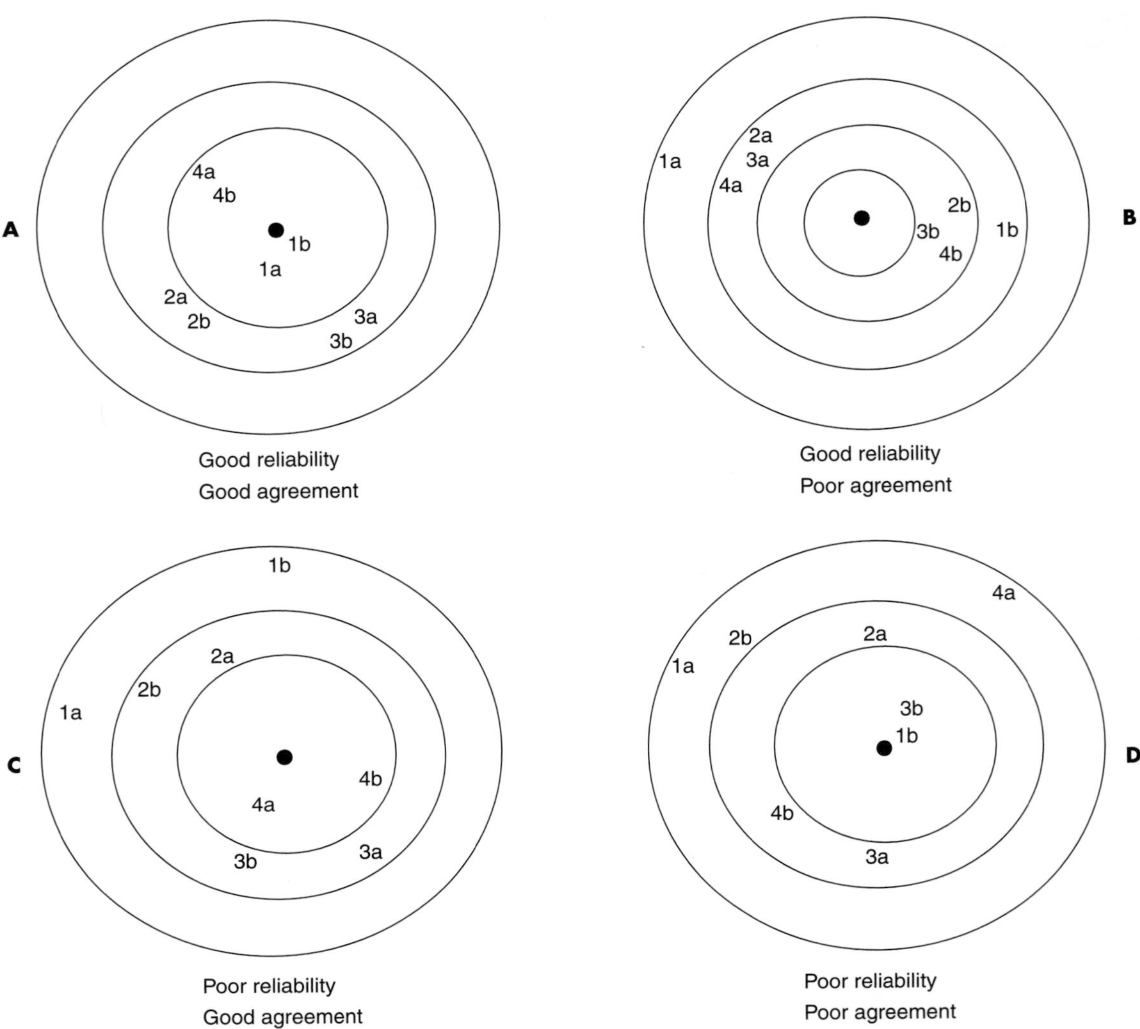

FIGURE 3–2
Reliability versus agreement. Within each target: *a,* initial score; *b,* retest or interrater; numbers indicate individual subjects rated.

the scores by the two therapists for each subject). However, the overall rank order of client performance (from best to worst) is identical for both therapists (i.e., there is high reliability between their rankings). Conversely, low reliability may not necessarily indicate poor rater agreement. Low reliability coefficients can occur with high agreement when the range of scores assigned by the raters is restricted or when the variability of the ratings themselves is inherently small (i.e., measuring a homogeneous population). In instances where the scores are fairly homogeneous, reliability coefficients lack the power to detect relationships and are often artificially depressed, even though agreement between ratings may be relatively high.[50]

Both reliability and agreement must be established on the target population or populations to which the measure will be applied, using typical examiners. The following five types of reliability and agreement will be discussed: *interrater, test-retest, intertrial, alternate form,* and *population specific.*

Interrater reliability and agreement

Interrater or *interobserver agreement* is the extent to which independent examiners agree exactly on a measurement score. In contrast, *interrater reliability* is defined as the degree to which the ratings of different observers are proportional when expressed as deviations from their means; that is, the ranking of one rated person to other rated people is the same, although the absolute numbers used to express the relationship may vary from rater to rater.[50] The independence of the examiners in the training they receive and the observations they make is critical when determining interrater agreement and reliability. When examiners have trained together or confer when performing a test, the interrater reliability or agreement coefficient calculated from their observations may be artificially inflated.

An interrater agreement or reliability coefficient provides an estimate of how much measurement error can be expected in scores obtained by two or more examiners who have independently rated the same subject. Determining interrater agreement or reliability is particularly important for test scores that largely depend on the examiner's skill or judgment. An acceptable level of interrater reliability or agreement (see below) is essential for comparison of impairment rating results obtained from different clinicians. Interrater agreement or reliability is a basic criterion to be fulfilled for a measure to be called objective. If multiple examiners consistently obtain the same absolute or relative scores, then it is much more likely that the score is a function of the measure, rather than of the collective subjective bias of the examiners.[44] "Pure" interrater agreement and reliability are determined by having one examiner administer the test measures and additional examiners independently score each subject at the same point in time. When assessing some parameters, where the skill of the examiner administering the test plays a vital role (e.g., sensory testing, range of motion testing), or where direct observation of each examiner is required (e.g., strength testing), it is impossible to assess pure interrater agreement and reliability. In these instances, each examiner must test the individual independently and may risk compromising agreement and reliability because of factors of time and variation in subject performance.

Test-retest reliability and agreement

Test-retest agreement is defined as the extent to which a subject receives identical scores during two different test sessions when rated by the same examiner. In contrast, test-retest reliability assesses the degree of consistency in how a subject's score is rank ordered relative to other subjects tested by the same examiner during different test sessions. Test-retest reliability is the most basic and essential form of reliability. It provides an estimate of the variation in subject scores over time when retested by the same examiner. Since some of the error in a test-retest situation also may be attributed to variations in the examiner's performance, it is important to determine the magnitude of expected day-to-day fluctuations so that true changes over time in the parameters of interest can be recognized. Frequent instrument recalibration may be required to maintain acceptable test-retest reliability. For example, if a functional capacity evaluation (FCE) is being used on repeat testing to measure severity of a client's work disability because of low back pain, it is essential that the FCE have sufficient test-retest reliability and agreement to reflect true variance in a client's work-related performance over time rather than artifacts caused by the test setting or examiners testing in each case.

The suggested test-retest interval is 1 to 3 days for most physical measures and 7 days for maximal-effort tests where muscle fatigue is involved.[7] The test-retest interval should not exceed the expected time for change to occur naturally. The purpose of an adequate, but relatively short interval is to minimize the effects of memory, practice, and maturation or deterioration on test performance.[9]

Intertrial reliability and agreement

Intertrial agreement provides an estimate of the stability of repeated scores obtained by one examiner within a test session. Intertrial reliability assesses the consistency of one examiner's rank ordering of repeated trials obtained from subjects within a test session. Intertrial agreement and reliability also are influenced by individual subject performance factors such as fatigue, motor learning, motivation, and consistency of effort. Consequently, tests designed to assess sincerity of client effort during impairment or disability evaluation (i.e., coefficient of variation on the Jamar dynamometer) must have high intertrial reliability and agreement at the outset. Intertrial agreement and reliability should not be confused with test-retest agreement and reliability. The latter involves test sessions usually separated by days or weeks as opposed to seconds or minutes for intertrial agreement and reliability. A higher level of association is expected for results obtained from trials within a test session than from those between different sessions.

Alternate form reliability and agreement

Alternate form agreement refers to the consistency of scores obtained from two forms of the same test. Equivalent or parallel forms are different test versions intended to measure the same traits at a comparable level of difficulty. *Alternate form reliability* refers to whether the parallel forms of a test rank order a subject's scores consistently relative to each other. A high level of alternate form agreement or reliability may be required if a subject must be tested more than once and a learning or practice effect is anticipated. This is particularly important when one form of the test will be used as a pretest and the second as a posttest.

Population-specific reliability and agreement

Population-specific agreement and reliability assess the degree of absolute and relative reproducibility, respectively, that a test has for a specific group being measured. A variation of this type of agreement and reliability refers to the population of examiners administering the test.[44]

Interpretation of Reliability and Agreement Statistics

Since measures of reliability and agreement are concerned with the degree of consistency or concordance between two or more independently derived sets of scores, they can be expressed in terms of correlation coefficients.[5] The reliability coefficient is usually expressed as a value between 0 and 1, with higher values indicating higher reliability. Agreement statistics can range from -1 to +1, with +1 indicating perfect agreement, 0 indicating chance agreement, and negative values indicating less than chance agreement. The coefficient of choice varies, depending on the type of data analyzed.[6, 21, 24, 33, 50] No definitive standards for minimum acceptable levels of the different types of reliability and agreement statistics have been established. Generally, agreement coefficients should exceed

.60 and reliability coefficients should exceed .75.[22] The acceptable level varies, depending on the magnitude of the decision being made, the population variance, the sources of error variance, and the measurement technique (e.g., instrumentation versus behavioral assessments). If the population variance is relatively homogeneous, lower estimates of reliability become more acceptable. In contrast, if the population variance is heterogeneous, higher estimates of reliability are demanded. Critical values of correlation coefficients, based on the desired level of significance and the number of subjects, are available in reference tables.[46, 51] Scores generated from instrumentation should be expected to have a higher level of reliability or agreement than scores obtained from behavioral observations.

It is important to note that a correlation coefficient that is statistically significant does not necessarily indicate that adequate reliability or agreement has been established because the significance level only provides an indication that the coefficient is significantly different from zero.

A test score actually consists of two different components: the true score and the error score.[5, 12] A person's true score is a hypothetical construct, indicating a test score that is unaffected by chance factors. The *error score* refers to unwanted variation in the test score.[11] All continuous scale measurements have a component of error, and no test is completely reliable. Consequently, reliability is a matter of degree. Any reliability coefficient may be interpreted directly in terms of percentage of score variance attributable to different sources.[44] A reliability coefficient of .85 signifies that 85% of the variance in test scores depends on true variance in the trait measured, and 15% depends on error variance.

In summary, reliability and agreement are essential components to any objective measurement. Measurements that do not have acceptable test-retest reliability can be considered so full of error as to be potentially useless because the numbers obtained may not reflect the variable measured.[44] Reliability is an important component of validity, but good reliability or agreement does not guarantee that a measure is valid. A reliable measurement is consistent, but not necessarily correct. A measurement that is unreliable, however, cannot be valid.

Validity

Validity is defined as the accuracy with which a test measures that which it is intended to measure. To use our target analogy, if a gun is aimed and fired at the target, validity is the ability to hit the target (Fig. 3–3, *A* and *B*). The higher the validity, the more closely you come to actually hitting the point at which you are aiming. Validity is initially investigated while a test or instrument is being developed and is confirmed through subsequent use. Four basic aspects of validity will be discussed, including *content, construct, criterion-related,* and *face validity.*

Content validity

Content validity is the systematic examination of the test content to determine if it covers a representative sample of the particular domain being measured. For example, digital amputation level, joint ankylosis and ROM, and sensory loss all contribute to hand impairment and presumably reflect functional losses, as the associated impairment ratings imply. Content validity generally is evidenced by the opinion of experts that the domain sampled is adequate. The AMA *Guides* is a classic example of a delphi (expert) panel that has endorsed a

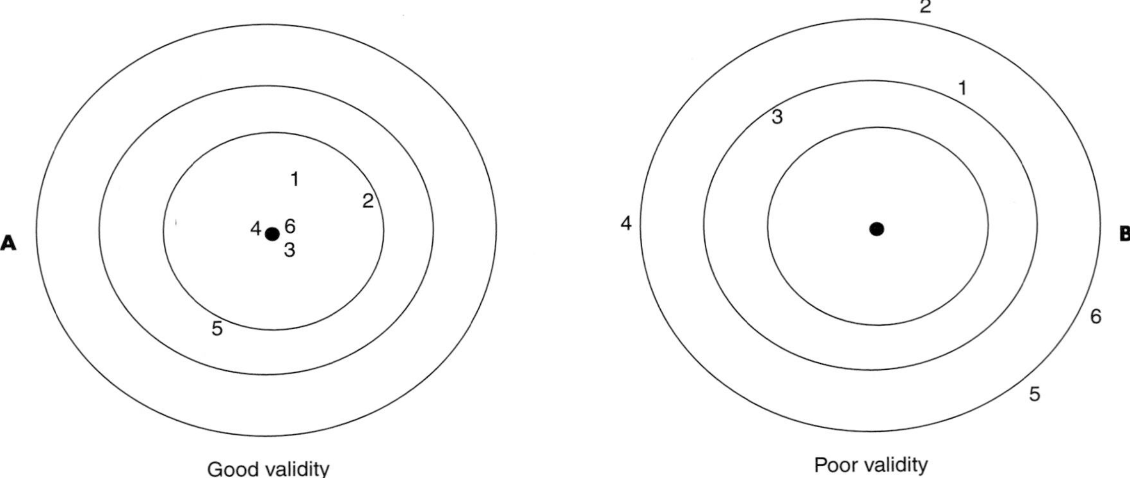

FIGURE 3–3
Validity conceptualized as the ability to hit the target.

traditional hand-impairment schedule in this manner and based on a sampling of anatomical criteria, including amputation, joint ROM or ankylosis, and digital sensory loss.[3] There are two primary methods that the developer of a test can use for obtaining professional opinions about the content validity of an instrument.[14] The first is to provide a panel of experts with the items from the test and request a determination of what the battery of items is measuring. The second method requires providing not only the test items but also a list of test objectives so that experts can determine the relationship between the two. Details of statistical analysis of content validity are described elsewhere.[49]

Construct validity

Construct validity refers to the extent to which a test measures a theoretical construct underlying the test. Construct validity should be obtained whenever a test purports to measure an abstract concept or theoretical aspect of human behavior, such as intelligence, self-concept, anxiety, pain and suffering, school or work readiness, or perceptual organization. The following five areas must be considered with regard to construct validity in test instruments[5, 14]:

1. **Age differentiation:** Any developmental changes in children or changes in performance caused by aging must be accounted for as part of the test development.

2. **Factor analysis:** Factor analysis is a statistical procedure that can be performed on data obtained from testing. The purpose of factor analysis is to simplify the description of behavior by reducing an initial multiplicity of variables to a few common underlying factors or traits that may be pertinent to the construct or constructs that the test was originally designed to measure.[11, 54, 56, 57] The more recent development of confirmatory factor analysis overcomes the relative arbitrariness of traditional factor analytical methods.[16, 34] Confirmatory factor analysis differs from traditional factor analysis in that the investigator specifies, before analysis, the measures that are determined by each factor and which factors are correlated. The specified relationships are then statistically tested for goodness of fit of the proposed model compared with the actual data collected. Confirmatory factor analysis is therefore a more direct assessment of construct validity than is traditional factor analysis.

3. Internal consistency: In assessing the attributes of a test, it is helpful to examine the relationship of subscales and individual items to the total score. This is especially important when the test instrument has many components. If a subtest or item has a very low correlation with the total score, the test developer must question the subtest's validity in relation to the total score. This technique is most useful for providing confirmation of the validity of a homogeneous test. A test that measures several constructs would not be expected to have a high degree of internal consistency. For dichotomous data, the Kuder-Richardson statistic is used to calculate internal consistency.[5] Cronbach's coefficient alpha is recommended when the measure has more than two levels of response.[5] The minimum acceptable level of alpha generally is set at .70.[31]

4. Convergent and divergent validity: Construct validity is evidenced further by high correlations with other tests that purport to measure the same constructs (i.e., convergent validity) and low correlations with measures that are designed to measure different attributes (i.e., divergent validity). It is desirable to obtain moderate levels of convergent validity, indicating that the two measures are not measuring identical constructs. If the new test correlates too highly with another test, it is questionable whether the new test is necessary because either test would suffice to answer the same questions. Moderately high, but significant correlations indicate good convergent validity, but with each test still having unique components. Good divergent validity is demonstrated by low and insignificant correlations between two tests that measure theoretically unrelated parameters.

5. Discriminant validity: If two groups known to have different characteristics can be identified and assessed by the test and a significant difference between the performance of the two groups can be shown, then incisive discriminant validity is present.

Criterion-related validity

Criterion-related validity includes two subclasses of validity—concurrent validity and predictive validity.[5, 9] The commonality between these subclasses of validity is that they refer to multiple measurement of the same construct. In other words, the measure in question is compared with other variables or measures that are considered to be accurate measures of the characteristics or behaviors being tested. The purpose is to use the second measure as a criterion to validate the first measure.

Criterion-related validity can be assessed statistically, providing clear guidelines as to whether a measure is valid. Frequently, the paired measurements from the tests under comparison have different values. The nature of the relationship is less important than the strength of the relationship.[44] Other workers have shown that the limits of agreement statistical technique provide the most accurate assessment of measurement error when comparing test results.[39]

Concurrent validity deals with whether an inference is justifiable at the present time. This is typically done by comparing results of one measure against some criterion (e.g., another measure or related phenomenon) that is the "gold standard." A frequently used example is the contrast venogram as the "gold standard" for diagnosis of deep venous thrombosis. A less invasive (presumably safer) and less costly alternative is the venous Doppler ultrasound. The ability of the Doppler to correctly diagnose deep venous thrombosis when compared with the venogram represents its concurrent validity. If the correlation is high, the measure is said to have good concurrent validity. Concurrent validity is relevant to tests used for diagnosis of existing status, rather than predicting future outcome. This aspect of validity has particular importance to the field of impairment ratings as the following example illustrates: A "diagnosis-based" approach to impairment ratings of the musculoskeletal system was introduced in the AMA *Guides*, third edition revised,[2] and carried forward with respect to spinal impairment ratings in the fourth edition[3] with the "diagnosis related estimates" (DRE) system. The DRE system is arguably simpler to apply than the ROM approach, and presumably has greater interrater reliability. The degree to which the DRE approach yields impairment estimates comparable to the ROM model is its concurrent validity.

Predictive validity involves a measure's ability to predict or forecast some future criterion. Examples include performance on another measure in the future, prognostic reaction to an intervention program, or performance in some task of daily living. Predictive validity is difficult to establish and often requires collection of data over an extended period after the test has been developed. Hence very few measures used in rehabilitation medicine, for example, have established predictive validity. A specific subset of predictive validity that is important to rehabilitation medicine practice is ecological validity. This concept involves the ability to identify impairments, functional limitations, and performance deficits within the context of the person's own environment. Measures with good concurrent validity sometimes are presumed to have good predictive validity, but this may not be a correct assumption. Unless predictive validity information exists for a test, extreme caution should be exercised in interpreting test results as predictors of future behavior or function.

Face validity

Face validity is not considered to be an essential component of the validity of a test or measure. It reflects only whether a test appears to measure what it is supposed to, based on the personal opinions of those either taking or giving the test.[5] A test with high face validity has a greater likelihood of being more rigorously and carefully administered by the examiner, and the person being tested is more likely to give his or her best effort. Although it is not essential, in most instances face validity is still an important component of test development and selection. Exceptions include personality and interest tests where the purpose of testing is concealed to prevent client responses from being biased.

Precision and Range

Instrument responsiveness to change is influenced by its precision and range. *Precision* refers to fineness of scale of an instrument, that is, the smallest unit of change that an instrument can distinguish. Sensitivity to change is critical to measures designed to detect the effects of treatment.[48] Measures that implement dichotomous or ordinal scales with limited rating levels tend to be less sensitive than measures utilizing interval or ratio scales. For example, a dichotomous functional outcome measure defined as "able" versus "not able" would be a gross indicator of performance ability and would fail to distinguish between clinically meaningful functional gradations of "able with adaptive equipment" or "able with helper assistance." By contrast, an interval measure of function such as time to distance ambulated would make it possible to detect differences of walking speed of a few feet per minute. Although such small differences might appear statistically significant among treatment groups with large numbers, they might not be clinically relevant. Instrument sensitivity should be appropriate to the level of precision required. For example, the Schober test is a useful but imprecise screening test for loss of spinal mobility (flexion/extension) of the lumbar region and can be administered simply by using a tape measure calibrated in centimeters.[35] By contrast, surface inclinometry is a more precise measure of lumbar spinal flexibility and is required where angular comparisons of degrees of motion are being made.[3]

Range refers to the distance between highest and lowest scores of a measure. A wide range can minimize the likelihood of "ceiling" or "floor" effects. Ceiling effects occur when initial test scores are high and leave little room for improvement. For example, the Barthel ADL Index is a commonly used measure of disability in stroke patients, sensitive to functional differences among moderately to severely impaired individuals.[53] However, ceiling effects are readily apparent among mildly impaired individuals who might otherwise show important differences in high-level activities such as balancing a checkbook or preparing a meal. Conversely, floor effects occur where initial scores are very low and there is little room for deterioration in performance.[48]

Feasibility and Practicality

A test or instrument should be practical (i.e., easy to use, insensitive to outside influences, inexpensive, and designed to allow efficient administration).[10] For example, it is not efficient to begin testing in a supine position, switch to a prone position, then return to supine. Test administration should be organized to complete all testing in one position before switching to another. Instructions for administering the test should be clear and concise, and scoring criteria should be clearly defined. If equipment is required, it must be durable and of good quality. Qualifications of the tester, and additional training required to become proficient in test administration, should be specified. The time to administer the test should be indicated in the test manual. The duration of the test and level of difficulty must be appropriate relative to the attention span and perceived capabilities of the subject being tested. Finally, the test manual should provide summary statistics and detailed guidelines for appropriate use and interpretation of test scores and be based on the test development data.

PRACTICAL APPLICATIONS

In view of the preceding discussions it appears fair to ask whether the measurement criteria employed by impairment and disability rating systems measure up with respect to the above criteria. This question will be addressed with a careful look at the AMA *Guides* approach to impairment ratings, and with particular attention to the musculoskeletal system.

With respect to measurement scales, both nominal-ordinal and interval-ratio data are used. Qualitative (i.e., nominal-ordinal) impairment measures include presence of amputation or joint ankylosis, sensory changes of the hand, and cosmetic disfigurement. The DRE approach to impairment of the spine is largely qualitative, with multiple categorical descriptors of level of severity, although the descriptors themselves (i.e., "segmental instability" according to angular or translational displacement) may be quantitatively derived. Quantitative (i.e., interval-ratio) impairment measures include loss of joint ROM (in degrees) and position of joint ankylosis. ROM assessment is carried out with accepted goniometric and surface inclinometric techniques for which normative data exists and reliability studies have been conducted.[3, 27, 37, 58]

The reliability of generally accepted anthropometric measurement techniques applicable to impairment ratings is suspect,[8] and the particular measurement techniques ascribed to by the AMA *Guides* have questionable reliability as well. To illustrate, surface inclinometry using single or dual inclinometer techniques is the preferred method for assessing spinal mobility,[3] and high interrater and intrarater reliability have been reported for cervical ROM[58] and for lumbar flexion and extension in the sagittal plane.[27] However, other work has yielded unacceptably low reliability estimates for these techniques based on intraclass correlations, even when applied by experienced observers with healthy, motivated, and fully compliant subjects.[43] Numerous potential sources of error exist and may include choice of surface reference landmarks from which actual measurements are taken, lack of uniform training and application of measurement techniques among raters, and differences inherent to different measurement instruments themselves.[43] Such errors may be further compounded during examination of a client who is symptomatic, apprehensive, and prone to self-inhibition.

In part, because of concerns about interrater reliability of measures of spinal ROM, the AMA *Guides* adopted the DRE approach as an alternative means of rating spinal impairment. The DRE uses categorical criteria as measures of severity, which are inherently easy to describe and identify and hence can be expected to show high interrater reliability and agreement. Examples include neurological findings of nerve-root tension (straight leg raise), muscle guarding, reflex changes or asymmetry, muscle atrophy, "long tract findings," bowel and bladder changes, and electrodiagnostic (EMG) findings. In addition, radiographic evidence of fracture or "segmental instability" in terms of translational and angular motion is accepted. Unfortunately, the reliability of many of these criteria is also highly questionable. To illustrate, there is no universal agreement in the literature as to what constitutes a positive "straight leg test,"[13] and this test is particularly prone to exaggeration during examination of the symptom magnifier.[52] Similarly, muscle guarding is highly subjective and prone to displays of exaggeration. Reflex assessment is also subjective insofar as it requires the examinee to relax and can easily be suppressed in the presence of muscle guarding. (The usefulness of the "Waddell's signs" themselves as indicators of invalid or unreliable performance is subject to debate because these signs offer a psychological "yellow flag" but are neither a complete nor sufficient psychological assessment.[36] Behavioral signs in and of themselves are not a test of credibility or faking.) Neurogenic muscle atrophy is not typically seen until a substantial reduction in anterior horn cell or motor unit function takes place, making this finding difficult to detect (less reliable?) in more subtle injuries. Studies from the old polio era demonstrate that in the vicinity of 40% of anterior horn cells must degenerate before the clinician can even detect any muscle weakness on manual muscle testing.[47] Although electrodiagnostic examination has definite value in the diagnosis of radiculopathic low-back pain, the criteria one should utilize to make this determination are less clear. Most electromyographers agree that positive sharp waves and fibrillation potentials are consistent with a clinical picture of radiculopathy and are highly specific. However, although criteria for abnormality of the S1 "H reflex" are relatively well defined, many electrodiagnostic consultants are hesitant to make the diagnosis of S1 radiculopathy based on this finding alone.[15] The radiographic criteria for loss of motion segment integrity within the AMA *Guides* are based on translational and rotational stability on flexion and extension views of lateral radiographs. Strangely, these criteria are not widely utilized by neuroradiologists, but are based on cadaveric studies with no known clinical correlate.[40] Although the DRE approach intuitively appears more reliable than the ROM approach, formal reliability studies of the various criteria employed would appear useful and desirable for future editions of the AMA *Guides*.

In terms of its concurrent validity, the AMA *Guides* has become the "gold standard" for impairment rating under Workers' Compensation, being mandated or recommended by law in 55% of jurisdictions and more frequently used than not in another 21% of jurisdictions not mandating or recommending by law.[3] Unfortunately, and in spite of this widespread acceptance, the lack of internal validity may be its most serious shortcoming with respect to the impairment rating process it is intended to serve.

To begin with, the lack of construct and criterion (i.e., predictive) validity of impairment ratings is an issue of fundamental concern. According to the AMA *Guides*, impairment ratings are intended to represent the degree to which physical capacity has been diminished. An expert panel of contributors to the AMA *Guides'* fourth and previous editions has relied largely on clinical experience, judgment, and consensus to derive its numerical ratings. The numbers themselves remain unsupported by rigorous and objective behavioral data to substantiate purported functional losses. This issue has received closest scrutiny with respect to functional loss directly associated with hand impairment. In one study, significant correlations between several valid and commonly accepted measures of hand function and associated impairment ratings were obtained[18]; however, the magnitude of these correlations was small in most cases, with fewer than 8% of correlations sufficient to explain 50% or more of the variance among impairment ratings derived.[41] In a separate study using simulated hand impairments of a mild-to-moderate degree of severity (equal to or less than 32% of hand impairment), no significant correlations between hand-impairment ratings and several quantitative measures of hand function were seen, and regression analysis showed that impairment failed to predict disability.[41] Clearly, more work is needed to address this fundamental issue in which the presumptive implications of construct and predictive validity can be so costly and misleading.

The relevance of anatomical criteria to functional loss (such as loss of ROM to loss of joint function) is also somewhat questionable and has been particularly problematic with respect to the spine. For example, the relation of surface inclinometry to underlying spinal mobility has been examined and seems apparent,[37] but the relation between spinal flexibility and functional loss caused by painful back conditions remains unclear.[17] In one study an inverse relationship between pain-associated disability and lumbar flexibility was even suggested.[30] A similar concern exists for the DRE approach to spinal impairment rating, for which comparative studies relating severity of injury (according to DRE criteria) to degree of resulting functional losses simply do not exist.

Throughout various sections of the AMA *Guides*, the functional basis of rating criteria remains suspect. Perhaps the most thorough and objective approach to functional impairment ratings based on objective testing exists for the respiratory and cardiovascular systems. For example, in the respiratory system the subjective history is functionally oriented with respect to exertional provocation of dyspnea, medications required (types and frequency), and degree of symptom relief and functional ability the client achieves while on medications. That history is substantiated by formal pulmonary function testing using commonly accepted, valid, and reliable indicators of pulmonary function, including the forced vital capacity (FVC), forced expiratory volume at one second (FEV1), and the diffusion of carbon monoxide test (DLCO) among others. Similarly, the client's history of cardiovascular functional impairment can be substantiated by performance on noninvasive studies (i.e., Bruce protocol or other exercise stress testing) and invasive studies (i.e., coronary angiography) where available. The client can then be classified in terms of functional Class I through IV pulmonary or cardiovascular impairment, respectively, to which an impairment rating can be assigned from the appropriate available range. A similar functionally based approach to the assessment of impairments to the musculoskeletal system is needed—perhaps based on ADL scales—to provide the construct validity desired and heretofore assumed of these measures. This problem and its potential solution were discussed in greater detail in Chapter 2.

Concerns regarding the content validity of commonly accepted impairment measures also abound. For example, the musculoskeletal system section of the AMA *Guides* makes no distinction between impairments affecting the dominant versus nondominant upper extremity, whereas the functional impact of the former would logically be expected to exceed the latter. In another example, impairment ratings affecting the male reproductive system are differentially weighted according to age categories. No adjustment is made for individuals whose age is between 40 and 65 years of age, whereas ratings are increased by 50% for individuals below 40 years of age and decreased by 50% for those over 65 years of age. Furthermore, no consideration is given to baseline fertility in regards to these ratings and with respect to any prior history of vasectomy or previous number of children fathered.

Instances can be shown in which the same impairment is rated differently in different sections of the AMA *Guides,* raising overall concerns about internal consistency. To illustrate, whole-person impairment associated with lower-limb gait derangement is rated to a maximum loss of 80% in the musculoskeletal system section, whereas the equivalent impairment related to station and gait is rated to a maximum of 60% in the nervous system section. Similarly, severe impairment of equilibrium caused by acoustic-nerve (VIII) dysfunction is rated to a maximum of 70% in the nervous system section, whereas the same result caused by vestibular dysfunction is rated up to 95% in the ear, nose, and throat section. The maximum impairment caused by loss of olfactory-nerve (I) function is rated as 5% in the nervous system section and 3% in the ear, nose, and throat section. As noted previously, for the musculoskeletal system section of the AMA *Guides,* no adjustment is made for losses to the dominant versus nondominant extremity, whereas in the nervous system section such adjustment for the "preferred extremity" is made.

Convergent validity is a concern whenever impairment ratings are applied to determine the economic loss associated with physical impairment. Although the AMA *Guides* provides a disclaimer against such applications, the fact is that many Workers' Compensation jurisdictions directly apply impairment ratings derived according to the AMA *Guides* to compute such economic losses. To illustrate, in Kansas (an "impairment rating" jurisdiction) the person as "a whole" is worth 415 weeks of compensation at a maximum weekly rate capped by statute at $319/week. At maximum medical improvement (MMI), a permanent partial impairment rating of 10% could result in a maximum direct payout equivalent to 415 weeks × $319/week × 10%, or $13,238.50 at case closure.[42] This practice clearly fails to take into account the various functional and socioeconomic complexities of the particular case, and consequently can be expected to have poor convergent validity. In addition, economic losses in terms of inability to perform other major life functions are frequently overlooked and may include needs for adaptive equipment or assistance to perform basic mobility and self-care activities and social and avocational pursuits. As such, additional research is needed to quantitatively assess nonvocational losses associated with various medical impairments and the concurrent validity of the AMA *Guides* to assess these losses.[41]

Several criteria for the evaluation of spinal impairment according to a DRE model appear to lack face validity. To illustrate, DRE categorical differentiators to the lumbosacral spine include "cauda equina syndrome without or with bowel or bladder impairment." By definition, cauda equina syndrome affects the lower motor neuron output to the sacral nerve roots innervating the bladder and bowel, making lumbosacral category VI a non sequitur. Furthermore, cauda equina syndrome is also assigned as a category VI or VII differentiator for cervicothoracic and thoracolumbar regions, respectively, and for which cauda equina syndrome does not exist. Similarly, "paraplegia" is an incorrect categorical differentiator (VIII) of the lumbosacral spine that is more appropriately assigned to the thoracolumbar region because paraplegia is a myelopathic condition brought about by injury or illness affecting the spinal cord at or above the conus medullaris and terminating at the L2 lumbar segment. Injuries to the lumbosacral spine typically affect the cauda equina to produce paralysis without paraplegia.

Finally, a few words about instrument precision and considerations of feasibility and practicality of the AMA *Guides* are in order. Precision levels vary considerably within and between sections of the AMA *Guides*. For the musculoskeletal section there is a high level of precision (measured in degrees of angular motion) associated with ROM determinations for the upper extremity. Goniometric techniques sensitive to angular change are defined and illustrated, and normative reference tables are provided corresponding to the multiple joints of the digits and hand, wrist, forearm, elbow, and shoulder. In addition, sensory impairments to the digits are precisely defined in terms of sensory loss (transverse or longitudinal). Sensory change is measured by sensitive calipers capable of detecting millimeter differences in two-point sensory discrimination. For the lower extremity, similar goniometric techniques are illustrated, and normative tables are provided for the hip, knee, ankle, hindfoot, and toes, although sensory loss is not counted. Spinal ROM is measured precisely (in angular degrees) by surface goniometry according to well-illustrated techniques. However, because of concerns over measurement reliability and validity, the latter techniques require an elaborate process of repetition and cross validation that requires the examiner to perform three separate repetitions of each spinal measurement, average the results, and reject the measurements outright if they differ from one another by more than 10% or 5°, whichever is greater! Such procedural encumbrance is, for all intent and purpose, impractical and not feasible to perform by most busy practitioners. The DRE approach discussed above obviates this problem.

In other sections of the AMA *Guides*, impairment criteria range from the very precise to the entirely imprecise. To illustrate, impairments to the visual system (e.g., loss of visual acuity in Snellen units or reduction of visual field in terms of deficits on perimetric charts or the Estherman Grid) and auditory system (e.g., deficits in tone detection and discrimination at 500, 1000, 2000, and 3000 Hz) can be precisely measured. In contrast, and perhaps out of necessity, impairments such as those affecting the brain are often imprecise because the complex array of factors comprising arousal level and emotional, psychomotor, and behavioral functioning cannot be precisely and feasibly reduced to unidimensional physical measurements in most cases. Indeed, under the section on psychiatric impairment, the AMA *Guides* states that available empiric evidence to support any method for assigning impairment is lacking and, consequently, guidelines for rating individual impairment cannot be feasibly provided at the present time.[3]

SUMMARY

The information presented above will hopefully provide the reader with a basis for critically assessing available tests and measures of impairment rating and disability determination. Ideally, the scale of the test or instrument selected should be sufficient to enable identification and discrimination of levels of impairment severity for the particular organ system of interest to the physician examiner. The measures selected should be practical from the standpoint of time, feasibility, and ease of application among trained examiners. Above all, the measures must have acceptable reliability, agreement, and validity for the specific applications selected, and that can be expected to include disability inference. The concerns raised and criticisms we have leveled toward the AMA *Guides* are, in the larger sense, indicative of shortcomings with the impairment rating process in general. It is likely that similar concerns and criticisms apply to most commonly accepted disability rating systems, including Workers' Compensation rating systems in which the AMA *Guides* is not applied, Social Security disability determinations, and compensation and pensioning within the Veterans Administration. It appears that further empirically based research is needed to provide improved measures of impairment of the various organ systems, and of the musculoskeletal system in particular, before the measurement criteria and ideals we have highlighted can be feasibly adhered to and acceptable scientific standards for disability evaluation can be met.

REFERENCES

1. American Educational Association, American Psychological Association, National Council on Measurement in Education: Standards for educational and psychological testing. Washington DC, American Psychological Association, 1985.
2. American Medical Association: Guides to the Evaluation of Permanent Impairment, 3rd ed (revised). Chicago, American Medical Association, 1990.
3. American Medical Association: Guides to the Evaluation of Permanent Impairment, 4th ed. Chicago, American Medical Association, 1993.
4. American Physical Therapy Association: Standards for tests and measurements in physical therapy practice. Phys Ther 71:589–622, 1991.
5. Anastasi A: Psychological Testing, 6th ed. New York, Macmillan, 1988.
6. Bartko JJ, Carpenter WT: On the methods and theory of reliability. J Nerv Ment Dis 163:307–317, 1976.
7. Baumgartner TA, Jackson AS: Measurement for Evaluation in Physical Education and Exercise Science, 4th ed. Dubuque, Iowa, William C Brown, 1991.
8. Bennett KA, Osborne RH: Interobserver measurement reliability in anthropometry. Hum Biol 58:751–759, 1986.
9. Bloom M, Fischer J, Orme JG: Evaluating Practice: Guidelines for the Accountable Professional. Boston, Allyn and Bacon, 1995.

10. Chaffin DB, Anderson GBJ: Occupational Biomechanics, 2nd ed. New York, John Wiley & Sons, 1991.
11. Cronbach LJ: Essentials of Psychological Testing, 5th ed. New York, Harper & Row, 1990.
12. Deitz JC: Reliability. Physical and Occupational Therapy in Pediatrics 9:125–147, 1989.
13. Deyo RA, Rainville J, Kent DL: What can the history and physical examination teach us about low back pain? JAMA 268: 760–765, 1992.
14. Dunn WW: Validity. Physical and Occupational Therapy in Pediatrics 9:149–168, 1989.
15. Dvorak J: Neurophysiologic tests in diagnosis of nerve root compression caused by disc herniation. Spine 21(suppl):39S–44S, 1996.
16. Francis DJ: An introduction to structural equation models. J Clin Exp Neuropsychol 10:623–639, 1988.
17. Frymoyer JW, Cats-Baril W: Predictors of low back pain disability. Clin Ortho Rel Res 221:89–98, 1987.
18. Gloss DS, Wardle MG: Reliability and validity of American Medical Association's Guide to ratings of permanent impairment. JAMA 248:2292–2296, 1982.
19. Granger CV, Gresham GE (eds): Functional Assessment in Rehabilitation Medicine. Baltimore, Williams & Wilkins, 1984.
20. Granger CV, Kelly-Hayes M, Johnston M, et al: Quality and outcome measures for medical rehabilitation. In: Braddom RL (ed): Physical Medicine & Rehabilitation. Philadelphia, WB Saunders, 1996, pp 239–253.
21. Hartmann DP: Considerations in the choice of interobserver reliability estimates. J Appl Behav Anal 10:103–116, 1977.
22. Hinderer SL, Hinderer KA: Principles and applications of measurement methods. In: DeLisa JA, Gans BM (eds): Rehabilitation Medicine: Principles and Practice, 3rd ed. Philadelphia, Lippincott-Raven, 1998, pp 109–136.
23. Hislop HJ, Montgomery J: Daniels and Worthingham's Muscle Testing: Techniques of Manual Examination, 6th ed. Philadelphia, WB Saunders, 1995.
24. Hollenbeck AR: Problems of reliability in observational research. In: Sackett GP (ed): Observing Behavior: Data Collection and Analysis Methods, vol 2. Baltimore, University Park Press, 1978, pp 79–98.
25. Janda V: Muscle Function Testing. Boston, Butterworths, 1983.
26. Johnston MV, Keith RA, Hinderer SR: Measurement standards for interdisciplinary medical rehabilitation. Arch Phys Med Rehabil 73(suppl):12–S, 1992.
27. Keeley J, Mayer TG, Cox R, et al: Quantification of lumbar function. Part 5. Reliability of range-of-motion measures in the sagittal plane and in vivo torso rotation measurement technique. Spine 11(1):31–35, 1986.
28. Kendall FP, McCreary EK, Geise PG: Muscle Testing and Function, 4th ed. Baltimore, Williams & Wilkins, 1993.
29. Krebs DE: Measurement theory. Phys Ther 67:1834–1839, 1987.
30. Lankhorst GJ, Van de Stadt RJ, Van der Korst JK: The natural history of idiopathic low back pain. Scand J Rehabil Med 17:1–4, 1985.
31. Law M: Measurement in occupational therapy: scientific criteria for evaluation. Can J Occup Ther 54:133–138, 1987.
32. Lawlis GF, Lu E: Judgment of counseling process: reliability, agreement, and error. Psychol Bull 78:17–20, 1972.
33. Liebetrau AM: Measures of Association. Sage University Paper Series on Quantitative Applications in the Social Sciences (Series No. 07-032). Newbury Park, Calif, Sage Publications, 1983.
34. Long JS: Confirmatory Factor Analysis. Sage University Paper Series on Quantitative Application in the Social Sciences (Series No. 07-033). Newbury Park, Calif, Sage Publications, 1983.
35. Magee DJ: Orthopedic Physical Assessment, 2nd ed. Philadelphia, WB Saunders Co, 1992.

36. Main CJ, Waddell G: Spine update: behavioral responses to examination: a reappraisal of the interpretation of "nonorganic signs." Spine 23:2367–2371, 1998.
37. Mayer T, Tencer A, Kristoferson S, Mooney V: Use of noninvasive techniques for quantification of spinal range of motion in normal subjects and chronic low-back dysfunction patients. Spine 9:588–595, 1984.
38. Merbitz C, Morris J, Grip JC: Ordinal scales and foundations of misinference. Arch Phys Med Rehabil 70:308–312, 1989.
39. Ottenbacher KJ, Tomchek SD: Measurement variation in method comparison studies: an empirical examination. Arch Phys Med Rehabil 75:505–512, 1994.
40. Posner I, White AA, Edwards WT, Hayes WA: Biomechanical analysis of the clinical stability of the lumbar and lumbosacral spine. Spine 7:374–389, 1982.
41. Rondinelli RD, Dunn W, Hassanein KM, et al: A simulation of hand impairments: effects on upper extremity function and implications toward medical impairment rating and disability determination. Arch Phys Med Rehabil 78:1358–1363, 1997.
42. Rondinelli RD, Katz RT, Hendler SL, Eisfelder B: Disability evaluation. In: Grabois M, Garrison SJ, Hart KA, Lemkuhl LD (eds): Physical Medicine and Rehabilitation: The Complete Approach. Malden, Mass, Blackwell Science Inc, 1999, pp 311–331.
43. Rondinelli R, Murphy J, Esler A, et al: Estimation of normal lumbar flexion with surface inclinometry. Am J Phys Med Rehabil 71:219–224, 1992.
44. Rothstein JM: Measurement and clinical practice: theory and application. In: Rothstein JM (ed): Measurement in Physical Therapy. New York, Churchill-Livingstone, 1985, pp. 1–46.
45. Rothstein JM, Echternach JL: Primer on Measurement: An Introductory Guide to Measurement Issues. Alexandria, Vir, American Physical Therapy Association, 1993.
46. Safrit MJ: Introduction to Measurement in Physical Education and Exercise Science, 2nd ed. St. Louis, Mosby, 1990.
47. Sharrard WJW: Distribution of the permanent paralysis in the lower limbs in poliomyelitis. J Bone Joint Surg 37B:540–558, 1955.
48. Studenski S, Duncan PW: Measuring rehabilitation outcomes. Clin Geriatr Med 9(4):823–830, 1993.
49. Thorn DW, Deitz JC: Examining content validity through the use of content experts. Occup Ther J Res 9:334–346, 1989.
50. Tinsley HE, Weiss DJ: Interrater reliability and agreement of subjective judgements. J Counsel Psych 22: 358–376, 1975.
51. Verducci FM: Measurement Concepts in Physical Education. St. Louis, Mosby, 1980.
52. Waddell G, McCulloch JA, Kummel E, Venner R: Nonorganic physical signs in low-back pain. Spine 5:117–125, 1980.
53. Wade DT, Collin C: The Barthel ADL index: a standard measure of physical disability. Disabil Studies 10:64–67, 1988.
54. Wilson M (ed): Objective Measurement: Theory Into Practice. Monterey, Calif, Ablex Publishing, 1991.
55. Wright BD, Linacre JM: Observations are always ordinal; measurements, however, must be interval. Arch Phys Med Rehabil 70:857–860, 1989.
56. Wright BD, Masters GN: Rating Scale Analysis. Chicago, Mesa Press, 1982.
57. Wright BD, Stone MH: Best Test Design: Rasch Measurement. Chicago, Mesa Press, 1979.
58. Youdas J, Carey J, Garrett T: Reliability of measurements of cervical spine range of motion: comparison of three methods. Phys Ther 71:98–106, 1991.

SECTION II

Assessment Tools for Rating Musculoskeletal Impairment and Work Disability

CHAPTER 4

Assessment Tools for Musculoskeletal Impairment Rating and Disability Assessment

Atul T. Patel, MD   Andrew J. Haig, MD   Mikel Cook, RPT, MPA

The AMA *Guides* encourages the disability physician examiner to utilize his or her "entire gamut of clinical skill and judgment in assessing whether or not the results of measurements or tests are plausible and relate to the impairment being evaluated."[2] The purpose of this chapter is to clarify the applications and limitations of physical tools and tests readily available to the clinician and typically used in the assessment of musculoskeletal impairment and disability. The three main areas of interest and discussion include measurement tools to assess joint range of motion (ROM) and muscle strength, radiographic assessment of bone and joint pathology, and electrophysiological assessment of neuromuscular function.

TOOLS FOR ASSESSING JOINT MOTION AND MUSCLE STRENGTH AND ENDURANCE

The disability examiner is frequently called on to objectively describe and identify impairment to the musculoskeletal system in terms of joint flexibility and muscle strength and endurance. There are a number of devices available to assist with the physical examination in this regard.

Range of Motion

Goniometers

Goniometers are used to measure joint ROM (flexibility). The most common and least expensive goniometer is the simple two-arm plastic or metal goniometer. The clinician can be trained to use this simple goniometer, and it remains by far the most widely used tool for measuring ROM. Electrogoniometers, computerized goniometers, and the bubble goniometer (also known as the *inclinometer*) are also used and have proved to be reliable.[23, 52] The simple goniometer is the primary tool used in extremity ROM testing, whereas the surface inclinometer (one inclinometer or two inclinometer methods) is primarily used in spine ROM testing.[42, 53, 54] The Back Range of Motion (BROM) device has also been used in lumbar ROM research.[9]

Evaluation of extremity range of motion

Extremity ROM evaluation is valuable when determining the level of impairment or baseline from which to monitor progress with therapy. The advantage in extremity ROM testing is that the majority of time the body has two joints that mirror each other (i.e., the right knee is mirrored by the left knee, right shoulder mirrored by the left shoulder), allowing for direct comparison of ROM. The nonaffected joint can serve as a normative baseline for comparison. In addition, normative ROM data are readily available for most of the extremity joints from which the reference tables of the AMA *Guides* are typically derived.[2, 23, 29, 52]

Evaluation of spine range of motion

Evaluation of spine ROM centers on the three spinal areas: cervical, thoracic, and lumbar. Thoracic ROM is limited because of rib attachments, and as such is evaluated much less than cervical and lumbar ROM. When measuring ROM in the lumbar and cervical spine, the evaluator must consider the multiple planes of motion. Flexion and extension, rotation, and lateral bending all play a role when considering normal ROM of the lumbar and cervical spine.

When evaluating an extremity joint, it is fairly easy to isolate a specific joint articulation. In the spine there are a number of joint articulations that contribute to ROM. Rotation and lateral bending can prove valuable because the motion to one side should mirror the motion to the opposite side. If motion is limited to one side it could be an indication of underlying pathology. Flexion of the lumbar spine should always exceed extension in the nonaffected spine.[2, 9, 42]

Reliability and validity of range of motion evaluation

Several studies have examined interrater and intrarater reliability of goniometric measurements to the spine[9, 42, 44, 53, 54] and extremities,[23, 52] and problems with interrater reliability have been identified.[53] Extremity ROM testing can be affected by excessive soft-tissue swelling, position of surrounding joints, instructions of the evaluator, different styles of goniometers, passive versus active movement, identification of bony landmarks, and cooperation of the client. These conditions can make it quite easy for measurements to vary by 5° or more, which could have a significant effect on an impairment rating. Research has also shown a difference in ROM of the dominant to nondominant extremity, the nondominant extremity having greater motion.[23] Gender may also significantly affect ROM measurements.

Unlike the extremities, the spine presents a particular normative problem when evaluating ROM because there is no mirror image for a comparative reference. In addition, normative data available for spine ROM are minimal when compared with the extremity joints. Studies show poor interrater reliability caused by difficulty with identification of bony landmarks, lack of training and/or inexperience of the examiner, using passive or active mode, and differences among testing devices.[53, 54] Cervical, thoracic, and lumbar ROM each have a number of joint articulations required to perform the motion, making it very difficult for the examiner to make accurate diagnostic assessments. In addition, validation procedures are cumbersome. These concerns have led the AMA to place decreased emphasis on spine ROM for impairment rating purposes.[2]

Summary of range of motion testing

ROM measurement is valuable in the assessment of permanent impairment and disability. The use of extremity ROM information is recommended over that of spine ROM because of the complexity of motion being measured, lack of "contralateral" joints for comparison, and complexity of validation procedures required of the examiner. It is further recommended that the occasional or less-experienced examiner seek the assistance of a trained and experienced therapist for joint ROM testing, and that each examiner choose the particular method of ROM testing that can be performed consistently to help minimize measurement errors that are prone to occur. When using ROM testing to determine permanent impairment, meticulous attention is warranted because a difference of 5° of motion measurement could significantly change the impairment rating.

Muscle Strength Testing

Testing of muscle strength and endurance may be valuable in determining impairment or developing a baseline for assessing improvement with medical care and rehabilitation. Manual muscle testing, isometric dynamometers, and isokinetic dynamometers are the most frequently used devices/methods for testing muscle strength and endurance.

Manual muscle testing

Manual muscle testing is probably one of the oldest methods of testing impairment in the musculoskeletal system.[38] The method originally used is to place a muscle or muscles performing a particular movement in a certain position and have the examiner apply resistance. The examiner then makes an assessment of the muscle strength. Different measurement methods use numbers, grades, or percentages as listed in Table 4–1.[43] A skilled and experienced examiner can perform a comprehensive assessment in a short period. Manual muscle testing has proved useful in assessing gross muscle deficits and guiding the evaluator in pursuing more precise diagnostic testing. However, in cases

TABLE 4–1 Systems of Muscle Strength Grading

Number	Work	Motor deficit (%)	Definition
5	Normal	0	Complete joint range of motion against gravity with full resistance
4	Good	1–25	Complete joint range of motion against gravity with moderate resistance
3	Fair	26–50	Full joint range of motion against gravity
2	Poor	51–75	Full joint range of motion with gravity eliminated
1	Trace	76–99	Visible or palpable muscle contraction; no joint motion produced
0	Zero	100	No visible or palpable muscle contraction

From McPeak L: Physiatric history and examination. In: Braddom RL (ed): Physical Medicine & Rehabilitation. Philadelphia, WB Saunders Co, 1996, pp 3–42. (Reproduced with permission from WB Saunders Co.)

where more precise measurement is required, the dynamometer has proved valuable.[7, 15, 35, 39, 46]

Isometric dynamometer

Use of the dynamometer over the past several years has increased the precision of muscle testing. Isometric dynamometers come in many different shapes, sizes, and uses. They are essentially force gauges that measure the maximum rate of force (torque) created by an isometric contraction about an axis of rotation. The measurement is generally displayed on a needle gauge or digital gauge, or is sometimes computerized. The isometric dynamometer reveals the maximum output of the tested muscle or muscles in contrast to using free weights to assess muscle strength. Dynamometers assess the maximum torque a muscle (or muscles) can produce throughout the ROM. In contrast, free weights do not provide an accurate assessment of muscle strength throughout ROM, as excursion of a free weight is limited by the weakest point within the joint arc.

Handgrip dynamometers have substantial normative data to draw upon.[37, 64, 66, 67, 68] Push/pull dynamometers[65] and multistation/task dynamometers[13, 19] have been used to assess manual handling tasks.

Isokinetic dynamometer

Many isokinetic devices are commercially available and applicable to an evaluation of permanent impairment, strength, and endurance deficits secondary to injury and/or disease. Isokinetic devices are designed to test the major joints in the body, including the hip, knee, ankle, shoulder, elbow, and wrist. A few isokinetic devices also have attachments to assess the lumbar and cervical spine. These devices are considered safe because they only resist in direct relationship to the speed and force the patient exerts. Most are also designed to switch immediately from extension to flexion or vice versa to more closely duplicate normal muscle activity. The majority of isokinetic devices are computerized, which allows a computer to graph and display the exact area of weakness through the arc of motion and to evaluate endurance deficits with repetitive trials. This display of information may be used to guide treatment, monitor progress, measure permanent impairment, and determine consistency and degree of client effort when assessing symptom magnification (see p. 59).

Evaluation of extremity muscle strength and endurance

Muscle strength and endurance testing for extremities has advantages similar to those of ROM testing because for each muscle tested there is a contralateral muscle with which to make comparisons. Manual muscle testing should precede isokinetic testing to determine if more precise measures, such as dynamometers, are indicated.

Handgrip dynamometers are the most frequently used isometric dynamometer for assessment of extremity strength. The handgrip dynamometer has normative data based on age and gender.[37, 66, 67, 68] Since the hands are frequently subject to an impairment determination, this normative data has proved to be clinically useful.

Isokinetic dynamometers are most frequently used for the assessment of knee impairment. The shoulder, elbow, wrist, hip, and ankle can also be tested with most isokinetic dynamometers.

Evaluation of spine strength and endurance

Manual muscle testing is used to evaluate gross strength of the cervical and lumbar spine. Since there are a number of muscles and joint articulations involved with cervical and lumbar movement, manual muscle testing of specific muscles cannot be done. Instead, the spinal movements of rotation, lateral bending, flexion, and extension are tested.[32] When deficits are noted, an isokinetic dynamometer evaluation can be done. Dynamometers are rarely used for evaluation of cervical strength and endurance. Isokinetic testing for the lumbar spine has been evaluated, but is not commonly done in clinical practice, in part because of a lack of consistent testing methodology.[40]

Evaluation of manual handling tasks

Range of motion, muscle strength, and muscle endurance are usually tested in isolation and, consequently, may not provide sufficient information about a client's ability to perform specific functional tasks. Manual handling tasks are function specific, not muscle or joint specific, and hence require further evaluation of performance.[13, 19, 65]

Dynamometers are frequently used in an attempt to improve the assessment of manual handling tasks. Available choice of equipment includes simple push/pull isometric dynamometers, as well as multistation/function isometric, dynamic, and isokinetic dynamometers. Normative data are available through the *Dictionary of Occupational Titles* to enable direct comparisons between dynamometer measurements and the predictability of task performance. Applications to return-to-work determinations are discussed in Chapter 5.

Reliability and validity of muscle strength and endurance evaluation

Manual muscle testing is not a precise measurement but rather a gross evaluation of muscle strength that greatly reduces the interrater and even intrarater reliability.[8, 29, 32, 38] Both the isometric dynamometer and the isokinetic dynamometer are more precise instruments, for which higher interrater reliability has been reported.[4, 6, 7, 15, 36, 39, 40, 46, 66, 67, 70, 71, 72] However, many factors can affect the reliability of isokinetic testing, including age (forces decline with increasing age), weight (increased body weight tends to produce higher torque), interaction between gender and weight (males generally produce torque measurements exceeding those of females), athletic background (athletes do better), and limb dominance (the dominant limb is stronger).[35] Other factors include inherent variability within testing equipment and among examiners. Testing validity also depends on correct positioning of the joint to be tested,[71] stabilization of the surrounding joints to avoid accessory movement, degree of client effort, and the presence of confounders such as pain.

Symptom magnification during maximal-effort testing

Symptom magnification (the display of exaggerated pain behavior and self-inhibition of effort out of proportion to observable pathology) is of concern because it may affect the validity of strength and endurance test results. The clinician may wish to examine the degree and consistency of effort using isometric or isokinetic testing equipment. The Jamar dynamometer has been frequently used to clinically examine degree of effort according to grip pressure measurements using the 5-position test.[11, 64, 68] The logic and application are as follows: grip strength measures vary in direct relation to the hand position and mechanical advantage. The 5-position hand dynamometer allows handgrip testing from smaller to larger grip and usually reveals greatest strength measurement with the middle position. The subject is tested in all five positions, with resulting grip pressures recorded on a graph, which is expected to be bell shaped. If the bell-shaped curve is not generated, submaximal effort is suggested.[68] This approach has been refined by examining peak and average force-time curves generated with side-to-side and gender-specific comparisons for normative data[64] and for subjects with unilateral hand injuries.[11] However, the utility of hand-held dynamometers to determine maximal effort has been critically reviewed,[51, 69] and results should be interpreted with considerable caution by the clinician.

Computerized isometric and isokinetic dynamometers have also been used to assess consistency of effort. When performing a task, a strength curve is generated. In the normal or affected subject, this curve should remain consistent from test to test. If the affected subject shows marked weakness at a certain ROM, it should be consistently reproducible. The computer program can calculate a "coefficient of variation" (COV) as the standard deviation among trials, divided by the mean × 100 as a unitless measure of consistency of effort.[41] However, the range of acceptable COV varies by anatomical region, test mode (isometric versus isokinetic), and according to specificity of strength test (i.e., whole body lift versus isolated muscle testing).[61]

Since there is no uniform agreement on norms and acceptable range of COVs, they should also be used only with considerable caution in interpreting consistency of effort during isometric or isokinetic testing.

Summary of muscle strength and endurance testing

Muscle strength and endurance testing is a key element of musculoskeletal assessment. The use of manual muscle testing and dynamometers can help the evaluator to objectively assess impairment and disability. Isokinetic and isometric dynamometers are available to assist with strength and endurance assessments of complex movement and functional performance abilities. The application of such objective testing to the assessment of symptom magnification (in terms of degree and consistency of effort) warrants considerable caution on the part of the clinician at this time.

Radiological Assessment of Bone and Joint Pathology

It is a common attorney strategy to show a radiograph at trial. The public puts stock in radiological examinations, and attorneys utilize that confidence to promote their cases. At face value, one might assume a strong correlation between disease, radiographic impairment, and disability or handicap. If this were true, however, then a simple interpretation of radiographic tests would often be sufficient evidence for a disability determination. In reality, disability determination is a complex process that remains highly subjective, and the functional significance of radiographic and other objective indicators of impairment is likely to be debated in any given case.

The purpose of this section is to review common radiographic procedures as they apply to musculoskeletal impairment rating and to examine functional interpretations that may be drawn from radiographic findings when making disability determinations.

Plain-film radiographs are obviously useful in documenting the precise level of amputation, fracture, nonunion, ankylosis, severe sprain, surgical intervention such as rods or screws, and heterotopic ossification. The relationship between these medical diagnoses and impairment is rather direct and unchanging. Still, when asked about disability or handicap, the physician must use other factors to modulate the effect of these diagnoses on the tasks at hand.

A number of other diagnoses can be proved with radiography, but the relationship between the severity of radiographic findings and function is more variable. For example, radiographic findings of recurrent patellar subluxation have a highly variable relationship with actual function.[14] Various arthritides are also diagnosed with radiography. Although the extent of erosion, joint-space narrowing, or bony spurring correlates somewhat with functional disability, the relationship is not direct. For example, in rheumatoid arthritis (RA), there are three common schemas for rating radiological findings: the Steinbrocker Stage, Kaye Modified Sharp Score, and the Larsen Score.[46] The Larsen system appears to correlate with elbow disability[59] and total disability,[34] but not hand function.[57] Although these scales provide similar quantitative data concerning radiographic damage in patients with RA, weak correlations are seen between radiographic scores and joint count scores for tenderness.[47] It is for this reason that indications for joint replacement surgery in arthritis include pain and dysfunction.

The presence of radiographic findings alone is often not sufficient to predict extent of functional limitations. Radiographs may reveal disorders or conditions that put an individual at risk for future injury or illness despite adequate current function. For example, severe osteopenia may be a relative contraindication to heavy lifting or repetitive activity, regardless of current function. The extent to which osteopenia warrants restrictions to protect the individual from trauma is further modulated by the individual's body habitus and strength, the particular activity in question, and other factors that are difficult to measure, such as the physician's personal belief regarding acceptable risk. Joint disruptions, such as fractures through cartilage, spondylolisthesis, or avascular necrosis of the femoral head, are thought to degenerate more quickly with increased weight bearing and activity. Although radiographs can demonstrate these findings effectively, the relationship between future activity and joint degeneration is variable.

Even with similar radiographs and levels of function, the extent of disability may demonstrate an inverse relationship to age. Younger persons with hip replacements will likely wear out the artificial joints, leading to multiple joint replacements and possibly a girdlestone procedure requiring modified weight bearing or wheelchair use; older persons, in contrast, are likely to retain ambulatory function with a single prosthesis for the duration of their life.

Radiographic findings can be used to document spinal impairment from fracture, instability, or degenerative arthritis. Radiographs are less applicable in assessing spinal disability. For example, most research shows little correlation between more subtle spinal radiographic findings and pain (let alone disability or handicap). Functional outcome after surgical fusion has been shown to be similar whether successful fusion or pseudoarthrosis occurs.[20] Population-based studies have demonstrated little correlation between degenerative changes shown on radiographs and pain[21, 45]; however, some notable exceptions occur. Radiographic findings that correlate somewhat with back pain include disc-space narrowing at L4 without changes at L5, high-degree scoliosis (greater than 60° in an adult), large leg-length discrepancies (5 cm or more), and severe multilevel degenerative changes. These findings reflect statistical significance of risk factors in a sample population that are insufficient criteria to "prove" pain or disability in the individual case, and are perhaps more useful to support the probability that an objective pain generator exists.

Radiological imaging during motion can determine instability in some extremity joints. Radiological assessment of spinal instability is much more complex. The AMA *Guides*[2] gives criteria for spinal instability, which it calls *loss of motion segment integrity* (LOMSI). This is based on comparison of flexion and extension views of lateral radiographs. Vertebral injury related to translational (anterior-posterior) motion that is 5 mm or greater than that seen at an adjacent intervertebral segment is the first diagnostic indicator of LOMSI. Angular motion is the second indicator. If comparing adjacent levels such as L4–L5 or above, any angular motion 11° or greater at one level over another also implicates LOMSI. When comparing the L5–S1 interspace with L4–L5, the difference must be greater than 15°. Strangely, these criteria are not widely utilized by neuroradiologists, but are based on cadaver studies with no known clinical correlate.[49, 55] Simply put, the association between instability and pain is yet undefined.[48]

Advanced radiologic imaging tests, including computerized tomography (CT), magnetic resonance imaging (MRI), and myelograms, are subject to additional concern because they are highly sensitive to conditions of questionable clinical significance. There is a great potential for these tests to reveal soft-tissue lesions, but the clinical significance of these findings is variable. Although lesions such as supraspinatus tendon tear are fairly reliable findings on MRI,[26] it is well documented that MRI, CT, and myelogram can demonstrate disc pathology in one third to two thirds of asymptomatic individuals studied.[5, 28] Clearly, imaging test results require clinical correlation, and the examiner should avoid inappropriate weighting of nonspecific findings that are likely to occur as a result of developmental changes or the normal aging process.[2]

Bone scans are useful indicators of ongoing bone repair, thus providing evidence of a fracture up to 1 year after an injury. They may be useful to document the presence or absence of a fracture (including hairline fractures) or to determine that fracture healing is complete, and thus a permanent impairment rating of the healed fracture can be assigned. Other potentially useful tests involve the injection of radiopaque agents under fluoroscopy for diagnostic provocation or palliation. Such tests include discography,[62] facet injection,[16] sacroiliac joint injection,[31] and selective nerve root block.[63] For all of these tests, the actual photographic evidence of an abnormality is not considered pathognomonic for a disabling lesion. Instead, they all rely on the client's report that the test reproduced his or her symptoms. Some progress has been made in protocols with placebo injections, injections at other "control" levels, blinded observers, etc., to avoid suggesting responses to the client, but the clinical applications of tests to document impairment and disability appear limited at this time.

Summary of radiological testing

Radiographic procedures provide objective evidence of bone and joint pathology useful to the diagnosis of musculoskeletal impairment. However, the disability examiner must exercise due caution when drawing functional inferences from radiographic findings as they pertain to disability in the particular case. Clinical correlation of radiographic findings to appropriate subjective complaints, a plausible history of associated functional losses, and supportive findings on physical examination appear necessary and warranted.

Neuromuscular Function

Electrodiagnostic testing is perhaps one of the most useful tests in assessing impairment related to the peripheral neuromuscular system. There is little research on electrodiagnosis (EDX) and impairment ratings per se, but a standard reference[17] is available to support evidence presented here. EDX consists of several components, and the ones that are most commonly used to assess the peripheral neuromuscular system include electromyography (EMG), nerve conduction studies (NCS), and somatosensory evoked potentials (SEPs). Electrodiagnostic abnormalities objectively demonstrate the existence and location of a neuromuscular deficit and can help in documenting the causation, severity, and permanence of a neurological lesion. As opposed to MRI, CT, and myelogram, EDX has very few false positives when done in a standardized fashion.[26]

Electromyography

EMG can be performed with either surface or needle electrodes. There is very limited information obtained by surface electromyography, and at this point there is no evidence to support its value in assessing patients with neuromuscular dysfunction.[24] Needle electromyography can be performed using several types of needles. The two types of needle most commonly used are concentric and monopolar.

Two major components are assessed during needle EMG, spontaneous and voluntary activity. Spontaneous activity consists of insertional activity, the presence or absence of positive sharp waves and fibrillation potentials and other spontaneous activity. Positive sharp waves and fibrillation potentials denote denervation. Voluntary activity involves the assessment of motor unit potentials and their duration, amplitude, morphology, and firing rate or recruitment.

One important point to keep in mind with regard to EMG is that it may take 14 to 21 days after nerve injury for the full evolution, and hence detection, of positive sharp waves and fibrillation potentials. This has several implications, one being that if someone is injured and assessed by electrodiagnosis within the first few days, evidence of abnormalities on needle examination may point to premorbid involvement. An EMG would support causation if it was initially normal and, subsequent to an exposure or event, became abnormal. Similarly, normal-looking motor units (albeit with decreased recruitment in severe cases) become larger and polyphasic over a longer period as a result of repair and regeneration. Thus in the rare cases when it is important to do so, repeated EMGs (with the first one early after the injury) can show a progression of findings that can retrospectively pinpoint the onset of nerve damage in time.

Positive waves and fibrillation potentials as signs of denervated muscle also get smaller over time as the muscle cell atrophies.[18] Thus there is some EMG evidence that can be gathered to support the presence of a new lesion superimposed on an old one, or the onset of a new lesion in temporal proximity to an event. EMG can often determine the severity of a neurological lesion. The distribution of spontaneous activity (positive waves and fibrillation potentials) in an extremity correlates with the distribution of the deficit and thus its severity. This has been better quantified in the paraspinal region, where quantitative EMG protocols such as MiniPM[25, 60] are actually sampling a number of separately innervated muscles (getting a sense of how widespread the lesion is).

The amount of spontaneous activity in a given single extremity muscle does not correlate well with the severity of neurological deficit. The recruitment rate of motor units (e.g., the firing rate of the first recruited motor unit at the point when a second motor unit begins to fire) indicates the number of intact nerve cells and reflects the severity of a lesion. This finding is present from the very onset of neurogenic paresis and improves with neurogenic recovery. It does not change with exercise, anxiety, or lack of effort (assuming minimal cooperation), thus it is a valid reflection of the nerve damage.

Nerve Conduction Studies

Nerve conduction studies assess the peripheral motor and sensory nervous system. The usual setup includes a site of stimulation and a site for recording. An electrical stimulation is provided that depolarizes the nerve under study and sets up a propagating action potential, which is recorded some distance away from the stimulation site. This can be performed for pure motor nerves, pure sensory nerves, or mixed nerves (motor and sensory). These studies allow for further functional assessment and classification of disorders, namely motor versus sensory involvement, demyelinating versus axonal involvement, and focal versus generalized involvement. The major limitations are that only accessible portions of the peripheral nervous system can be assessed. There is a wide range of "normal," making if difficult to detect early or mild changes, and these techniques assess primarily the large myelinated fibers. When nerve conduction studies are done according to a careful protocol, the amplitude of the evoked response, whether motor or sensory, reflects the number of nerve cells left intact and thus the severity of the lesion. This technique may be the most useful EDX technique for quantifying nerve deficits. A caution exists, however, that placement of the active and reference electrodes in different locations, lack of temperature control, lack of supramaximal stimulation, and other technical issues can interfere with interpretation.

Motor nerve conduction studies

Motor nerve conduction studies involve supramaximal stimulation of a motor or mixed nerve at two or more points, with recording over a distal muscle innervated by the same nerve. The response is usually recorded from the motor point of the muscle and is represented as a compound muscle action potential (CMAP). Most commonly, this study is performed with surface stimulation and surface recording. The parameters that are recorded include latency, amplitude, and duration. Nerve conduction velocity is calculated indirectly by using the distance between the proximal and distal stimulating sites. Prolongation of the distal latency or reduction in the conduction velocity would suggest a demyelinating process; however, it is important to note that some slowing in conduction velocity can occur with pure axonal degeneration involving primarily the large-diameter, fastest conduction fibers.

The latency of a nerve conduction study (e.g., a very slow conduction across the carpal tunnel) does not reflect the severity of a lesion functionally, but merely demonstrates the existence of a lesion.[33] The amplitude of the CMAP is an estimation of the summated activity of the muscle fibers in the muscle innervated by the axons and motor units being depolarized. Hence the CMAP provides a physiological assessment of the motor axons in the pathway distal to the stimulation, the neuromuscular junction between the axons and the muscle, and the muscle fibers. The CMAP can be used to assess disease at the axon, the neuromuscular junction, and muscle. CMAPs can provide objective measurement of the extent and type of weakness and can help differentiate self-inhibition and submaximal effort from an upper motor neuron disorder or a peripheral neuromuscular disease. Changes in amplitude of the CMAP between sites of stimulation can also help localize focal nerve lesions such as conduction block. One must, however, keep in mind that motor response amplitude is an insensitive measure of mild neurogenic lesions because of the wide variation in normal subjects. The duration and shape reflect the synchrony of contraction of muscle fibers, and marked variation in the shape or duration occurs when some of the axons are conducting more slowly, for example, in a demyelinating process.

Sensory nerve conduction studies

Sensory function is usually assessed via nerve action potentials (NAP). This is achieved by stimulation of a nerve and recording a potential over the nerve at a different site. This can be done over a mixed nerve (motor and sensory), in which case either the recording or stimulation involves only the sensory axons or a pure sensory nerve. Usually, surface electrodes are used for stimulation and recording. The parameters that are usually recorded are the amplitude and latency. Conduction velocities, as in motor nerve conduction studies, can be calculated using the latencies and distance measurements of nerve length. Focal neuropathies are characterized by involvement of a single nerve, whereas abnormalities in multiple nerves point toward a more generalized process. Localization of focal nerve lesions is best achieved by examining short segments of the nerve and maintaining short distances between stimulating and recording electrodes. On the other hand, detection of diffuse nerve conduction slowing requires examination of long segments of nerve with long distances between the stimulating and recording electrodes. Prolonged distal latencies and slowed conduction velocities in the presence of normal NAP amplitudes suggest a demyelinating process; reduced or absent NAP amplitudes can be due to an axonal process, a combination of an axonal and demyelinating injury, or a primary demyelinating process with conduction block. Finally, sensory nerve conduction studies can help localize the lesion proximal or distal to the dorsal root ganglion (DRG). With lesions involving the DRG or distal elements of the sensory fibers, there is a reduction in or loss of the NAP. A lesion that is proximal to the DRG preserves the sensory cell bodies and distal elements, and hence sensory nerve action potentials, in spite of clinical sensory loss.

Sensory nerve conduction studies are very useful in detecting peripheral neuropathies, primarily sensory and sensorimotor neuropathies. Abnormalities when assessing sensorimotor neuropathy may be seen earlier in the sensory studies compared with the motor studies.[10] Sensory studies are the most sensitive for detecting mononeuropathies, such as carpal tunnel syndrome, and may be the only way to document cutaneous neuropathy.[33] In assessing the brachial plexus, sensory nerve conduction studies can be helpful in determining preganglionic and postganglionic injury (i.e., root avulsion versus brachial plexus injury). Sensory NAP studies are limited in that there is a wide range in the “normal” distal latencies and amplitudes, making it difficult to detect mild abnormalities.

Late responses

Late responses consist of F-waves and H-reflexes. F-waves are recorded over the muscle belly that is being tested by supramaximal stimulation of the nerve innervating that muscle, allowing for conduction proximal to the site of stimulation to the spinal cord and then back to the muscle. This allows the assessment of the most proximal aspects of the peripheral nervous system. The limitations are that it only assesses about 1% to 2% of the available motor fibers and that there is a variability from response to response in the latency because different fibers are depolarized each time. In general, this test has limited value in the diagnosis of radiculopathy or nerve entrapment syndromes.

The H-reflex is the electrophysiologic counterpart of the deep tendon reflex. It is present in almost all the skeletal muscles of an infant but only a few in the adult. The two most frequently assessed are the flexor carpi radialis and gastrocnemius-soleus muscles. This waveform is recorded by stimulating the nerve supplying these muscles, allowing for conduction proximally along the sensory fibers to the spinal cord, and then synaptically activating the motor pathway back to the muscle. Compared with the F-wave response, the H-reflex requires submaximal stimulation. Both these techniques for assessing late responses allow for the evaluation of the proximal nervous system. However, it is important to keep in mind that both techniques are technically involved and require someone experienced to perform them. Currently, there is very limited use of these responses in assessing common peripheral nerve system disorders.

Repetitive studies

The recording of CMAP as described earlier assesses motor nerve function in peripheral neuromuscular disorders. Repetitive stimulation studies help assess the function of the neuromuscular junction (the point of connection between the nerve and the muscle). It involves repeated supramaximal stimuli given in a short train at a constant frequency (usually 2 to 4 Hz) to a motor or mixed nerve, and the CMAP is recorded from the corresponding muscle. Changes in the size of the CMAP are measured between responses to provide an indirect but objective assessment of the neuromuscular function. A great deal of attention to detail and technical expertise are required to avoid false positive and false negative results. The type of diseases that this test can help diagnose are rare and seldom seen among the patients being evaluated for disability determination and include myasthenia gravis, myasthenic syndrome (Lambert-Eaton syndrome), and botulism.[30] These tests can be helpful in excluding these rare diseases in patients presenting with common symptoms such as fatigue, vague weakness, ptosis, or diplopia.

Somatosensory evoked potentials

There are several types of evoked potentials, including somatosensory evoked potentials (SEPs), dermatomal somatosensory evoked potentials, visual evoked potentials, brainstem auditory evoked responses, and motor evoked potentials. The most commonly used evoked potentials in assessing the peripheral nervous system are the SEPs. Motor evoked potentials that use magnetic stimulation are still being researched and may become more useful after further research. SEPs are recorded by stimulating a mixed nerve distally in the extremity and then recording the responses proximally along the nerve and then centrally over the spine and the scalp. Because the recording is across the proximal peripheral nervous system and the spinal cord, it allows for the assessment of very proximal lesions of the peripheral nervous system. However, the limiting factor is that it only assesses the posterior columns or the sensory fibers and not the motor fibers in the anterior portion of the spinal cord.

The value of this is questionable in disease affecting the peripheral nervous system (i.e., peripheral neuropathy or radiculopathy). SEPs are known to be less sensitive than electromyography in the detection of cervical radiculopathy.[73] In the detection of lumbosacral radiculopathy, there is conflicting evidence in the usefulness of somatosensory and dermatomal somatosensory evoked potentials compared with electromyography.[2, 58] SEPs are helpful in detecting central demyelinating lesions such as those found in multiple sclerosis and leukodystrophies.[12, 22]

Autonomic nervous system testing

The autonomic nervous system is a complex neural network maintaining internal physiological homeostasis. There are several tests to assess this system, including cardiovascular responses, heart-rate variation with respiration, blood-pressure changes with Valsalva maneuver, thermal regulatory function, and sympathetic skin responses (SSRs). Of these, only the SSR is assessed electrophysiologically. SSRs are indicated in assessing the integrity of peripheral sympathetic cholinergic (sudomotor) function. They can be helpful in assessing patients with progressive autonomic failure syndromes and peripheral neuropathies (especially with autonomic or small-fiber involvement), and can possibly be used in patients with sympathetically mediated pain.

Responses are usually recorded after a startling stimuli, either by electrical stimulation or an auditory stimulus, and recording electrodermal activity from the skin. Electrodermal activity reflects sympathetic cholinergic sudomotor functions that include changes in the resistance of the skin to electric conduction. The SSR is a sensitive and reproducible test that can be carried out simply; however, it has disadvantages because it is only semiquantitative and not all investigators advocate the value of this test in assessing sudomotor function.[56] At present, this test is infrequently used and may be of greater use in the future as more research is done in this area.[50]

Summary of electrodiagnostic testing

Nerve conduction studies help with determining the presence or absence of disease when sorting out demyelinating versus axonal involvement and with localization of the lesion (e.g., entrapment syndrome such as carpal tunnel syndrome, or superimposed problems such as peripheral neuropathy). The limitations of nerve conduction studies include a large range of normal and difficulty assessing the severity of involvement based only on nerve conduction studies. EMG helps to identify and confirm the presence of nerve involvement, differentiating between chronic versus acute neuropathic versus myopathic processes, and localizing the lesion and extent of involvement. Table 4–2 summarizes the usefulness of the various components of electrodiagnostic tests in the diagnosis of some of the commonly encountered clinical syndromes. These are functional and dynamic tests versus an anatomic or static test such as a radiograph. Hence these studies are examiner-dependent and should be performed by a physician (generally a neurologist or a physiatrist) who is a specialist in electrodiagnostic medicine. There are two examinations specifically emphasizing electrodiagnostic medicine in the United States that are available

TABLE 4–2 Usefulness of Electrodiagnostic Tests in the Diagnosis of Commonly Encountered Clinical Syndromes

Clinical syndrome	MNCS	SNAPs	H-reflex	F-wave	Needle EMG	SEPs
Nerve entrapment (e.g., CTS)	++	++	–	–	++	+/–
Radiculopathy	+	+	+/–	+/–	++	+/–
Plexopathy	+	++	+/–	+/–	++	+/–
Polyneuropathy	++	++	+	+	+	+/–
Myopathy	+	++	–	–	++	–

MNCS, Motor nerve conduction studies; *SNAPs,* sensory nerve action potentials; *SEPs,* somatosensory evoked potentials. ++, Very helpful in supporting or rejecting the diagnosis; +, helpful in supporting or rejecting the diagnosis; +/–, complementary in supporting the diagnosis; –, not helpful in supporting or rejecting the diagnosis.

to physicians who are qualified by training and experience: The American Board of Electrodiagnostic Medicine examination and the American Board of Psychiatry and Neurology's Added Qualifications in Clinical Neurophysiology examination.[1] Finally, a good study should be a good consultation; looking at the report to make sure that a "shotgun" approach was not used can assess this. A report should include certain elements: documentation of all the individual nerves tested by nerve conduction studies and information about the parameters measured; documentation of all the muscles tested by needle EMG examination and information about spontaneous and voluntary activity; and an impression that summarizes the electrophysiologic findings in correlation with the clinical findings, reports the diagnoses that are confirmed or excluded, and qualifies the degree of the severity and acuteness of the involvement when possible.

REFERENCES

1. American Association of Electrodiagnostic Medicine: Proposed Policy for Electrodiagnostic Medicine, Rochester, Minn, American Association of Electrodiagnostic Medicine, 1997.
2. American Medical Association: Guides to the Evaluation of Permanent Impairment, 4th ed. Chicago, American Medical Association, 1993.
3. Aminoff MJ, Goodin DS, Parry GJ, et al: Electrophysiologic evaluation of lumbosacral radiculopathies: Electromyography, late responses, and somatosensory evoked potentials. Neurology 35:1514–1518, 1985.
4. Anderson H: Reliability of isokinetic measurements of ankle dorsal and plantar flexors in normal subjects and inpatients with peripheral neuropathy. Arch Phys Med Rehabil 77:265–268, 1996.
5. Boden SD, Davis DO, Dina TS, et al: Abnormal magnetic resonance scans of the lumbar spine in asymptomatic subjects. J Bone Joint Surg 72A:403–408, 1990.
6. Bohannon RW: Hand-held dynamometer measurements obtained in a home environment are reliable but not correlated strongly with function. Int J Rehabil Res 19:345–347, 1996.
7. Bohannon RW: Reference values for extremity muscle strength obtained by hand-held dynamometry from adults aged 20 to 79 years. Arch Phys Med Rehabil 78:26–32, 1997.
8. Brandsma JW, Schreuders Ton AR, Birke JA, et al: Manual muscle strength test-

ing: intraobserver and interobserver reliabilities for the intrinsic muscles of the hand. J Hand Ther 8(3):185–190, 1995.

9. Breum J, Wiberg, J, Bolton JE: Reliability and concurrent validity of the BROM II for measuring lumbar mobility. J Manipulative Physiol Ther 18(8):497–502, 1995.
10. Buchtal F, Rosenfalck A: Sensory potentials in polyneuropathy. Brain 4:241–262, 1971.
11. Chengalur SN, Smith GA, Nelson RC, Sadoff AM: Assessing sincerity of effort in maximal grip strength tests. Am J Phys Med Rehabil 69(3):148–153, 1990.
12. Chiappa KH: Short-latency somatosensory evoked potentials: Interpretation. In: Chiappa KH (ed): Evoked Potentials in Clinical Medicine. New York, Raven Press, 1990, pp 399–437.
13. Cooke C, Dusik LA, Menard MR, et al: Relationship of performance on the ERGOS work simulator to illness behavior in a workers' compensation population with low back versus limb injury. J Occup Med 6(7):757–762, 1994.
14. Dandy DJ: Chronic patellofemoral instability. J Bone Joint Surg Br 78(2): 328–335, 1996.
15. Davies GJ, Heiderscheit BC: Reliability of the lido linea closed kinetic chain isokinetic dynamometer. J Sports Phys Ther 25(2):133–136, 1997.
16. Dreyfuss P, Dreyer S: Lumbar facet joint. In: Gonzalez EG, Materson RS (eds): Nonsurgical Management of Acute Low Back Pain. New York, Demos Vermande, 1997, pp 123–136.
17. Dumitru D: Electrodiagnostic medicine. Philadelphia, Hanley & Belfus, 1995.
18. Dumitru D, King JC: Fibrillation potential amplitude after denervation. Am J Phys Rehabil 77:483–489, 1998.
19. Dusik LA, Menar MR, Cooke C, et al: Concurrent validity of the ERGOS work simulator versus conventional functional capacity evaluation techniques in a workers' compensation population. J Occup Med 35(8):759–767, 1993.
20. Frymoyer JW, Hanley EN, Howe J, et al: A comparison of radiolographic findings in fusion and nonfusion patients ten or more years following lumbar disc surgery. Spine 4(5):435–440, 1979.
21. Frymoyer JW, Newberg A, Pope MH, et al: Spine radiographs in patients with low-back pain: An epidemiological study in men. J Bone Joint Surg 66A(7): 1048–1055, 1984.
22. Guerit JM, Argiles AM: The sensitivity of multimodal evoked potentials in multiple sclerosis: A comparison with magnetic resonance imaging and cerebrospinal fluid analysis. Electroencephalogr Clin Neurophysiol 70:230–238, 1988.
23. Gunal I, Kose N, Erdogan O, et al: Normal range of motion of the joints of the upper extremity in male subjects, with special reference to side. J Bone Joint Surg 78A(9):1401–1404, 1996.
24. Haig AJ: AAEM practice topics in electrodiagnostic medicine: Technology assessment: The use of surface EMG in the diagnosis and treatment of nerve and muscle disorders. Muscle Nerve 19(3)392–395, 1996.
25. Haig AJ: Clinical experience with paraspinal mapping II: MiniPM: A simplified technique. Arch Phys Med Rehabil 78:1185–1190, 1997.
26. Haig AJ, LeBreck DB, Powley SG: Quantified needle electromyography of the paraspinal muscles in persons without low back pain. Spine 20(6):715–721, 1995.
27. Herzog R: Magnetic resonance imaging of the shoulder. J Bone Joint Surg 79A: 934–953, 1997.
28. Hitselberger WE, Witten RM: Abnormal myelograms in asymptomatic patients. J Neurosurg 28:204–206, 1968.
29. Hoppenfeld S: Physical Examination of the Spine and Extremities. Norwalk, Conn, Appleton-Century-Crofts, 1976.
30. Howard JF, Sanders DB, Massey JM: The electrodiagnosis of myasthenia gravis and the Lambert-Eaton myasthenic syndrome. Neurol Clin 12:305–330, 1994.
31. Huston C: The sacroiliac joint. In: Gonzalez EG, Materson RS (eds): Nonsurgical

Management of Acute Low Back Pain. New York, Demos Vermande, 1997, pp 137–150.

32. Ito T, Shirado O, Suzuki H, et al: Lumbar trunk muscle endurance testing: an inexpensive alternative to a machine for evaluation. Phys Med Rehabil 77:75–79, 1996.
33. Jablecki CK, Andary MT, So YT, et al: Literature review of the usefulness of nerve conduction studies and electromyography for the evaluation of patients with carpal tunnel syndrome. AAEM Quality Assurance Committee. Muscle Nerve 16(12):1392–1414, 1993.
34. Kaarela K, Sarna S: Correlations between clinical facets of outcome in rheumatoid arthritis. Clin Exp Rheumatol 11(6):643–644, 1993.
35. Keating JL, Matyas TA: The influence of subject and test design on dynametric measurements of the extremity muscles. Phys Ther 76(8):866–899, 1996.
36. Kellis E, Baltsopoulos V: Isokinetic eccentric exercise. Sports Med 19(3):202–222, 1995.
37. Kellor M, Frost J, Silberberg N, et al: Hand strength and dexterity. Am J Occup Ther 25(2):77–83, 1971.
38. Kendall FP, McReary EK, Provance PG: Muscles: Testing and Function, 4th ed. Baltimore, Williams and Wilkens, 1993.
39. Leggin BG, Neuman RM, Iannotti JP, et al: Intrarater and interrater reliability of three isometric dynamometers in assessing shoulder strength. J Shoulder Elbow Surg 5:18–24, 1996.
40. Madsen OR: Trunk extensor and flexor strength measured by the Cybex 6000 dynamometer. Spine 21(23):2770–2776, 1996.
41. Matheson L: How do you know that he tried his best? Industr Rehabil Q 1:82–84, 1988.
42. Mayer TG, Kondraske G, Beals SB, et al: Spinal range of motion. Spine 22(17): 1976–1984, 1997.
43. McPeak L: Physiatric history and examination. In: Braddom RL (ed): Physical Medicine & Rehabilitation. Philadelphia, WB Saunders Co, 1996, pp 3–42.
44. Nilsson N: Measuring passive cervical motion: A study of reliability. J Manipulative Physiol Ther 18(5):293–297, 1995.
45. Phillips RB, Frymoyer JW, MacPherson BV, et al: Low back pain: A radiographic enigma. J Manipulative Physiol Ther 9(3):183–187, 1986.
46. Pincivero DM, Lephart SM, Karunakara RA: Reliability and precision of isokinetic strength and muscular endurance for the quadriceps and hamstrings. Int J Sports Med 8(2):113–117, 1997.
47. Pincus T, Larsen A, Brooks RH, et al: Comparison of three quantitative measures of hand radiographs in patients with rheumatoid arthritis: Steinbrocker stage, Kaye modified Sharp score, and Larsen score. J Rheumatol 24(11):2106–2112, 1997.
48. Pitkanen M, Manninen HI, Lindgrer KA, et al: Limited usefulness of traction-compression films in the radiographic diagnosis of lumbar spinal instability: comparison with flexion-extension films. Spine 22(2):193–197, 1997.
49. Posner I, White AA, Edwards WT: Biomechanical analysis of the clinical stability of the lumbar and lumbosacral spine. Spine 7:374–389, 1982.
50. Ravits J: AAEM Minimonogram #48: Autonomic nervous system testing. Muscle Nerve 20:919–937, 1997.
51. Rheault W, Beal JL, Kubik KR, et al: Intertester reliability of the hand-held dynamometer for wrist flexion and extension. Arch Phys Med Rehabil 70: 907–910, 1989.
52. Rome K, Cowieson F: A reliability study of the universal goniometer, fluid goniometer, and electrogoniometer for the measurement of ankle dorsiflexion. Foot Ankle Int 17(1):28–32, 1996.
53. Rondinelli R, Murphy J, Esler A, et al: Estimation of normal lumbar flexion with surface inclinometry: a comparison of three methods. Am J Phys Med Rehabil 4:219–224, 1992.

54. Samo DG, Chen SPC, Chen EH, et al: Reliability of three lumbar sagittal motion measurement methods: surface inclinometers. J Occup Environ Med 39(3):217–223, 1997.
55. Schaffer WO, Spratt K, Weinstein J: Consistency and accuracy of roentgenograms for measuring sagittal translation in the lumbar vertebral motion segment: An experimental model. Spine 15:741–750, 1990.
56. Schondorf R, Gendron D: Evaluation of sudomotor function in patients with peripheral neuropathy. Neurology 40:386, 1990.
57. Scott DL, Coulton BL, Bacon PA, et al: Methods of X-ray assessment in rheumatoid arthritis: a re-evaluation. Br J Rheumatol 24(1):31–39, 1985.
58. Sedgwick EM, Katifi HA, Docherty TB, et al: Dermatomal somatosensory evoked potentials in lumbar disc disease. In: Morocutti C, Rizzo PA (eds): Evoked Potentials: Neurophysiological and Clinical Aspects. Amsterdam, Elsevier Science Publishers, 1985, pp 77–88.
59. Shigeyama Y, Inoue H, Hashizume H, et al: Muscle strength in rheumatoid elbow: quantitative measurement and comparison to Larsen's X-ray grade. Acta Medica Okayama 51(5):267–274, 1997.
60. Sihvonen T, Herno A, Paljarvi L, et al: Local denervation atrophy of paraspinal muscles in postoperative failed back syndrome. Spine 18(5):575–581, 1993.
61. Simonsen JC: Coefficient of variation as a measure of subject effort. Arch Phys Med Rehabil 76:516–520, 1995.
62. Slipman CW: Discography. In: Gonzalez EG, Materson RS (eds): Nonsurgical Management of Acute Low Back Pain. New York, Demos Vermande, 1997, pp 103–114.
63. Slipman CW: Diagnostic nerve root blocks. In: Gonzalez EG, Materson RS (eds): Nonsurgical Management of Acute Low Back Pain. New York, Demos Vermande, 1997, pp 115–124.
64. Smith GA, Nelson RC, Sadoff SJ, Sadoff AM: Assessing sincerity of effort in maximal grip strength tests. Am J Phys Med Rehabil 68(2):73–80, 1989.
65. Snook S: The design of manual handling tasks. Ergonomics 21(12):963–985, 1978.
66. Stephens JL, Pratt N, Michlovitz S: The reliability and validity of the Tekdyne hand dynamometer: Part II. J Hand Ther 9(1):18–26, 1996.
67. Stephens JL, Pratt N, Parks B: The reliability and validity of the Tekdyne hand dynamometer: Part I. J Hand Ther 9(1):10–17, 1996.
68. Stokes J: The seriously uninjured hand: weakness of grip. J Occup Med 25(9): 683–684, 1983.
69. Su CY, Lin JH, Chien TH, et al: Grip strength in different positions of elbow and shoulder. Arch Phys Med Rehabil 75:812–815, 1994.
70. Tin CR, Wu Y, Maffuli N, et al: Eccentric and concentric isokinetic knee flexion and extension: a reliability study using the Cybex 6000 dynamometer. Br J Sports Med 30:156–160, 1996.
71. Tis LL, Maxwell T: The effect of positioning on shoulder isokinetic measures in females. Med Sci Sports Exerc 28(9):1188–1192, 1996.
72. Wilson GJ, Murphy AJ: The use of isometric tests of muscular function in athletic assessment. Sports Med 22(1):19–37, 1996.
73. Yiannikas C: Short-latency somatosensory evoked potentials in peripheral nerve lesions, plexopathies, radiculopathies, and spinal cord trauma. In: Chiappa KH (ed): Evoked Potentials in Clinical Medicine, ed 2. New York, Raven Press, 1990, pp 439–468.

CHAPTER 5

Functional Capacity Evaluation for Impairment Rating and Disability Evaluation

Glenn Dabatos, RPT   Robert D. Rondinelli, MD, PhD   Mikel Cook, RPT, MPA

The physician disability examiner is empowered and entrusted to determine the nature and degree of medical impairment and associated severity of disability, and draws largely on traditional methods of medical examination to make such determinations. Among the resources available to assist in this task, the AMA *Guides* provides a reference manual for assigning percentages of impairment caused by anatomical or functional losses of the various organ systems of the body. The process and outcomes of this approach are problematic insofar as the impairment ratings derived are highly subjective, have limited reliability, and are not strongly predictive of associated disability.[28] As discussed in Chapter 2, there is a need for more systematic and objective functional assessment in impairment ratings and disability evaluations. Most physicians do not have specific training, access to proper office equipment, or sufficient time to feasibly and empirically address and verify the degree of functional loss relating to impairment in each case. However, because of the medicolegal and financial implications of disability ratings, physicians are becoming increasingly responsible under managed-care systems and the Americans with Disabilities Act (ADA) for generating objectively based disability determinations regarding a client's return-to-work potential.[30]

Therapeutic functional assessment is integral to the process of disability evaluation because it enables the physician to obtain objective functional measures of performance in a work setting to substantiate work-related disability associated with medical impairment. Such assessment is helpful during the initial evaluation of an injured worker to determine his or her ability to return to modified or transitional duty; it is also a useful tool for devising treatment and monitoring progress during the recovery phase. It can aid the physician in deciding when treatment benefits are exhausted and functional recovery has plateaued. When rating and releasing a client from treatment, it can provide objective indicators of physiological performance (or lack thereof) and a more valid indication of work disability and fitness for duty than is otherwise possible.

The purpose of this chapter is to outline the procedures and methodologies whereby therapeutic functional assessment is carried out, and to highlight the direct applications of this approach to impairment rating and work-disability determination.

DEFINITION AND PURPOSE

Functional capacity evaluation (FCE) is a systematic, comprehensive, and objective measurement of an individual's maximum work abilities.[11] FCE provides a detailed evaluation of an individual's functional level and performance abilities with respect to the physical demands of the workplace. The evaluation is carried out in a therapeutic setting simulating the physical demands of the workplace and usually lasts for 4 hours. FCE generally includes tests of strength and flexibility, cardiovascular endurance, neuromuscular coordination and reaction speed, and functional performance and safety. Functional activities tested include materials handling (e.g., lifting, carrying, pushing, and pulling), sitting, standing, walking, reaching, stooping, squatting, crouching, and climbing. In addition, the evaluation of hand activities such as gripping, finger manipulation, and dexterity may be assessed. FCEs may extend over a 2-day period as a practical and objective means of determining reproducibility of specific task performances and stability of test results and/or work conditions over time.

Job-site evaluation (JSE) is a related process designed to evaluate the individual's ability to meet critical job demands and, where applicable under the ADA, to successfully perform the essential functions of the job at the worksite.

HISTORICAL BACKGROUND

The historical origins of FCE are rooted in post-World War II U.S. industrial developments. In 1944 the American Medical Association introduced the notion of systematic medical examinations in industry to promote and maintain health among workers. At that time the U.S. Civil Service Commission was preparing a classification of physically disabling conditions to be matched with compatible positions of employment available within the federal government. This represented, perhaps, the first attempt to define work activities of the job, and ultimately gave rise to the U.S. Department of Labor's *Dictionary of Occupational Titles*.[7] During the next decade, in a series of papers by Dr. B. Hanman, the traditional medical examination was scrutinized as a means of determining fitness for work. Hanman introduced concepts of physical-demands analysis (PDA) and functional-capacity assessment (FCA). PDA provided details of the physical requirements of job-related tasks such as lifting, carrying, standing, walking, and stooping. FCA became a series of assessment procedures designed to examine an individual's capacity to perform the physical tasks listed in a PDA and involved two components: evaluation of medical fitness and evaluation of work capacity.[7]

The process of FCE has evolved with contributions from occupational and physical therapists and vocational analysts, while drawing on principles of physics, physiology, kinesiology, biomechanics, and more recently, ergonomics. FCE developed partly out of the needs of the insurance industry and legal professionals to seek more objective information on which to base return-to-work decisions. During the past two decades, FCE has emerged as *the* objective measurement approach to matching physical abilities with critical job demands, targeting treatment goals to justify work-hardening therapy, identifying job modifications to enhance worker safety, and delineating functional capacities in cases of litigation and disability determination.[11] Further applications toward behavior management and the detection of submaximal effort (i.e., nonphysiological performance) have also been promoted.[11] With the recent advent of the ADA, FCE has become readily applicable to testing an individual's capacity to meet or exceed the essential functions of his or her job.[30]

AVAILABLE TESTING TOOLS

A number of testing tools for FCE are available.[14] Several of these are listed in Table 5–1 for comparison. Many involve the purchase of special equipment and payment of license costs and ongoing utilization fees. Normative data or reference criteria are generally available for each system to assist the therapist in interpreting individual test performance against expectations, which may vary according to age, gender, and the specific job in question. Many facilities opt for an individually tailored approach, creating test programs based on their individual experience, specialized needs, and available equipment. Some facilities include equipment available to and used by the injured worker at the workplace, with the cooperation of the employer.

COMPONENTS OF A FUNCTIONAL CAPACITY EVALUATION

FCEs are typically administered by a specially trained physical or occupational therapist. The choice of measures included in the test battery should be individually tailored, with consideration to safety, reliability, practicality, and relevance to the stated purpose of the test.[31] FCEs generally include a clinical interview, vocational history, physical capacity testing, functional capacity testing, and performance validation.

Clinical Interview

At the outset, the therapist must gain a subjective understanding of the client's perceived problem and how it impacts on his or her ability to function. An opportunity is afforded to empathize with the client to gain cooperation and trust.[30] Attention should be paid to the client's perception of disability as well as his or her willingness to cooperate and give full effort to a test situation. Any physician-imposed restrictions or activity precautions must be noted to help gauge performance expectations with regard to test feasibility, client safety, and compliance. Any prior history of injury should be noted because frequent or recurrent injuries may reflect undue or excessive exposure to high-risk work activity, inattention to or noncompliance with preventive measures, or inherent weakness or instability of the involved body parts. Baseline activity levels, including athletic ability and exercise routine, should also be noted and can help set expectations for activity tolerance during testing.

A subjective history regarding the nature, location, and severity of pain and its association with activity should be noted. Individual pain tolerance varies considerably and may dictate the client's willingness and ability to participate in testing or training. Because pain is subjectively reported, it is not possible to measure objectively.[6] Various methods and tests have been created to assess an individual's perception of pain and the behavioral responses to it, and these are discussed in detail in Chapter 6.

TABLE 5–1 A Sample of Functional Testing Tools Available

Tool	Length of assessment	Validity and reliability	Equipment/license costs	Ongoing costs	Norm or criterion*
Arcon	<2 hr	No	$40,000	No	Both
AccessAbility	2 hr	Based on research	$400 + computer	$30/client	Criterion
Blankenship	2–4 hr	Based on medical research	$19,950–$75,000	$25/evaluation	Both
ERGOS	4 hr	Testing being done	$20,000–$100,000	No	Criterion
ErgoScience (PWPE)	3–4 hr	Yes	$6500–$8500	50 forms for $75	Criterion (some hand dexterity uses norm data)
IWS	5 hr/2 day 3 hr/2 parts	No	$9000–$10,000	No	Criterion (some norm data for select items)
Key	3.5–4 hr	Yes	$20,000	$60/assessment $10/job placement	Both
West-EPIC (Cal-FCP)	2 hr	Yes, of lifting capacity only	$23,500	No	Mainly criterion
WorkAbility Mark III	2–4 hr	No	$10,400	No	Criterion
WorkHab	2–3.5 hr	No	$1500	$75/yr fee	Criterion

*Normative data is based on repeated trials to establish where the average person would perform. Criterion uses a baseline or criteria to establish an expectation (that could vary depending upon the specific job).

For more information on the above tools contact the specific designer (see Appendix 5–1).

From King PM, Tuckwell N, Barrett TE: A critical review of functional capacity evaluations. Phys Ther 78(8):852–866, 1998. Reprinted with permission from American Physical Therapy Association.

Vocational History

Vocational information should be obtained directly from the client and employer. Client information should include duration of present employment, job satisfaction, job activity level and physical demands, and perceptions of employer expectations and flexibility. Employer information should include a job description (JD) that lists the essential functions of the job in terms of physical task demands and frequencies of performance required during the normal work shift. If a formal JD is unavailable, the U.S. Department of Labor's *Dictionary of Occupational Titles*[39] may provide useful information on the job requirements. However, accurate information regarding the physical demands of the job can best be obtained by a job-site evaluation, where critical task demands can be measured and verified. The employer's satisfaction with a client's job performance should also be noted. Positive or negative perceptions between employer and client may affect the client's incentive to return to work. Recovery and outcomes can be confounded by existing or perceived animosities between employer and client, including the employee's fear of losing his or her job, or aversion of a stressful or punitive situation.[29] In such instances, communication with the employer is helpful and should address whether job retraining and alternative job placement are being contemplated. Furthermore, an employer's flexibility and willingness to accommodate and availability of options, including modified duty or transitional return to work, can help define the most appropriate testing venue in each case.

Physical Capacity Testing

Strength

Assessment of strength according to capacity to lift is critical to safe placement of workers with a history of back injury. Protocols have been developed to address maximal acceptable weight limits and frequency of lifting applicable to industrial workers[36, 37] and provide comparative data for lifting capacity of uninjured workers versus those with low-back pain.[20, 21] Static strength testing has been used to predict the likelihood of injury or treatment outcome for healthy potential industrial workers.[3] It remains questionable whether parameters for healthy unimpaired workers apply adequately to physically impaired workers.[42] Dynamic testing of lifting and carrying has gained favor over static or isokinetic modes because it more closely approximates the actual demands of the job.[31]

Maximum effort testing is the evaluation of the individual's capacity to perform specific tasks correctly to his or her maximum level without increasing complaints of pain. The results are then measured against normative data. Maximum effort testing is performed in a static or dynamic mode as follows.

The *static strength test* is measured using a dynamometer while the client performs various tasks. The client is instructed to perform a task at maximum isometric effort. The following method is adopted by the National Institute of Occupational Safety and Health (NIOSH) for strength prediction methodology[24]: The client is placed in the position to be tested and then instructed to perform the task with sustained force for about 6 seconds. Care should be taken that the client does not alter his or her posture while performing the test. The various activities tested include a full squat (10 cm from floor), half squat (30 cm from floor), knuckle level reach, overhead arm reach, horizontal push, and horizontal pull. It is important to document if there is any increase in pain or symptoms during testing, or the level at which the client fails to perform the test.

The *dynamic strength test* is measured while doing functional and dynamic activities in various positions. The client is instructed to perform the task using his or her preferred posture. The activities evaluated are floor to knuckle, 30 cm to knuckle, knuckle height to shoulder height, shoulder height to arm reach, carrying, pushing, and pulling. To compare the values with the norms, it is ideal to use equipment with standard dimensions.[35] For lifting and carrying, the equipment is a box with measurements that are 36 cm, 49 cm, or 75 cm, with handle heights at 10 cm and 30 cm from the floor. Pushing and pulling are tested using a sled with handle heights at 64 cm, 95 cm, and 144 cm from the floor. A force gauge must be used to determine the effort applied to move the sled. The individual's capacity is measured by adding weight to the box or sled until it is heavy enough that the individual fails to perform the task. The data are compared to the recommended maximum acceptable weight limits.[35]

Testing isolated muscle strength is also important. Upper and lower extremities are manually tested using a grading system of 0 to 5.[12] However, manual muscle testing above grade 3 (full movement within available range against gravity) may be invalid, and it is preferable to use objective devices, such as the Chatillon dynamometer, that measure isometric strength of the extremity. Trunk strength can be measured using repetitive movement such as partial sit-ups for the abdominal muscles, or computerized equipment such as the Isostation B200 and the MedX. The data collected from strength testing can be used to guide a specific strengthening program for the spine or extremities.

Grip strength is a major factor in an individual's ability to perform daily tasks. Gripping and hand manipulation are required in the majority of materials handling tasks, during the operation of heavy equipment, and in the performance of daily activities such as pulling the handle of a heavy door. The Jamar hand dynamometer has been shown to give the most accurate measurement of grip strength.[18] It is designed with five slots to measure the grip strength in various handle positions. Two common tests performed to measure grip strength are the five-position grip test and the position-2 sustained grip test.

The five-position grip test is performed with the client in sitting position with the elbows at 90° flexion. The client is instructed to grip the dynamometer with maximal force. The amount of maximal effort of each of the five levels of the dynamometer is measured and graphed. With maximum grip effort, there will be a slightly skewed bell curve showing the weakest grip force at positions 1 and 5, and maximum force at position 3. It is ideal to get a comparison of the injured hand and the unaffected hand. The patient with true hand weakness will demonstrate the same skewed bell curve, but with diminished force, on the affected side compared with the uninvolved side. If the graph shows a straight line, the patient may not apply a maximum grip by exerting the same force in all five positions.

The *position-2 sustained grip test* is performed with the client positioned similar to that of the five-position grip test. The dynamometer handle is placed in position 2 for both males and females, and the client is instructed to grip the dynamometer with maximum force while data is collected. The patient's maximum grip force measured is compared with age and gender-based norms.[17] The disadvantage of this test is the difficulty in evaluating the patient's true effort to provide maximum grip force (see p. 83).

Flexibility

An assessment of joint mobility and flexibility is often needed to help understand limitations in the functional ability of an individual. Ideally, the evaluation should include active range of motion (ROM) measurements of all joints involved with the functional restriction. However, this method is painstaking and generally not practical for routine evaluations. To facilitate assessment, upper and lower extremities are examined during performance of quick and functional movements. In the upper extremities, examples of functional movements are reaching forward, reaching across, reaching overhead, and hand behind back (reaching behind). Examples of lower-extremity functional movements are squatting, kneeling, half-kneeling, and sitting with the leg crossed in a figure of four. If the individual shows difficulty in performing a particular movement, then a more thorough evaluation of the affected extremity becomes necessary.

ROM of an affected region should be measured as accurately as possible, with active ROM determinations generally being preferable to passive ROM for safety reasons. The quality of motion (e.g., ratchety, guarded) should also be considered along with the range. Goniometry is the preferred method of measuring joint ROM for the extremities. A two-arm goniometer is usually sufficient and is placed on the joint surface parallel to the plane of movement while measurement is taken of the available active range. Spinal measurements are more complicated, in part because of the combined joint motions being measured. The preferred method to measure spinal mobility is surface inclinometry using a single or dual inclinometer technique.[22] In some cases, computerized equipment such as the Isostation B200, Biodex, or Cybex is also used. To minimize errors and help maintain intrarater reliability, it is preferable that the evaluator performs spinal measurements consistently, using his or her preferred method and equipment rather than varying equipment and technique.[27]

Positional tolerance

Although a JD may indicate the various positions and activities of a particular job, it may not include the length of time required to maintain a position or activity. A job analysis (JA) can provide information on the various positions required and the average duration held at each position during an individual's specific work. This is important in understanding the positions that aggravate or provide relief of the individual's symptoms, whether in standing, sitting, lying prone, side lying, squatting, crouching, or crawling. Once an aggravating position is identified, it is important to know how long that position is held before symptoms arise. Finally, the time it takes for the symptoms to disappear or decrease to a tolerable level when returning to a comfortable position can be noted. Such information may help the therapist to design an individualized treatment program of appropriate intensity or to suggest a modified duty program that is suitable for the employee. For example, if the client can only tolerate 30 minutes of sitting, it would not be ideal to assign extended desk-work activities such as computer work or clerical work.

Aerobic capacity

Aerobic capacity is an important determinant of an individual's fitness for metabolically demanding occupational activity.[31] Depending on the individual's physical activity before injury, he or she may demonstrate significant ease or difficulty in performing even the most basic activities such as walking or climbing up and down stairs. If the client was following a regular exercise routine before injury, either at home or by participating in a gym, he or she may be motivated to return to the prior exercise and cardiovascular routine. Response to materials-handling activities may be well tolerated because of the client's baseline physical fitness. Often, individuals do not give serious consideration to their aerobic and cardiovascular fitness or conditioning until after injury. A deconditioned patient may need more intensive aerobic training to prepare for materials-handling activities.

A common and safe practice to measure aerobic fitness is the use of a bicycle ergometer or a treadmill. The test is done for 3 minutes, and the individual's heart rate, blood pressure, and breathing pattern are measured before and after the test. An individual with a good cardiovascular response will have a post-test heart rate return to a level identical to the pre-test heart rate after 3 minutes. Evaluation of walking tolerance can also be performed using a treadmill or an oval circuit. The distance ambulated can be modified to the amount of walking that is required at work. Vital signs before and after testing are similarly documented. Facilities vary in their approach to evaluating climbing activities. Depending on the job requirements of the patient, climbing is usually evaluated using several flights of stairs. Some facilities may not have access to stairs and will use steps or stair climbers instead. The test should be modified if the job requires climbing on a ladder or pole.

Aerobic capacity assessment allows direct comparison of a client's exercise tolerance level with the estimated requirements of a variety of jobs[8] and may help predict maximum continuous performance of aerobic tasks without undue fatigue.[31]

Functional Capacity Testing

The U.S. Department of Labor has reported the physical demands and environmental conditions encountered for a large variety of occupations.[39] The physical demands (PD) listings reflect the physical requirements of each occupation and the physical capacities that a worker must demonstrate to meet the standards. The PD descriptions include the following factors: strength, climbing, balancing, stooping, kneeling, crouching, crawling, reaching, handling, fingering, feeling, talking, hearing, tasting and smelling, near acuity, far acuity, depth perception, visual accommodation, color vision, and field of vision. Most FCEs address the following:

1. **Strength:** Strength can be expressed according to level of activity and frequency of performance at that level (Table 5–2). The frequency is measured based on length of time in a workday. *Occasionally* means activities or conditions that exist up to 33% of the time; *frequently* means activities or conditions that exist from 34% to 66% of the time; and *constantly* means activities or conditions that exist 67% or more of the time. There are five possible activity levels defined as follows:

Sedentary (S): If the object to be moved requires exerting no greater than 10 lb of force occasionally and less (negligible) weight frequently or constantly. This involves performance mostly from a seated position (at least 6 hours of an 8-hour shift) and may involve brief periods of walking and standing.

Light work (L): If the object to be moved requires exerting no greater than 20 lb of force occasionally, and/or no greater than 10 lb frequently, and

TABLE 5–2 Level of Physical Activity According to U.S. Department of Labor

Level of activity	Occasional 0%–33%	Frequent 34%–66%	Constant 67%–100%
Sedentary	≤10 lb	Negligible	Negligible
Light	≤20 lb	≤10 lb	Negligible
Medium	≤50 lb	≤20 lb	≤10 lb
Heavy	≤100 lb	≤50 lb	≤20 lb
Very heavy	>100 lb	>50 lb	≥20 lb

negligible amounts constantly. Light work requires more standing or walking than sitting (at least 6 hours of an 8-hour shift), and it requires more use of the arm or leg when in a seated position.

Medium work (M): If exerting no greater than 50 lb of force occasionally, and/or no greater than 20 lb of force frequently, and/or no greater than 10 lb of force constantly to move an object.

Heavy work (H): If exerting no greater than 100 lb of force occasionally, and/or no greater than 50 lb of force frequently, and/or no greater than 20 lb of force constantly to move an object.

Very heavy work (VH): If moving an object requires exertion greater than 100 lb of force occasionally, and/or greater than 50 lb of force frequently, and/or greater than 20 lb of force constantly.

Functional activities traditionally measured according to frequency include lifting, carrying, pushing and pulling, standing, walking, sitting, and operating controls. Controls includes the use of one or both arms or hands, or one or both feet or legs to operate machines or equipment. Lifting strength can be measured in terms of the various activities listed in Table 5–3.

2. **Climbing:** Involves ascending and descending ladders, stairs, scaffoldings, ramps, poles, and similar objects, using the arms, hands, legs, or feet.
3. **Balancing:** Involves maintaining equilibrium of the body to avoid falling while performing tasks such as walking, standing, crouching, or running on a narrow or moving platform or slippery surfaces.
4. **Stooping:** Requires bending of the spine at the waist forward and downward.
5. **Kneeling:** Bending the legs at the knees, resting on one knee or both knees.
6. **Crouching:** Bending the trunk forward and downward by bending at the legs and spine.
7. **Crawling:** Moving around while on hands and knees.
8. **Reaching:** The use of hand(s) and arm(s), extending the extremity in various directions.
9. **Handling:** With the use of one hand or both hands, while seizing, holding, grasping, or turning.
10. **Fingering:** Manipulation of an object using the fingers to pick or pinch an object, without the use of the whole arm or hand. Employers benefit with this information to find the appropriate work or restrictions when assigning modified duty assignments.

FCE in conjunction with the U.S. Department of Labor job analysis approach

TABLE 5–3 Functional Task Measures

Floor to Knuckle Lift

This test is similar to a full-squat lift in which the object is picked up from floor level. The client performs the task by squatting until the buttocks are close to straddling the heels. The test begins with grabbing the lowest handle (10 cm from the floor), keeping the box close to the body. The box is lifted while keeping the elbows straight, and movement should be initiated by first extending the trunk, followed by the lower extremities. After lifting the box and standing erect, the client is instructed to lower the box.*

30 cm to Knuckle Lift

This test simulates lifting objects from the knee level. The client moves into a half-squat position, grabbing the handles that are 30 cm from the floor, and is then instructed to lift the box while keeping the elbows straight until the trunk is fully extended. After the lift, the client immediately lowers the box.*

Knuckle Height to Shoulder Height

The movement tested identical to working on multi-level shelves moving objects laterally from hip level to shoulder level. The test is performed with the client standing in front of the box and instructed to lift the box, move laterally, and place it on a platform that is at shoulder level. The client then replaces the box to its original position.*

Shoulder Height to Arm Reach

This test simulates overhead activities such as stocking shelves overhead. The test is performed with the client standing in front of the box, lifting the box, and moving laterally before placing it on a platform about 30 cm above shoulder level. The client replaces the box to its original position.*

Carrying

The object of this test is to evaluate the ability of the client to carry a box for a specific distance according to the client's work activity. Standard norms are available for heights of 72 cm and 105 cm, and distances from 2.1 m, 4.3 m, and 8.5 m.† The test is performed with the patient carrying a box and walking the distance as specified by the job requirements.*

Pushing and Pulling

These tests are measured using a weighted sled. The heights of the handles of the sled are specified.† The distance measured to push the sled can be 2.1 m, 7.6 m, 15.2 m, 30.5 m, 45.7 m, or 61.0 m, whereas pulling is measured at a distance of 2.1 m. In both tests, care should be taken that the individual maintains a safe posture. A dynamometer is used to measure the forces to push or pull the sled, with the results compared with the data collected from the workplace (if available).*

*Testing is stopped when the weight being tested is heavy enough that the client mechanically substitutes to achieve the lift (i.e., use of the hips and knees to lift instead of the trunk extensor muscles).
†Data from Snook SH: The design of manual handling tasks. Ergonomics 21(12):963–985, 1978.

has been used to evaluate an injured worker's ability to return to work.[34] Ideally, FCE should be combined with a JSE, in which actual measurements of the critical job demands can be obtained. An example of an FCE evaluating and reporting form is provided (Table 5–4), which was developed with input from a physical therapist and vocational analyst. The form can be tailored to the essential functions of a particular job if a job description, job analysis, or JSE results are available. This will directly assist the physician in generating a set of return-to-work recommendations or restrictions that are compatible with the ADA, specific to the essential functions of the job, and which enable accommodation needs to be identified precisely and quantitatively.[29] The form can also be used to identify a client's functional baseline in preparation for a conditioning exercise program, work hardening, or transitional return-to-work program. It is equally useful to identify incremental treatment goals, monitor functional progress during treatment, and identify when treatment has plateaued and maximum medical improvement (MMI) has been reached.

Performance Validation With Implications for Symptom Magnification and Sincerity of Effort

The injured client who is motivated to return to work is a good candidate for FCE, and his or her performance on physical and functional capacity testing is generally straightforward, as described earlier. However, the most compelling reason for FCE may be to objectively assess the injured worker experiencing delayed recovery with respect to his or her return-to-work options. Such a client often poses a challenge to overcome various motivational and situational confounders, including attorney involvement. Consequently, the assessment of the client's level of effort in relation to objective findings is critical.

Clients subjected to FCE may display signs and symptoms of pain or other distress, which can impede performance in predictable or unpredictable ways. Performance limitations in the presence of an organic nociceptive focus are predictable and can be expected to occur consistently with mechanical provocation during task repetitions. Self-inhibition because of pain or apprehension in the absence of, or out of proportion to the degree of organic nociception (i.e., symptom magnification) may invalidate test results obtained. To help distinguish performance limitations from a physiological versus nonphysiological cause, the following approaches may be useful.

A simple screening test includes examination of five physical signs listed in Table 5–5. A score of three or more positive signs is considered significant and suggests nonphysiological performance limitations that may warrant further evaluation.[40]

The assessment of maximal effort and reproducibility during strength testing has been carried out for the upper extremity using the Jamar dynamometer[4, 13, 33, 38] and BTE work simulator,[13] for the lower extremity using the KinCom II,[5] and for various trunk and back lifting activities using the ERGOS Work Simulator[32] and isokinetic equipment (e.g., Cybex, Liftask),[10] among others. Reproducibility of maximal effort testing is often measured in terms of the *coefficient of variation (COV),* defined as the variance in repeat maximal effort testing divided by the mean effort × 100%. A COV of less than 10% for males and 12% for females has been suggested to reflect maximal effort during testing.[15] However, the acceptable range of COVs may vary by test procedure and region examined,[32] making their interpretation suspect. Consequently, the clinician is advised not to rely on the COV as the sole basis of determining degree of subject effort.

The COV has been used to assess sincerity of effort[4, 32, 33] where "sincere" refers to maximum effort during testing. *Sincerity* has to do with honesty and lack of pretense or deceit. Application of the term to maximal effort testing is problematic insofar as it implies knowledge of the client's motivation, which may be impossible to determine and also irrelevant. However, it is possible for the clinician performing the FCE to determine if the client performed in a physiological (i.e., maximal) manner. Performance in a nonphysiological (i.e., submaximal) manner allows one to deduce that the client withheld effort but does not indicate the motivation for doing so.

TABLE 5–4 Job Analysis and Physical Demand Comparison

Job Title: Name of individual:
Who/how information obtained:
Key: N=Never O=Occasionally (0–2.5 hr/day) F=Frequently (2.5–5.5 hr/day) C=Constantly (5.5+ hr/day)

	JOB REQUIREMENT				EMPLOYEE STATUS				COMMENTS
1. **Lifting**									
≤10 lb	N____	O____	F____	C____	N____	O____	F____	C____	____
11–20 lb	N____	O____	F____	C____	N____	O____	F____	C____	____
21–50 lb	N____	O____	F____	C____	N____	O____	F____	C____	____
51–100	N____	O____	F____	C____	N____	O____	F____	C____	____
>100 lb	N____	O____	F____	C____	N____	O____	F____	C____	____
2. **Carrying**									
≤10 lbs	N____	O____	F____	C____	N____	O____	F____	C____	____
11–20 lb	N____	O____	F____	C____	N____	O____	F____	C____	____
21–50 lb	N____	O____	F____	C____	N____	O____	F____	C____	____
51–100 lb	N____	O____	F____	C____	N____	O____	F____	C____	____
>100 lb	N____	O____	F____	C____	N____	O____	F____	C____	____
3. **Pushing/Pulling**									
≤10 lbs	N____	O____	F____	C____	N____	O____	F____	C____	____
11–20 lb	N____	O____	F____	C____	N____	O____	F____	C____	____
21–50 lb	N____	O____	F____	C____	N____	O____	F____	C____	____
51–100 lb									
>100 lb	N____	O____	F____	C____	N____	O____	F____	C____	____
4. **Reaching** (list weights):									
Below knees	N____	O____	F____	C____	N____	O____	F____	C____	____
Knee/Waist	N____	O____	F____	C____	N____	O____	F____	C____	____
Waist/Chest	N____	O____	F____	C____	N____	O____	F____	C____	____
Chest/Shoulder	N____	O____	F____	C____	N____	O____	F____	C____	____
Above Shoulder	N____	O____	F____	C____	N____	O____	F____	C____	____
5. **Functions** (list distance):									
Walking	N____	O____	F____	C____	N____	O____	F____	C____	____
Standing	N____	O____	F____	C____	N____	O____	F____	C____	____
Sitting Twisting	N____	O____	F____	C____	N____	O____	F____	C____	____

6. **Climbing**									
Stairs	N____	O____	F____	C____	N____	O____	F____	C____	________
Ladders	N____	O____	F____	C____	N____	O____	F____	C____	________
Scaffolds	N____	O____	F____	C____	N____	O____	F____	C____	________
7. **Balancing**									
Narrow	N____	O____	F____	C____	N____	O____	F____	C____	________
Slippery	N____	O____	F____	C____	N____	O____	F____	C____	________
Moving	N____	O____	F____	C____	N____	O____	F____	C____	________
8. **Stooping**	N____	O____	F____	C____	N____	O____	F____	C____	________
9. **Kneeling**	N____	O____	F____	C____	N____	O____	F____	C____	________
10. **Squatting**	N____	O____	F____	C____	N____	O____	F____	C____	________
11. **Crawling**	N____	O____	F____	C____	N____	O____	F____	C____	________
12. **Handling/Fingering** (list weights when applicable):									
Simple grasping	N____	O____	F____	C____	N____	O____	F____	C____	________
Power grasping	N____	O____	F____	C____	N____	O____	F____	C____	________
Pushing/Pulling	N____	O____	F____	C____	N____	O____	F____	C____	________
Wrist twisting	N____	O____	F____	C____	N____	O____	F____	C____	________
Fine motor	N____	O____	F____	C____	N____	O____	F____	C____	________

Recommended Job Category: **Sedentary** ____ **Light** ____ **Medium** ____ **Heavy** ____ **Very Heavy**____

Notes: ____

____

____

Job Analyzer: ____________________ **Date** ____________________

Therapist: ____________________ **Date**____________________

Modified from Rondinelli RD, Robinson JP, Scheer SJ, Weinstein SM: Occupational rehabilitation and disability determination. In: DeLisa J, Gans BM (eds): Rehabilitation Medicine: Principles and Practice, 3rd ed. Philadelphia, Lippincott-Raven Publishers, 1998, pp 213–230. Reprinted with permission from Lippincott-Raven Publishers.

TABLE 5–5 "Nonorganic" Physical Signs of Low-Back Pain

1. *Tenderness* that is superficial or nonanatomically localized. Superficial tenderness occurs when the client reports tenderness to light pinch or palpation across the lumbar region. *Nonanatomic* refers to deep tenderness to palpation over a wide area extending past the lumbar region toward the sacrum, pelvis, or thoracic region.
2. *Simulation* of mechanical provocation of nociception through sham maneuvers such as "axial loading" (provocation of low-back pain complaints when the examiner applies vertical pressure to the top of the skull) and "rotation" (provocation of lumbar pain with passive rotation of the torso as a unit at the hips while shoulders and pelvis are fixed in the same plane).
3. *Inconsistencies* with distraction, such as the response to a straight leg raise (SLR) performed in seated position while checking strength of the quadriceps or anterior tibial muscle groups versus testing SLR in the supine position.
4. *Regional disturbances* of sensory deficit or motor weakness that do not reflect a neuroanatomical pattern, such as numbness over the entire leg or half the body, or "giving way" of the lower extremity to manual muscle testing.
5. *Overreaction* to the examiner, with disproportionate pain behavior in relation to clinical presentation.

Finally, the assessment of subject effort using isomachines in general has been shown to be problematic on a number of levels, including the following:

1. Inferences toward symptomatic individuals have been drawn largely from tests on "normal" individuals and may not be valid.
2. Complex statistical manipulations are often needed to achieve discrimination criteria with desired sensitivity and specificity.
3. Consistency measures using static isometric (i.e., grip strength) data are generalized to complex isokinetic or isoinertial (i.e., trunk strength) data.
4. Maximal versus submaximal effort cannot always be distinguished based on performance consistency.[25]

In view of the above, the clinician must exercise due caution in interpreting consistency of effort based on isometric, isokinetic, or isoinertial testing.

When nonphysiological performance is suspected to invalidate FCE, the test results obtained should not be used as the primary basis for return-to-work restrictions. In such cases, the physician disability examiner must rely on clinical judgment and may opt for more conservative and restrictive recommendations than might otherwise appear warranted.

SAFETY ISSUES

FCE has the potential to cause harm and, consequently, must be individually tailored and self-directed to some extent. Maximum-effort testing can be designed to lessen probability of further injury if it meets the criteria listed in Table 5–6.[16]

Possible reasons for terminating FCE testing include any of the criteria listed in Table 5–7. The therapist must continually exercise good clinical judgment and common sense because complaints of increased symptoms during the test itself are common and do not preclude thorough and complete testing in most cases.

TABLE 5–6 Recommended Safety Measures During Maximum-Effort Testing

1. Cardiovascular effort does not exceed 65% predicted maximal heart rate.
2. Testing avoids or minimizes direct mechanical involvement of an impaired functional unit.
3. Testing is controlled by the client being evaluated.
4. Test measures have high internal consistency and low error variance.
5. Testing allows short-term replication of effort and brief rests between trials.
6. During testing, visual and proprioceptive feedback to client are limited with respect to effort.

APPLICATIONS OF FCE TO IMPAIRMENT RATINGS AND DISABILITY EVALUATIONS

The applications of therapeutic functional assessment are varied. FCEs are used to obtain objective, accurate, and reproducible information on a client's abilities to perform physical activities. The data thereby collected can be used to establish functional baselines and treatment goals, monitor progress during treatment, demonstrate nonphysiological performance and symptom magnification, determine current ability to return to work safely, and support the physician's assessment regarding MMI and the need for case closure.[29] Although an FCE might ideally be performed on every injured worker, it is expensive and usually unnecessary because most injured workers return to work safely and without incident. At a minimum, FCE should be considered in those cases in which the injured worker has experienced delayed recovery, enlisted legal counsel, or suffered permanent physical impairment and return-to-work potential is in question.

FCE has several specific uses to the physician disability examiner, including impairment ratings, work disability determinations, and ADA accommodation studies.

Impairment Ratings

The difference between impairment and disability ratings is discussed in detail in Chapter 2. Impairment ratings may establish a medical (i.e., anatomical or physiological) basis to explain loss of functioning at the workplace. The formal linkage of low-back impairment ratings to work disability has previously been attempted[41] but remains entirely unsubstantiated by scientific inquiry. A limited number of studies have examined correlations between impairment ratings and function of the hand[9, 26] and lower extremity[23]; however, no correlational studies currently exist between impairment rating and residual functional

TABLE 5–7 Possible Reasons for Terminating the FCE

1. The client complains of increased symptoms.
2. The client is unable to demonstrate the movement safely.
3. The client refuses to perform the task.
4. The evaluator deems it to be unsafe to perform the task.

capacity according to FCE.[30] Shortcomings of the AMA approach with respect to validity and reliability are highlighted in Chapter 3, and many of these are likely to be reduced or eliminated by a more functionally and diagnosis-based approach (see Chapter 2). In this context, the major application of FCE is to determining functionally based impairments of the cardiac and pulmonary organ systems,[1] and similar applications to the musculoskeletal and nervous systems are needed. Standard application of FCE to the impairment rating process in general has been recommended,[19] and the routine inclusion of FCEs into permanent impairment ratings may ultimately affect a valid linkage between impairment and disability ratings.

Work Disability Determinations

Functionally based work disability determinations are becoming increasingly important to treatment protocols emphasizing return to work.[28] As managed care's influence within Workers' Compensation increases and ADA compliance is reinforced through litigation, the role of FCE in disability evaluation protocols is also likely to increase.[30] FCEs provide the physician with access to valid and reliable information concerning the injured worker's residual physical capacities when authorizing modified duty or transitional return to work during treatment, or sanctioning permanent activity restrictions at MMI. Restrictions that are not functionally based (hence of questionable validity) may be needlessly restrictive, leading to significant economic loss and negatively impacting the individual's work identity and sense of independence.[30] Alternatively, work disability determinations based on FCEs can facilitate the return-to-work transition during treatment and enable less restrictive outcomes at case closure.

Americans With Disabilities Act Accommodation

Where applicable, the ADA prohibits discrimination by employers against individuals with disabilities and may require accommodation of an otherwise qualified individual with a disability. The concept of essential functions applies, and for a given job functions can be considered essential for several reasons. In general, functions listed in a job description are essential if they must be performed for the job to exist. However, a function does not have to be the reason the job exists to be essential. A function would be considered essential if no other employee is available to whom that function could be assigned, even though it might be a minor function. For example, turning on a light switch in the morning might be done only once and seemingly be a marginal function. However, if no one else is available to whom the function could be assigned, it would be considered an essential function. Failure to perform the essential functions of a job is grounds for termination of an employee "for cause." Under ADA, an *otherwise qualified individual with a disability* is considered employable if he or she can meet or exceed the performance of these essential functions with or without *reasonable accommodation*. Accommodation is reasonable if it enables the disabled individual to perform the essential functions of a job, without posing *undue hardship* (logistical and/or financial) on the employer or posing a *direct threat* to the health and safety of co-workers at the job site.[2] Where applicable, ADA accommodation is the employer's and not the physician examiner's responsibility. However, FCE-based decisions on fitness for work are inherently

ADA compatible and can be used by physicians to assist the employer in achieving reasonable accommodation by specifically addressing the disabled worker's residual ability to meet or exceed the critical physical demands associated with the essential functions of a particular job in question, and identifying those functions where accommodation is medically necessary and appropriate in each case.

ACKNOWLEDGEMENTS

Mr. Robert King, RPT (King Consulting, Silverthorne, Colorado) reviewed this manuscript and provided many helpful criticisms and comments. Mr. Donald Harkins, MA (Director of Vocational Services) and Ms. Jane Duebler-White, MEd (Manager of Consulting Services) of The Rehabilitation Institute, Kansas City, Missouri, helped develop the job analysis and physical demands comparison chart presented in this chapter.

REFERENCES

1. American Medical Association: Guides to the Evaluation of Permanent Impairment, 4th ed. Chicago, American Medical Association, 1993.
2. Americans with Disabilities Act. 29CFR, Part 1630. Equal Opportunity for Individuals with Disabilities. Fed Reg 56(144):21–32, 1991.
3. Chaffin DB, Herrin GD, Keyserling WM: Pre-employment strength testing: an updated position. J Occup Med 20:403-408, 1978.
4. Chengalur SN, Smith GA, Nelson RC, Sadoff AM: Assessing sincerity of effort in maximal grip strength tests. Am J Phys Med Rehabil 69:148–153, 1990.
5. Dvir Z, David G: Suboptimal muscular performance: measuring isokinetic strength of knee extensors with new testing protocol. Arch Phys Med Rehabil 77: 578–581, 1996.
6. Fordyce WE (ed): Back Pain in the Workplace. Seattle, IASP Press, 1995.
7. Fraser TM: Fitness for Work. London, Taylor & Francis, 1992.
8. Garg A, Chaffin DB, Herrin GD: Prediction of metabolic rate for manual materials handling jobs. Am Ind Hyg Assoc J 39:661–674, 1978.
9. Gloss DS, Wardle MG: Reliability and validity of American Medical Association's Guide to ratings of permanent impairment. JAMA 248:2292–2296, 1982.
10. Hazard RG, Haugh LD, Reid S, et al: Early prediction of chronic disability after occupational low back injury. Spine 21:945–951, 1996.
11. Isernhagen SJ: Functional capacity evaluation. In: Isernhagen SJ (ed): Work Injury: Management and Prevention. Rockville, Md, Aspen Publishers, Inc., 1988, pp 139–194.
12. Kendall FP, McReary EK, Provance PG: Muscles: Testing and Function, 4th ed. Baltimore, Williams & Wilkins, 1993.
13. King JW, Berryhill BH: Assessing maximum effort in upper-extremity functional testing. Work 1(3):65–76, 1991.
14. King P, Tuckwell N, Barrett T: A critical review of functional capacity evaluations. Phys Ther 78(8):852–866, 1998.
15. Matheson LN: How do you know that he tried his best? The reliability crisis in industrial rehabilitation. Indus Rehab Q 1(1):11–12, 1988.
16. Matheson LN: Work Capacity Evaluation: Interdisciplinary Approach to Industrial Rehabilitation. Anaheim, Employment and Rehabilitation Institute of California (ERIC), 1984.
17. Mathiowetz V, Kashman N, Volland G, et al: Grip and pinch strength: normative data for adults. Arch Phys Med Rehabil 66:69–74, 1985.

18. Mathiowetz V, Weber K, Volland G, Kashman N: Reliability and validity of hand strength evaluation. J Hand Surg 9A:222–226, 1984.
19. May VR, Taylor D, Brigham C, Washington C: Functional capacity evaluation, impairment rating, and applied certification processes. Neuro Rehabil 11:13–27, 1998.
20. Mayer TG, Barnes D, Kashino ND, et al: Progressive isoinertial lifting evaluation. I. A standardized protocol and normal database. Spine 13:993–997, 1988.
21. Mayer TG, Barnes D, Kashino ND, et al: Progressive isoinertial lifting evaluation. II. A comparison with isokinetic lifting in a disabled chronic low back pain industrial population. Spine 13:998–1002, 1988.
22. Mayer T, Tencer A, Kristoferson S, Mooney V: Use of non-invasive techniques for quantification of spinal range-of-motion in normal subjects and chronic low back dysfunction patients. Spine 9:588–595, 1984.
23. McCarthy ML, McAndrew MP, MacKenzie EJ, et al: Correlation between measures of impairment, according to the modified system of the American Medical Association, and function. J Bone Joint Surg 80-A(7):1034–1042, 1998.
24. National Institute for Occupational Safety and Health: Work Practices Guide for Manual Lifting. Technical Report 81-122. Cincinnati, NIOSH, 1981, pp 129–144.
25. Newton M, Waddell G: Trunk strength testing with iso-machines. Part 1. Review of a decade of scientific evidence. Spine 18:801–811, 1993.
26. Rondinelli RD, Dunn W, Hassanein KM, et al: A simulation of hand impairments: effects on upper extremity function and implications toward medical impairment rating and disability determination. Arch Phys Med Rehabil 78:1358–1363, 1997.
27. Rondinelli R, Murphy J, Esler A, et al: Estimation of normal lumbar flexion with surface inclinometry: a comparison of three methods. Am J Phys Med Rehabil 71:219–224, 1992.
28. Rondinelli RD, Robinson JP, Scheer SJ, Weinstein SM: Industrial rehabilitation medicine. 4. Strategies for disability management. Arch Phys Med Rehabil 78:S21–28, 1997.
29. Rondinelli RD, Robinson JP, Scheer SJ, Weinstein SM: Occupational rehabilitation and disability determination. In: DeLisa J, Gans BM (eds): Rehabilitation Medicine: Principles and Practice, 3rd ed. Philadelphia, Lippincott-Raven Publishers, 1998, pp 213–230.
30. Sawyer H: Functional capacity evaluations: impact of the Americans with Disabilities Act and managed care. Neuro Rehabil 11:3–12, 1998.
31. Scheer SJ, Wickstrom RJ: Vocational capacity with low back pain impairment. In: Scheer SJ (ed): Medical Perspectives in Vocational Assessment of Impaired Workers. Gaithersburg, Md, Aspen Publishers Inc, 1991, pp 19–63.
32. Simonsen JC: Coefficient of variation as a measure of subject effort. Arch Phys Med Rehabil 76:516–520, 1995.
33. Smith GA, Nelson RC, Sadoff SJ, Sadoff AM: Assessing sincerity of effort in maximal grip strength tests. Am J Phys Med Rehabil 68:73–80, 1989.
34. Smith SL, Cunningham S, Weinberg R: The predictive validity of the functional capacities evaluation. Am J Occup Ther 40:564–567, 1986.
35. Snook SH: The design of manual handling tasks. Ergonomics 21(12):963–985, 1978.
36. Snook SH, Irvine CH: Maximum acceptable weight of lift. Am Indust Hyg Assoc J 28:322–329, 1968.
37. Snook SH, Irvine CH: Maximum frequency of lift acceptable to male industrial workers. Am Indust Hyg Assoc J 29:532–536, 1968.
38. Stokes HM: The seriously uninjured hand: weakness of grip. J Occup Med 25(9): 683–684, 1983.
39. US Department of Labor, Employment and Training Administration: Dictionary of Occupational Titles, 4th ed. Washington, DC, US Government Printing Office, 1977.

40. Waddell G, McCulloch JA, Kummel E, Venner RM: Nonorganic physical signs in low-back pain. Spine 5(2):117–125, 1980.
41. Wiesel SW, Feffer HL, Rothman RH: Industrial Low Back Pain, Charlottesville, Va, The Michie Company, 1985, pp 662–665.
42. Zeh J, Hansson T, Bigos S, et al: Isometric strength testing: recommendations based on a statistical analysis of the procedure. Spine 11:43–46, 1986.

APPENDIX 5–1

Contact Designer Information for Functional Testing Tools*

Arcon
Attn: Dana Rasch
University of Michigan
475 East Jefferson, Rm 2354
Ann Arbor, MI 48109-1248
Phone (313) 936-0435
Fax (313) 936-1330

AccessAbility
Attn: Michael Coupland
1166 Jamestown Rd.
Williamsburg, VA 23185
(757) 221-8134

BIODEX
Biodex Medical Systems, Inc.
Brookhaven R&D Plaza
20 Ramsay Road
Box 702
Shirley, NY 11967-0702
Phone (800) 224-6339
(516) 924-9000
Fax (516) 924-9338
email: sales@biodex.com

Blankenship
Attn: Keith Blankenship
Blankenship System
3620 Eisenhower
Suite 7
Macon, GA 31206
Phone (912) 788-3488
Fax (912) 781-8566

* From King PM, Tuckwell N, Barrett TE: A critical review of functional capacity evaluations. Phys Ther 78(8):852-866, 1998.

CYBEX
Cybex International, Inc.
10 Trotter Drive
Medway, MA 02053

ERGOS
Work Recovery, Inc.
2341 S. Friebus, Suite 14
Tucson, AZ 85713
Phone (502) 322-6634
Internet address: www.ergos.com

ErgoScience
Attn: Deborah Lechner
PWPE
Users Guide
Birmingham, AL
email: dlechner@uab.edu

ISOSTATION B200
Isotechnologies, Inc.
Elizabeth Brady Rd.
PO Box 1239
Hillsborough, NC 27278
Phone (919) 462-1776
Fax (919) 462-1780

IWS
Susan Isernhagen
Isernhagen Work Systems
2202 Water Street
Duluth, MN 55812
Phone (218) 728-6455
Fax (218) 728-6454

Key
Attn: Glenda Key
Key Method
619 10th St. South
Minneapolis, MN 55404-1475
Phone (612) 333-1191
Fax (612) 333-2366
email: c.bodway@keymethod.com

West-EPIC
Attn: Leonard Matheson
WEST-EPIC
Roy Matheson and Associates
PO Box 492
Keene, NH 03431-0492
Phone (603) 358-6525

WorkAbility
Attn: GC Heyde and J Shervinton
WorkAbility Mark III
Users Guide
New South Wales, Australia

WorkHab
Attn: David Roberts and Sam Bradbury
WorkHab
Users Guide
Queensland, Australia

CHAPTER 6

Psychological, Social, and Behavioral Assessment Tools

William Stiers, PhD *Raymond C. Tait, PhD*

Impairment ratings and disability evaluations are complicated by the fact that there is considerable variation between objectively measured impairment and subjectively reported disability. Impairment has to do with anatomical, physiological, or psychological abnormality or loss, whereas disability has to do with inability to perform usual tasks or assume usual obligations.[122] Although disability is related to impairment, it is also subject to modulation by numerous other factors, such that identical types of measured impairments may result in widely different levels of reported disability. In fact, even among individuals without measured impairments, disability may be reported and demonstrated. This variable relationship is a significant problem in medico-legal evaluations.

Psychological, social, and behavioral factors must be recognized as significant contributors to the relationship between impairment and disability. These factors can produce significant disability alone, or in combination with physical impairment.[41] Understanding the role of these non-medical factors can aid in evaluation and treatment.

Intractable pain is used here to illustrate the complex relationship between impairment and disability. Pain is often the presenting condition for medical impairment evaluation and disability determination, yet its relationship to tests of objective impairment remains poorly understood.[90] It has been estimated that objective impairment accounts for only about 25% of the variance in low-back pain–related disability.[125] For a given level of impairment, pain can lead to significant disability for an individual with severe psychosocial stressors, limited coping skills, and little positive experiences or hopes. However, the same level of impairment and pain may result in only mild disability for an individual with significant psychosocial supports, good coping skills, and numerous positive experiences and hopes.

The contribution of psychological, social, and behavioral factors to disability ranges from mild to severe. Many clients have minor elements of symptom magnification, if only in an attempt to express the seriousness of their concerns, or perhaps because of other problems in their lives. Other clients may have severe elements of symptom magnification related to significant psychological dysfunction or even overt malingering. This chapter discusses the broad range of these contributions.

Psychosocial assessment in impairment ratings and disability evaluations is directed toward answering two questions:

1. Is the patient at maximum medical improvement (MMI), or are there

psychological, social, or behavioral factors contributing to disability that should be treated (i.e., should a final disability rating be postponed)?
2. Given appropriate treatment, are there remaining psychological, social, or behavioral contributions to disability of such magnitude that a separate estimate of psychological disability should be conducted?

Although many physician examiners already use an organizational schema to evaluate psychological, social, and behavioral factors contributing to disability, the process of data collection and interpretation often lacks standardization. To the extent that these factors can be systematically and accurately evaluated, the validity and reliability of impairment ratings and disability evaluations may be enhanced. This chapter provides a conceptual and practical guide to physicians for standardized psychological, social, and behavioral assessment of clients with musculoskeletal complaints. Of course, some clients may require more formal psychological evaluation.

The information that follows is presented for the three domains of psychological, social, and behavioral functioning. Within each domain, the general concepts are discussed, followed by a description of basic items appropriate to the physician, as well as detailed assessment items and instruments appropriate to the psychologist. Because pain is a frequent medical complaint that can have significant psychological, social, and behavioral components, we will emphasize the assessment of pain-related disability.

ASSESSMENT OF PSYCHOLOGICAL FACTORS

There are a number of psychological factors that mediate the relationship between impairment and disability, including the following:

1. **Mood:** Sensory information causes affective responses, and preexisting affective states modify perceptions of sensory information.
2. **Cognition:** Cognitive processes assign meaning to sensory information and affective responses.
3. **Personality:** Overall psychological adjustment and coping skills modify processing of sensory information, affective responses, and cognitions.
4. **Motivation:** Sensation, affect, cognition, and personality interact with environmental contingencies (direct and indirect gains and losses).

Mood: Depression and Anxiety

Concepts

Emotions interact with sensory stimuli in several ways. The most direct involves emotional responses to sensory stimuli. For example, some level of emotional distress can be expected in response to painful stimuli. In addition, preexisting affective disturbance can lower one's threshold and tolerance for noxious or disturbing stimuli. Anxiety and depression are the affective elements that most often interact with experiences of pain and impairment. This complex relationship is well illustrated in research on affective responses to pain.

Painful stimuli, as well as the anticipation of pain, produce anxiety. Reduction of pain is followed by reduction of anxiety.[37] On the other hand, higher anxiety is associated with lower pain tolerance.[24] Both state (acute) and trait (chronic) anxiety are correlated with amount of reported postoperative pain, with greater pain reported in response to experimental stimuli.[37]

Reduction of anxiety is followed by reduction in reported pain, whether anxiety is reduced by medication, reassurance, or perceived control of the noxious stimuli. Anxiolytic medication may be roughly equal in pain relief to analgesics in some situations.[37]

Depression is another common symptom in individuals with chronic pain,[94] and reduction of pain is followed by reduction of depression.[127] On the other hand, higher depression is associated with lower pain tolerance, and reduction of depression is followed by reduction of reported pain.[71]

Both depression and anxiety are responses to pain and also serve to modulate it. Moreover, each has shown associations to self-perceived disability.[109] Clearly, assessment of both anxiety and depression can provide valuable information in assessment of impairment and its relation to disability.

Assessment

Several measurement instruments are widely used for assessment of depression and anxiety.

Depression. The Beck Depression Inventory (BDI) is a 21-item self-report inventory, with each item scaled from 0 (not at all) to 3 (severe). This instrument asks clients to respond to questions about the following three mood-related characteristics:

1. Feeling sad, being discouraged about the future, crying, irritability, thoughts of suicide
2. Feeling like a failure, loss of interest in activities, not being able to work
3. Sleep and appetite disturbance

This scale measures overall level of depression, and has also been found to have three subscales: negative attitudes/suicide, performance difficulty, and physiological manifestations.[85] Although the physiological and performance items in this scale (e.g., fatigue, sleep and appetite disturbance) may inflate depression scores for persons with physical illness, research has shown that these items discriminate among pain patients with and without depression.[35] Overall level of depression on this scale is associated with psychosocial functioning, and the specific somatic symptoms on this scale are associated with physical functioning.[40]

The total BDI score is rated in the following categories:

0–9 = minimal
10–16 = mild
17–29 = moderate
30–40 = severe
41–63 = extreme

Anxiety. The Beck Anxiety Inventory (BAI) is also a 21-item self-report instrument, with items scaled from 0 (not at all) to 3 (severe). This instrument asks clients to respond to questions about the following four mood-related characteristics:

1. Nervous, terrified, scared
2. Wobbly, shaky, unsteady, faint
3. Heart pounding, difficulty breathing, choking
4. Sweating, flushing, numbness, or tingling

This scale assesses overall level of anxiety, and has also been found to have four subscales: subjective (fearfulness), neurophysiological (unsteady and shaky), autonomic (e.g., flushing, sweating), and panic (e.g., heart pounding, choking). The BAI can be used with patients of all diagnoses.

The total BAI is rated in the following categories:

0–7 = minimal
8–15 = mild
16–25 = moderate
26–40 = severe
41–63 = extreme

There are also a number of pain-specific measures of fear and avoidance (e.g., Pain Anxiety Symptom Scale,[73] Fear and Avoidance Beliefs Questionnaire,[126] and Tampa Scale for Kinesiophobia[59]).

Distress. Verbal descriptor scales contain lists of adjectives that describe the characteristics of pain, ordered from low to high severity. The most commonly used of these, the McGill Pain Questionnaire, has 78 words grouped into 20 lists. Patients choose one word from each list that best describes their pain. This scale asks patients to describe the following three types of subjective pain characteristics:

1. Sensory (e.g., sore, pounding, sharp, burning)
2. Affective (e.g., sickening, punishing, killing)
3. Evaluative (i.e., mild to excruciating)

This scale has good reliability, validity, and sensitivity to change.[79] The affective descriptors from this scale can be used to evaluate the overall level of distress an individual reports regarding his or her pain.

Summary

Basic instruments: Beck Depression Inventory and Beck Anxiety Inventory.
Advanced instruments: McGill Pain Questionnaire, affective subscale.

Cognition: Attitudes and Beliefs

Concepts

Attitudes and beliefs are important in an individual's interpretation and understanding of sensory information and affective responses. Attitudes have to do with feelings about events (e.g., that one cannot possibly cope with adversity, or that one is "tough" and not to be deterred by an impairment, or that solicitous responses from others are appropriate). Beliefs have to do with information about events, such as understanding the cause of an impairment, its future course, and what treatments are appropriate. In addition, beliefs about self-efficacy, locus of control, and helplessness are critical because they have to do with the belief that one can achieve desired outcomes. These types of beliefs are related to the level of depression individuals experience and to the level of effort and/or persistence they will produce toward a goal.[19]

Attitudes and beliefs influence perceptions of experience. They influence the level of perceived demands through evaluations about what the level of demands "should be." They also influence the level of perceived resources through evaluations about personal capability and social support. Stress occurs when perceived demands exceed perceived resources.[61] Thus attitudes and beliefs influence the extent to which an individual perceives himself or herself as "not so bad off" or "very bad off," and are uniquely individual.

Attitudes and beliefs have been shown to correlate with adjustment to pain, including levels of disability associated with pain[48, 103] and with response to treatment.[13, 19, 104]

Attitudes and beliefs are different from active coping responses and other behaviors purposefully done to manage or lessen the negative consequences of stress.[46] These active coping behaviors are discussed in the next section.

Assessment

The Survey of Pain Attitudes (SOPA)[48] is the most widely used measure of pain-related attitudes. It is a 57-item self-report instrument, with each item rated on a scale ranging from 0 (not at all) to 4 (very much). The SOPA asks patients to respond to questions about the following seven attitudes:

1. Expect others to treat them with special concern because of their pain, and to make them feel better
2. Think emotional states such as depression and anxiety affect their pain
3. Expect a cure
4. Can influence or moderate their pain level
5. Think exercise is beneficial or dangerous
6. Think the pain is disabling
7. Think medication is the best treatment

The SOPA has been found to be associated with psychosocial functioning,[40, 48] levels of physical activity,[43] utilization of medical services,[44] and physical disability.[48] The main drawback of the SOPA is its length; it can be time consuming to administer and score. A brief version (30 items) has recently been developed that has good reliability and validity,[107] and in which all seven subscales are preserved. As yet, there are limited research data regarding this brief version.

The Pain Belief and Perceptions Inventory (PBPI)[131, 132] is a 16-item self-report instrument, with each item rated on a scale ranging from –2 (not at all true) to +2 (very true) (with no zero point). The PBPI asks patients to respond to questions about the following four beliefs:

1. Pain is confusing, of unknown origin, hard to understand (mystery)
2. Pain was caused by the client, is his or her fault (self-blame)
3. Pain is temporary or permanent, and whether client expects a cure (permanence)
4. Pain varies in intensity and frequency, or is constant and continuous (constancy)

These beliefs have been found to have important associations with other client factors: belief in pain constancy is associated with greater reported pain; permanence is associated with anxiety; mystery is associated with greatest overall distress; and self-blame is associated with depression.[132]

Summary

Basic instruments: SOPA, short form (30 items); PBPI.

Personality: Adjustment and Coping

Concepts

Personality is the spectrum of an individual's emotional and behavioral traits.[130] The characteristics and response patterns that express personality directly determine adjustment and coping and have strong influences on the relationship between impairment and disability. Some clients may have preexisting maladaptive personality traits, whereas others may have been functioning relatively well until the stress of injury and pain led to increased maladaptive responses.

Personality encompasses a broad range of psychological features. For purposes of this discussion, two categories will be considered. The first, adjustment, refers to the client's overall management of internal affective and cognitive states. The second, coping, refers to the client's overall management of external environmental conditions given available resources.

Adjustment. Overall psychological characteristics and response patterns, including specific psychological symptoms, reflect an individual's ability to achieve internal harmony among different affective and cognitive states. In assessing an individual's overall level of adjustment, the total number of reported symptoms are the clearest indicator. However, in addition there are a number of specific personality patterns and response styles that significantly influence impairment and disability.

Of the response styles relevant to pain, somatization is probably the one with greatest application. True somatization disorders are quite rare, with multiple unexplained and disabling physical complaints involving at least four pain symptoms from different sites, two gastrointestinal symptoms other than pain, one sexual symptom or dysfunction other than pain, and one pseudoneurologic symptom other than pain. True conversion disorders, with unexplained deficits in sensory functioning or voluntary motor control, are also quite rare, as are true hypochondriacal disorders, with disabling fears of having a serious disease based on misinterpretation of bodily symptoms, persisting despite appropriate medical evaluation and reassurance.

Unlike hypochondriacal and conversion disorders, undifferentiated somatoform disorders are more common, requiring only one unexplained and disabling physical complaint. However, this is potentially subject to over-diagnosis, and can be made in patients for whom objective diagnosis has yet to occur.[38] Thus when physicians examine patients with unexplained disabling pain, more is needed to make the diagnosis of undifferentiated somatoform disorder than the absence of objective evidence for the complaints. In particular, it is important to establish a persistent pattern of physical complaints, lasting at least 6 months, as well as significant psychosocial stressors relevant to the client.

However, many clients who do not meet the above criteria may still have characteristics and response patterns that result in psychological symptoms. Measurement of overall level of psychological symptoms can identify the overall level of adjustment.

Coping. Coping involves purposeful efforts to minimize or manage the effects of stressful situations or events.[46] Obviously, pain and impairment can be significant stressors. Individuals engage in a variety of coping behaviors in response to such stressors. The actions taken to cope with impairment and disability are important in determining functional abilities.

Coping behaviors generally are of two types: (1) actions taken to deal with the internal aspects of the stressful situation (i.e., affective management and regulation of stress-related tension and distress, and cognitive redefinition of the environmental demands and opportunities or of the individual's capacities and goals) and (2) actions taken to deal with the external aspects of the stressful situation (i.e., direct problem-solving actions).

Specific coping behaviors may be adaptive or maladaptive (i.e., they may lead to greater or lesser distress and/or disability).[29] Coping behaviors such as affective regulation and self-soothing, cognitive reinterpretation or diverting attention, and appropriate pacing and scheduling of activities can be important modifiers in reducing pain and disability. Inappropriate coping behaviors, such as blaming others for the impairment and for mistreatment, can lead to greater disability and interfere with treatment.[18] Clients with dysfunctional coping are likely to present with levels of disability that exceed available medical evidence, to exhibit perceptions of disability that exceed those of the examiner, and to blame the examiner for discrepancies between these perceptions.

Assessment

Adjustment. Simple structured reporting of psychological symptoms can be a useful means of identifying current problems. The Symptom Check List-90 (SCL-90) is a 90-item self-report instrument, in which individuals rate the degree to which they are distressed by symptoms on a 0 (not at all) to 4 (extremely) scale. These 90 items sum to a global distress index, and cluster into the following nine subscales:

1. Somatization
2. Obsessive-compulsive symptoms
3. Interpersonal sensitivity
4. Depression
5. Anxiety
6. Hostility
7. Phobia
8. Paranoid symptoms
9. Psychotic thinking

Although this instrument is designed to have a number of different subscales, with pain patients it appears to function as a single overall measure of severity of psychological symptoms.[7, 57] It is known to be sensitive to change in pain patients.[99, 127]

The PRIME-MD (Primary Care Evaluation of Mental Disorders) is a 26-item self-report instrument, in which individuals respond "yes" or "no" to questions about the following five types of symptoms:

1. Mood: sadness or anxiety
2. Panic
3. Somatoform: pain, dizziness, fainting, gastrointestinal upset, and worry about health
4. Alcohol-use disorders
5. Eating disorders

The PRIME-MD is structured to provide DSM-IV–related diagnoses of these five types of mental disorders. There are two parts to this evaluation: a client self-report questionnaire regarding symptoms and signs within the past month, and a clinician evaluation to follow up on clients' positive self-reports. The identification of these specific mental-health disorders by the PRIME-MD has been found to be equivalent with identification by mental-health professionals and has been found to be associated with functional impairment and health-care utilization.[100–102]

More detailed and structured assessment of psychological characteristics can add greater precision in identifying less obvious symptoms and response styles and can control for reporting bias (under-reporting, over-reporting, social desirability). The Minnesota Multiphasic Personality Inventory-2 (MMPI-2) is the most widely used personality inventory. Its main disadvantage is its length

(567 items), so it requires considerable time for the client to complete and the examiner to interpret. Clients are asked yes/no questions regarding their interests and enjoyments, moods and thoughts, attitudes and beliefs about self and others, and physical sensations and experiences.

One advantage of this scale is that it assesses validity and response bias in a number of different ways. Another advantage is its established use with pain patients. Four factors identified with pain patients include psychological dysfunction, interpersonal isolation, psychomotor retardation, and physical dysfunction.[17] These factors have been found to be related to health-care utilization and function.[10, 76] It also shows sensitivity to change with reductions in pain,[4, 26, 34, 84] indicating that this measure is sensitive to the current situation. Finally, because it is widely used, the MMPI-2 is readily accepted in medico-legal settings, such as those involved in disability determinations.[122]

Coping. The most widely studied measure of individual coping behaviors is the Coping Strategies Questionnaire (CSQ).[96] It was originally a 50-item self-report instrument, designed to have seven rationally derived subscales regarding coping behaviors and several items regarding efficacy of coping. However, two large factor-analytic studies have identified 27 items that load reliably on the following six factors:

1. **Distraction:** think of something else, do something else pleasant
2. **Catastrophizing:** feel it's awful and overwhelming, worry all the time, can't stand it
3. **Ignoring:** don't think about it, don't pay attention
4. **Distancing:** try to feel distant from the pain, pretend it's not part of me
5. **Coping self-statements:** tell myself I can overcome the pain, tell myself I can't let it stand in the way
6. **Prayer:** pray for the pain to stop, rely on faith in God

Studies have shown that individuals who catastrophize and feel helpless tend to be more disabled and depressed. However, use of distraction, distancing, and praying is also associated with high levels of pain and disability.[52] Although a number of coping activities have been associated with poor adjustment, unfortunately none have been associated with good adjustment.

Additional factor-analytic studies of the CSQ have identified two higher-order factors: active coping versus passive coping. Active coping has to do with distraction, ignoring, coping self-statements, and distancing, and is related to better outcomes. Passive coping has to do with catastrophizing and praying, and is related to poorer outcomes.[11, 39] The dimensions of active and passive coping have also been assessed with the Vanderbilt Pain Management Inventory.[12] Hence the disability examiner may want to be sensitive to these general coping styles (active versus passive) in assessing whether the client is coping with pain and impairment in ways likely to minimize or magnify pain-related disability.

The West Haven-Yale Multidimensional Pain Inventory (WHYMPI)[56, 98] is a 52-item self-report instrument, with each item rated on a scale from 0 (not at all) to 6 (very much). This instrument asks questions about the following four factors:

1. **Activity interference:** pain interferes with activities, work, satisfaction, relationships
2. **Social support:** spouse or significant other is supportive or worried
3. **Pain intensity**

4. **Emotional distress:** suffering, able to deal with problems, irritable, or anxious

The utility of this instrument is that these subscales can be jointly considered to determine one of three general response styles: dysfunctional coping, interpersonally distressed, and adaptive coping.[118, 119] These response styles have been shown to be correlated with use of medication, physician visits, number of hospitalizations, work, and sleep disturbance.[42] Again, the disability examiner should be sensitive to these general response styles to evaluate whether the client is likely to minimize or magnify the functional impact of pain.

Summary

Basic instruments: SCL-90, PRIME-MD.
Advanced instruments: MMPI-2, CSQ, WHYMPI, family response style.

Motivation: Satisfaction, Secondary Gain, Factitious Disorders, and Malingering

Concepts

Satisfaction. The extent to which individuals enjoy their work, as well as other aspects of their lives, is an important factor in the development of illness symptoms and behavior. Work dissatisfaction has been found to be associated with psychological strains such as boredom, irritation, and low self-esteem, with physical symptoms of strain such as increased blood pressure, serum cholesterol, and gastric acidity, and with behavioral symptoms of strain such as increased smoking and absenteeism.[87] Bigos et al.[9] found job satisfaction to be an important predictor of subsequent industrial back-pain injury claims, even after controlling for previous back problems and other psychological factors. A single question regarding whether workers enjoy what they do provided significant predictive power for subsequent injury claims.

Secondary gain. *Secondary gain* is a term much used in the clinical discussion of impairment and disability. This has been defined as having both legitimate and illegitimate aspects, for example, as "acceptable or legitimate interpersonal advantages that result when one has the symptom of a physical disease"[5] and "the gain achieved from a conversion symptom in avoiding a particular activity that was noxious to the patient and/or in enabling the patient to get support from the environment that might not be otherwise forthcoming."[2]

Although secondary gain is well recognized, it is critical to acknowledge that physical and/or mental disorders also carry secondary losses. Although some individuals may find that being dysfunctional provides some secondary benefits, almost all individuals with dysfunction also have significant secondary losses, such as financial problems, social isolation, etc. These losses tend to increase as pain and impairment persist, adding further to the psychosocial components of disability and maintaining a "sick role."[88]

In regard to issues about possible gain caused by disability, there is a long history of opinions stating that disability is often increased by possible compensation for impairment. Although some authors have stated that symptoms are usually resolved after successful litigation or compensation,[55, 83] there is considerable evidence that this view is inaccurate. In regard to chronic pain, for example, patients' symptoms do not resolve on resolution of litigation, and such individuals remain with significant disabling symptoms over the course of their lives.[81, 82] In addition, symptoms of pain and distress are not different for patients who have compensable versus noncompensable injuries, although levels of disability are higher for patients with compensable injuries, and treatment outcomes often are poorer.[36, 62, 80, 89, 111] Therefore compensation status appears to contribute to level of disability, and through channels other than magnification of symptoms.[32]

In addition to environmental contingencies related to job satisfaction or receipt of benefits, behaviors related to impairment itself are subject to modification by environmental contingencies. For example, solicitous reactions to pain behavior are known to increase the frequency of these behaviors.[105] Punishing reactions to pain behaviors are known to decrease their frequency, although punishing responses also increase interpersonal conflict and overall affective distress.[69] To some extent, disability can become a conditioned response, serving to avoid undesirable activities, maintain self-esteem (by displacing the responsibility for failure to perform on the impairment), exert control over others, gain special considerations, or satisfy socially unacceptable needs (e.g., extreme dependency).[33]

Factitious disorders and malingering. Both factitious disorders and malingering involve the intentional production or feigning of physical or psychological signs or symptoms. *Factitious disorder* is defined as the intentional production of symptoms to assume the sick role when obvious external incentives (e.g., money) are not evident. *Malingering* is defined as the intentional production of symptoms motivated by external incentives. This is a fine distinction, which often cannot be determined by a physician in an office visit. In fact, the determination of these "diagnoses" often can only be accomplished with outside evidence (e.g., that provided by private investigators). Physician evaluators must be aware that they will meet some clients whose presentation is consciously and deliberately deceptive. However, this does not describe the majority of individuals presenting for evaluation.

Assessment

Satisfaction. Job satisfaction is a critical psychological modifier between impairment and disability. The wish to return to or avoid one's job acts as an important behavior modifier. Assessment of job satisfaction through interview can be done using questions such as the following:

- Do you enjoy your job?
- Do you miss working?
- Do you feel you have been treated fairly by your employer?
- Would you return to your job if you were able?

Alternatively, job satisfaction has been assessed in the modified Work Apgar, an instrument that has been correlated with return-to-work.[9] This is a 7-item self-report instrument, with each item scaled on a 3-point scale from "almost always" to "hardly ever." This instrument asks patients to respond to questions about the following:

1. Emotional support from co-workers
2. Acceptance from co-workers
3. Enjoyment of job tasks
4. Relationship with supervisor

Secondary gain. The identification of subtypes of family responses to individuals with impairment can help in understanding the reinforcement contingencies under which client behaviors operate. Family members may respond with greater or lesser amounts of solicitousness, anger and impatience, or withdrawal and ignoring. The WHYMPI asks questions about the following additional significant behaviors:

- **Solicitousness:** tries to help, takes over duties, gets pain medication
- **Punishment:** ignores, gets angry or frustrated
- **Distraction:** reads or talks to the individual, tries to involve him or her in an activity

Factitious disorders and malingering. Although additional outside evidence may be necessary for identification of factitious disorder or malingering, there are a number of physician-observable behaviors that are suggestive of these diagnoses, including proven exaggeration of symptoms, invariable relapse after improvement, self-manipulated worsening of condition, resisting communication with prior health-care providers, poor continuity of care, and lack of cooperation during diagnostic evaluation or with treatment regimen.[28]

Summary

Basic instruments: Work Apgar, questions regarding satisfaction with treatment and expectations for compensation.

Advanced instruments: WHYMPI, family response style.

ASSESSMENT OF SOCIAL HISTORY AND PRESENT CIRCUMSTANCES

There are a number of social factors that act as important modifiers of disability. The examiner will want to assess both historical and current factors.

Concepts

History. Sexual and/or physical abuse are known to be more frequent in patients reporting chronic pain, and are known to have negative effects. The rates of reported sexual and/or physical abuse among chronic-pain patients, ranging from 25% to 65%, is two to five times higher than in the general population. A history of abuse is associated with increased health-care utilization (especially emergency room visits), emotional distress, and poor coping.[116] No other historical conditions have been identified as having consistent relationships with impairment or disability.

Present circumstances. Stress occurs in situations in which perceived demands exceed perceived resources, such that the individual experiences an inability to meet the demands. Stress can occur in several areas.

Job stress has been shown to be a significant factor in the occurrence of both physical and psychological disorders. Work stressors include underutilization of skills and abilities, machine-paced and/or simple and repetitive work, low participation in decisions affecting one's work, job insecurity, and poor social support at work.[87]

Similar effects are likely to occur with family/marital stress, although the nature of these stressors, as noted previously, is different.[69]

In addition to job or family stress, there are stresses associated with impairment and job disability. It is known that involuntary job loss results in increased depression, anxiety, blood pressure, serum cholesterol, and norepinephrine levels.[15] Demotions have been found to be related to increased diagnosed illness.[50] Other unfavorable or loss events (not just occupational) have been found to be associated with physical illness, depression, cardiac disease, and accidents.[23, 91, 123] Involuntary and unanticipated changes in roles caused by impairment result in shifts in norms, obligations, and responsibilities among family members, and also result in significant stress.[97]

Assessment

History. The Sexual-Physical Abuse History Questionnaire[25] is a 12-item self-report instrument in which clients respond to six yes/no items, four 4-point ("never" to "often") items, and two items regarding whether these events have been discussed with others or whether help has been sought. It has been found to be acceptable to patients and to have good reliability and validity.[63] This scale asks whether anyone has ever done any of the following to the client:

- Exposed his or her sex organs to the client
- Touched the client's sex organs when he or she did not want them to
- Forced the client to have sex
- Insulted and humiliated the client
- Hit, kicked, or beat the client

Present circumstances. Although we do not recommend specific measurement scales here, clinicians should inquire regarding a number of potential life stressors that may be complicating the client's situation, including the following:

- Job stress, including underutilization of skills and abilities, machine-paced and/or simple and repetitive work, low participation in decisions affecting one's work, job insecurity or demotions, and poor social support at work
- Family and marital stress, including involuntary and unanticipated changes in roles
- The overall levels of perceived demands, rewards, and abilities (overall perceived "balance sheet" for the individual)

Summary

Basic instruments: Sexual-Physical Abuse History Questionnaire, clinical questions regarding general stressors.

ASSESSMENT OF BEHAVIORAL FACTORS

There are a number of behavioral factors that mediate the relationship between impairment and disability, including the following:

1. **Social communication behaviors:** communicative expressions to others regarding the state of the individual
2. **Function:** specific levels and types of disability

Social Communication Behaviors

Concepts

Clients enact two forms of social communication behavior: they report their experience and they demonstrate their experience. One of the important ways they report their experience is through reports of pain intensity, quality, and distribution. One of the important ways they demonstrate their experience is through vocal, verbal, and physical behaviors. In this section, reports and demonstrations regarding impairment will be considered. Reports and demonstrations of disability will be considered in the next section.

Client reports. Client-reported symptom intensity, frequency, and distribution is a fundamental aspect of client-physician interaction. These factors have been studied most when impairment is predominantly reported as pain. Clients report intensity of pain, as well as its location and frequency.

Vocal and physical demonstrations. Clients also demonstrate information regarding their condition. Such behaviors include facial expressions, nonverbal vocalizations, physical actions, behavioral actions, and social actions. These behaviors have been found to be related to verbal descriptors and function.[54, 95]

Assessment

Client reports. Pain intensity has been examined in a number of ways. The most common are visual analog scales (VAS) and numeric rating scales (NRS). VAS assessment involves the client marking a point on a line, usually anchored by "no pain" and "pain as bad as it can be." The distance along the line can be measured to gauge pain intensity. NRS involve choosing a number on a scale anchored by 0 (no pain) and 10 (pain as bad as it can be). VAS, NRS, and other measurement scales have been shown to be valid, reliable, and sensitive to change.[44]

An important question with measurement of pain intensity regards the number of gradations that result in the best instrument performance. Measurement of pain intensity has been examined using instruments with as little as 4 or as many as 101 gradations. Clients appear unable to conceptualize greater than 20 gradations, and less than 10 gradations results in loss of information.[47, 66] The authors recommend using a "1–10" scale because it is familiar and allows easy comparison with the research literature.

In addition to general pain intensity, variability in pain should be assessed. It is the experience of the authors that the evaluator should ask a sequence of questions as follows:

- What is the worst your pain has been in the past 2 weeks?
- What is the least your pain has been in the past 2 weeks?
- What is the average your pain has been in the past 2 weeks?

This first question allows clients to communicate their distress. The second question is important in evaluating clients' tendency to over-report symptoms, because all types of pain would be expected to have some variation in intensity. Clients who report their worst pain and least pain as nearly identical may be over-reporting. The third question allows clients to give a report of pain after having removed the need to communicate how bad it gets sometimes. As compared with daily diary recording, "least" and "usual" pain are most highly correlated with actual average level of pain ($r = .81$ and $r = .78$, respectively).[49] In general, the examiner can most accurately assess pain intensity by averaging the client's estimates of least and usual pain.

The sensory subscale of the McGill Pain Questionnaire[77, 78] can also be used to generate a pain intensity severity indicator, the Pain Rating Index, by adding the ranks of the selected descriptors. This 32-item sensory subset of the McGill Pain Questionnaire has been found to have good statistical properties.[117]

In addition to pain intensity, pain distribution drawings are a quick means of collecting data regarding location and extent of pain, and can be used to quantify this type of information. Such assessment provides information different from that provided by intensity measures, and allows reliable identification of the anatomical distributions of pain, weakness, and numbness. The total percentage of painful body surface is a method of summarizing pain drawings that has good reliability and validity.[68, 70, 110, 115] Additional interpretation of pain drawings has been proposed, such as the "penalty-point" system developed by Ransford, Cairns & Mooney,[92] which assigns points to drawing elements thought to reflect psychological involvement (e.g., markings outside the body outline, nondermatomal distributions). However, these penalty points are highly correlated with simple measures of pain extent,[70] and do not appear to add additional information.

Vocal and physical demonstrations. Demonstrated pain behaviors include the following:

- Facial expressions (grimace, furrowed brow, squinting, pursed lips)
- Nonverbal vocalizations (moans, groans, gasps, sighs)
- Physical actions (rubbing, guarding, bracing, limping, position shifts)

These can be coded for grimacing, sighing, rubbing, guarding, and bracing.[51, 53] This measure has significant correlations with self-reported pain, function and depression,[95] with guarding having the strongest association.

The University of Alabama Pain Behavior Rating Scale[93] is an observational record of patients' behavior, and includes 10 subscales, including verbal complaints, vocal complaints, down-time, grimacing, standing posture, mobility, body language, use of supportive equipment, stationary movement, and medication use. Items separate into two factors: facial/audible, and motor.[93] The scale has been found to be associated with disability and functional capacity.[30, 109]

Summary

Basic instruments:

- Numeric rating scale
  - Ask for pain intensity on "1-10" scale
  - Ask for worst, least, average pain during last 2 weeks
- Visual analog scale
  - Use with patients who have hearing/speech impairment
- Pain diagrams
  - Compute percentage of painful body surface
- Observed Pain Behaviors
  - Grimacing, sighing, rubbing, guarding, and bracing

Advanced instruments: University of Alabama Pain Behavior Rating Scale.

Function

Concepts

Disability has been defined in terms of both limitation of function and limitation of role performance. Limitation of function can be assessed in relation to the function of other individuals of the same age and gender[124]. However, this fails to account for differences in previous and expected function. Therefore limitation of usual role performance has been proposed as more relevant to measuring disability in any particular individual. The Institute of Medicine[41] has proposed the following definition of disability: "A disadvantage for an individual (resulting from an impairment or functional limitation) that limits or prevents the fulfillment of a role that is normal for that individual."

Unfortunately, impairment (based on objective medical evidence) and disability (based on limitations in role performance) correlate poorly.[1] Thus the rating physician can face a dilemma in which relatively little impairment is associated with considerable disability. The challenge for the physician is to accurately quantify those role limitations that arise from physical versus psychological, social, or behavioral factors and to recommend either psychological treatment or, if thought to be at MMI, psychological disability evaluation.

Assessment

Client reports of functional abilities and the effects of impairments on function can be objectified through use of standardized reporting scales. In addition, such scales allow comparison across impairment types, such as individuals with arthritis, limb loss, and chronic pain, to evaluate client function in relation to others with similar or dissimilar conditions.

The Medical Outcomes Study Short Form-36 (SF-36)[129] contains 36 items regarding eight areas of functioning:

1. Physical function
2. Physical role function
3. Emotional role function
4. Pain
5. Social function
6. Mental health
7. Energy
8. General health perceptions

Responses are either yes/no, or on a six-point scale. These eight areas collapse into three factors: functional status, perceived well-being, and overall health.

The SF-36 has been shown to be useful in assessing pain patients.[60, 86] It allows comparison with a number of other disability groups, and thus could be used to compare the functional level of a specific client with other individuals with similar diagnoses.[128] However, because it assesses overall function, it may be affected by a wide variety of medical problems.

The Sickness Impact Profile (SIP) is the most widely used measure of functional status in individuals with impairment or illness.[6] It is composed of 136 yes/no items asking about the impact of health problems on 12 areas of functioning. This scale asks questions about ability to function in areas such as:

- Ambulation, mobility, body care, and movement
- Social interaction and communication
- Emotional behavior
- Sleep and eating
- Work and home management
- Recreation and leisure activities

These 12 areas can be aggregated into three factors: physical, psychosocial, and total (physical plus psychosocial plus additional items related to instrumental activities of daily living). It is known to be valid and sensitive to change.[21, 22, 64, 65, 67] The Roland Disability Scale is a 24-item instrument derived from the SIP and focuses only on physical function. It has been shown to have good reliability and validity and to be a sensitive measure of function.[8, 20, 45]

Summary

Basic instruments: Roland Disability Questionnaire and Medical Outcomes Study Short Form-36.
Advanced instruments: Sickness Impact Profile.

PSYCHOLOGICAL ASSESSMENT DURING PHYSIATRIC EXAMINATION

Physicians can incorporate assessment of many of these important psychological, social, and behavioral factors into routine examination. Although assessment using the instruments described earlier can be performed, many of the important factors discussed can also be incorporated through use of some basic questions.

Mood

- Do you feel sad?
- Do you cry?
- Do you feel like giving up?
- Have you lost interest in usual activities?
- Is there anything that makes you smile or laugh?
- Do you feel worried and nervous?
- Do you ever feel like you're in a panic?
- Do you have times when your body becomes tense, your heart pounds, your hands sweat, etc.?

Cognition

- What do you understand about the cause of your symptoms?
- What do you think the best treatment is?
- How do you think these symptoms affect your functional abilities?
- Do you think you can cope successfully with this problem?
- What do you think the future will bring for you?

Motivation

- Do you enjoy your job?
- Do you miss working?
- Did your employer treat you fairly?
- Would you go back to work if you could?
- How does your family react to your problems?
  - Do they: get irritated or mad
    - try to help or protect
    - try to distract you
- Are you generally happy at home?
- What do you miss most that you can't do now?

Social history and present circumstances

- Have you ever been forced to have any type of sexual activity you did not want?
- Has anyone ever physically hit, kicked or beat you?
- Has anyone ever repeatedly insulted and shamed you?
- How much stress do you have at work?
- How much stress do you have at home?
- Do you have people to count on if you need help?

Communication

- Tell me how strong your pain has been during the last 2 weeks on a scale of

0–10, with 0 being no pain, and 10 being the worst pain any human being could ever have
What is the worst it has been in the past 2 weeks?
What is the least it has been in the past 2 weeks?
What has been your average pain in the past 2 weeks?
Where is the pain (diagram)?
What activities are you unable to do at all that you used to do?
What activities are you limited in that you used to do?

These questions do not require use of specific psychological measurement instruments, but do allow the physician to identify the major psychological, social, and behavioral factors involved in the client's situation. Concerns raised during this questioning may lead to referral for more detailed psychological assessment.

PREEXISTING VERSUS IMPAIRMENT-RELATED PSYCHOLOGICAL FACTORS

It is important to differentiate preexisting from impairment-related psychological factors. There are a number of psychological problems that arise as a result of pain and impairment and decrease when pain and impairment decrease. Again considering pain as a prototype for other impairment conditions, depression is more commonly seen in patients with chronic pain than in the general population.[3, 27, 120] There has been evidence to support both a pain-to-depression effect, as well as a depression-to-pain effect, although predisposition to depression is more likely to result in pain-related depression.[31]

PHYSICIAN JUDGMENT FACTORS

Physicians performing impairment ratings and disability evaluations operate in an inherently "noisy" environment, with data that are seldom fully quantifiable. They must integrate physical evidence with the assessment of psychological and environmental factors, which is a conceptually complex task with considerable ambiguity. They must do this in the context of a diagnostic interview and physical examination, which is an interactive, interpersonal task in which a client's self-presentation can influence judgments. In addition, physician evaluators themselves bring beliefs and attitudes to the setting.

It is important that physicians who operate in such contexts be aware of factors that may affect their judgments. For example, studies have shown that health-care providers are likely to underestimate pain intensity for individuals who report high levels of pain,[113, 121] who are older[16, 72] who are non-white,[74, 114] and who are female.[75] In addition, observers underestimate the pain of patients with emotional distress or other life stresses[106, 108] Chronic pain tends to be a problem that is viewed negatively by physicians, which is another factor that can be related to underestimation of symptom intensity.[58, 112] On the other hand, some factors lead to overestimation of symptoms, including the presence of medical evidence consistent with reported symptoms.[14] Thus the disability examining physician should be aware of a range of contextual factors that may operate to influence his or her judgments.

CONCLUSIONS

Impairment ratings and disability evaluations are complex activities, with considerable variation between objectively measured impairments and subjectively reported disabilities. Disability is related to impairment, but is also subject to modulation by numerous other psychological, social, and behavioral factors. Understanding these nonmedical factors that influence disability can help identify the causal linkages involved between impairment and disability and can aid in evaluation and treatment.

It is our contention that most clients have some nonmedical contribution to their presentation of impairment and disability. It is our hope that through improved evaluation of psychological, social, and behavioral factors, clients may be more accurately assessed, more effectively treated when indicated, and enabled to achieve their highest functional potential.

The strength of the contribution of psychological, social, and behavioral factors to a client's presentation during evaluation ranges from mild to severe. Assessment of these factors can help to answer two questions:

1. Is the client at MMI or are there psychological, social, or behavioral factors contributing to disability that should be treated (should a final disability rating be postponed)?
2. Given appropriate treatment, are there remaining psychological, social, or behavioral contributions to disability of such magnitude that a separate estimate of psychological disability should be conducted?

This chapter has provided an organizational and measurement structure for standardized psychological, social, and behavioral assessment of clients with musculoskeletal complaints. Physicians should be aware of the conceptual complexity, ambiguity and imprecision of available data, and of the client and physician characteristics that influence judgments about these symptoms and symptom-related disability. We hope that through increased awareness of these complex psychosocial factors, accuracy of judgment can be increased.

REFERENCES

1. Allen D, Waddell G: An historical perspective on low back pain and disability. Acta Orthop Scand 60(S234):1, 1989.
2. American Medical Association: Diagnostic and Statistical Manual of Mental Disorders, 3rd ed rev. Washington, DC, American Psychiatric Association, 1987.
3. Banks M, Kerns R: Explaining high rates of depression in chronic pain: a diathesis-stress framework. Psychol Bull 119:95, 1996.
4. Barnes D, Gatchel R, Mayer T, et al: Changes in MMPI profiles of chronic low back pain patients following successful treatment. J Spinal Disord 3:353, 1990.
5. Barsky A, Klerman G: Overview: hypochondriasis, bodily complaints, and somatic styles. Am J Psychiatry 140:273, 1983.
6. Bergner M, Bobbitt R, Carter W, et al: The Sickness Impact Profile: development and final revision of a health status measure. Med Care 19:787, 1981.
7. Bernstein I, Jaremko M, Hinkley B: On the utility of the SCL-(90)-R with low-back pain patients. Spine 19:42, 1994.
8. Beurskens A, deVet H, Koke A: Responsiveness of functional status in low back pain: a comparison of different instruments. Pain 65:71, 1996.

9. Bigos S, Battie M, Spengler D, et al: A prospective study of work perceptions and psychosocial factors affecting the report of back injury. Spine 16:1, 1991.
10. Bradley L, Van der Heide L: Pain-related correlates of MMPI profile subgroups among back pain patients. Health Psychol 3:157, 1984.
11. Broome M, Bates T, Lillis P, et al: Children's medical fears, coping behaviors, and pain perceptions during a lumbar puncture. Ontology Nurs Soc 17:361, 1990.
12. Brown G, Nicassio P: Development of a questionnaire for the assessment of active and passive coping strategies in chronic pain patients. Pain 31:53, 1987.
13. Carosella A, Lackner J, Feuerstein M: Factors associated with early discharge from a multidisciplinary work rehabilitation program for chronic low back pain. Pain 57:59, 1994.
14. Chibnall J, Tait R: Observer perceptions of low back pain: effects of pain report and other contextual factors. J Applied Soc Psych 25:418, 1995.
15. Cobb S, Kasl S: Termination: the consequences of job loss. (Pub No. 77-224). Cincinnati, US Dept of Health, Education, and Welfare, National Institute for Occupational Safety and Health, 1977.
16. Davits L, Pendleton S: Nurses' inferences of suffering. Nurs Res 18:100, 1969.
17. Deardorff W, Chino A, Scott D: Characteristics of chronic pain patients: factor analysis of the MMPI-2. Pain 54:153, 1993.
18. DeGood D, Kiernan B: Perception of fault in patients with chronic pain. Pain 64(1):153, 1996.
19. DeGood D, Shutty M Jr: Assessment of pain beliefs, coping and self-efficacy. In: Turk D, Melzack R (eds): Handbook of Pain Assessment. New York, The Guilford Press, 1992, p 214.
20. Deyo R: Comparative validity of the Sickness Impact Profile and shorter scales for functional assessment in low-back pain. Spine 11(9):951, 1986.
21. Deyo R: The early diagnostic evaluation of patients with low-back pain. J Gen Intern Med 1:328, 1986.
22. Deyo R, Centor R: Assessing the responsiveness of functional scales to clinical change: an analogy to diagnostic test performance. J Chronic Dis 39:897, 1986.
23. Dohrenwend BS, Dohrenwend BP (eds): Stressful life events: their nature and effect. New York, John Wiley and Sons, 1974.
24. Dougher M: Sensory decision theory analysis of the effects of anxiety and experimental instructions on pain. J Abnormal Psychol 88(2):137, 1979.
25. Drossman D, Leserman J, Nachman G, et al: Sexual and physical abuse in women with functional or organic gastrointestinal disorders. Ann Intern Med 113:828, 1990.
26. Dvorak J, Valach L, Fuhrimann P, et al: The outcome of surgery for lumbar disc herniation II: a 4–17 years' follow-up with emphasis on treatment response in chronic pain. Spine 13:1423, 1988.
27. Dworkin R: What do we really know about the psychological origins of chronic pain? Am Pain Soc Bull Oct:7, 1991.
28. Eisendrath S: Psychiatric aspects of chronic pain. Neurology 45(suppl 9):S26, 1995.
29. Fernandez E, Turk D: The utility of cognitive coping strategies for altering pain perception: a meta-analysis. Pain 38:123, 1989.
30. Fishbain D, Abdel-Moty E, Cutler R, et al: Measuring residual functional capacity in chronic low back pain patients based on the Dictionary of Occupational Titles. Spine 19:872, 1994.
31. Fishbain D, Cutler R, Rosomoff H, et al: Chronic pain-associated depression: antecedent or consequence of chronic pain? A review. Clin J Pain 13:116, 1997.
32. Fishbain D, Rosomoff H, Cutler R, et al: Secondary gain concept: a review of the scientific evidence. Clin J Pain 11:6, 1995.
33. Fordyce W, Fowler R Jr., Lehmann J, et al: Operant conditioning in the treatment of chronic pain. Arch Phys Med Rehabil 54:399, 1973.

34. Gatchel R, Mayer T, Capra P, et al: Quantification of lumbar function. Part IV. The use of psychological measures in guiding physical functional restoration. Spine 11:36, 1986.
35. Geisser M, Roth R, Robinson M: Assessing depression among persons with chronic pain using the Center for Epidemiological Studies Depression Scale and the Beck Depression Inventory: a comparative analysis. Clin J Pain 13:163, 1997.
36. Guest G, Drummond P: Effect of compensation on emotional state and disability in chronic back pain. Pain 48:125, 1992.
37. Hendler N: Diagnosis and nonsurgical management of chronic pain. New York, Raven Press, 1981.
38. Hendler N, Bergson C, Morrison C: Overlooked physical diagnoses in chronic pain patients involved in litigation. Part 2. The addition of MRI, nerve blocks, 3-D CT, and qualitative flow meter. Psychomatics 37:509, 1996.
39. Holmes J, Stevenson C: Differential effects of avoidant and attentional coping strategies on adaptation to chronic and recent-onset pain. Health Psychol 9:577, 1990.
40. Holzberg A, Robinson M, Geisser M, et al: The effects of depression and chronic pain on psychosocial and physical functioning. Clin J Pain 12:118, 1996.
41. Institute of Medicine Committee on Pain, Disability, and Chronic Illness Behavior, Os M, Kleinman A, Mechanic D (eds): Pain and disability: clinical, behavioral, and public policy perspectives. Washington, DC, National Academy Press, 1987.
42. Jamison R, Rudy T, Penzien D, et al: Cognitive-behavioral classifications of chronic pain: replication and extension of empirically derived patient profiles. Pain 57:277, 1994.
43. Jensen M, Karoly P: Control beliefs, coping efforts, and adjustment to chronic pain. J Consult Clin Psychol 59:431, 1991.
44. Jensen M, Karoly P: Pain-specific beliefs, perceived symptom severity, and adjustment to chronic pain. Clin J Pain 8:123, 1992.
45. Jensen M, Strom S, Turner J, et al: Validity of the Sickness Impact Profile Roland scale as a measure of dysfunction in chronic pain patients. Pain 50:157, 1992.
46. Jensen M, Turner J, Romano J: Self-efficacy and outcome expectancies: relationship to chronic pain coping strategies and adjustment. Pain 44:263, 1991.
47. Jensen M, Turner J, Romano J: Correlates of improvement in multidisciplinary treatment of chronic pain. J Consult Clin Psychol 62:172, 1994.
48. Jensen M, Turner J, Romano J, et al: Relationship of pain-specific beliefs to chronic pain adjustment. Pain 57:301, 1994.
49. Jensen M, Turner L, Turner J, et al: The use of multiple-item scales for pain intensity measurement in chronic pain patients. Pain 67:35, 1996.
50. Kasl S, French J Jr: The effects of occupational status on physical and mental health. J Soc Issues 18:67, 1962.
51. Keefe E, Block A: Development of an observational method for assessing pain behavior in chronic low back pain patients. Behav Ther 13:636, 1982.
52. Keefe E, Brown G, Wallston K, et al: Coping with rheumatoid arthritis pain: catastrophizing as a maladaptive strategy. Pain 37:51, 1989.
53. Keefe E, Crisson J, Trainor M: Observational methods for assessing pain: a practical guide. In: Blumenthal J, McKee D (eds): Applications in Behavioral Medicine and Health Psychology: A Clinician's Source Book, Sarasota, Fla, Professional Resources Exchange, 1987, p 67.
54. Keefe F, Williams D: Assessment of pain behaviors. In: Turk D, Melzack R (eds): Handbook of Pain Assessment. New York, The Guilford Press, 1992.
55. Kennedy F: The mind of the injured worker: its effect on disability periods. Comp Med 1:19, 1946.
56. Kerns R, Turk D, Rudy T: The West Haven-Yale multidimensional pain inventory. Pain 23:345, 1985.

57. Kinney R, Gatchel R, Mayer T: The SCL-90-R evaluated as an alternative to the MMPI for psychological screening of chronic low-back pain patients. Spine 16: 940, 1991.
58. Klein D, Najman J, Kohrman A, et al: Patient characteristics that elicit negative responses from family physicians. J Fam Pract 14:881, 1982.
59. Kori S, Miller R, Todd D: Kinesiophobia: a new view of chronic pain behavior. Pain Mgt 35–43, 1990.
60. Lansky D, Butler J, Waller F: Using health status measures in the hospital stetting: from acute care to "outcomes management." Med Care 30:57, 1992.
61. Lazarus R, Folkman S: Stress, Appraisal, and Coping. New York, Springer, 1984.
62. Leavitt F, Garron D, McNeill T, et al: Organic status, psychological disturbance, and pain report characteristics in low back pain patients on compensation. Spine 7:398, 1982.
63. Lesserman J, Drossman D, Li Z: The reliability and validity of a sexual and physical abuse history questionnaire among women patients with gastrointestinal disorders. Behav Med 59(2): 152, 1997.
64. Liang M, Larson M, Cullen K, et al: Comparative measurement efficiency and sensitivity of five health status instruments for arthritis research. Arthritis Rheum 28:542, 1985.
65. Liang M, Fossel A, Larson M: Comparisons of five health status instruments for orthopedic evaluation. Med Care 28:632, 1990.
66. Machin D, Lewith G, Wylson S: Pain measurement in randomized clinical trials: a comparison of two pain scales. Clin J Pain 4:161, 1988.
67. MacKenzie C, Charlson M, DiGioia D, et al: Can the sickness impact profile measures change? An example of scale assessment. J Chronic Dis 39:429, 1988.
68. Margolis R, Chibnall J, Tait R: Test-retest reliability of the pain drawing instrument. Pain 33:49, 1988.
69. Margolis R, Merkel W, Tait R, Richardson W: Evaluating patients with chronic pain and their families. Can Fam Physician 37:429, 1991.
70. Margolis R, Tait R, Krause S: A rating system for use with patient pain drawings. Pain 24:57, 1986.
71. Max M, Ksihore-Kumar R, Schafer S, et al: Efficacy of desipramine in painful diabetic neuropathy: a placebo-controlled trial. Pain 45:3, 1991.
72. McCaffrey M, Ferrell B: Patient age: does it affect your pain-control decisions? Nursing '91 21:44, 1991.
73. McCracken L, Zayfert C, Gross R: The Pain Anxiety Symptom Scale: development and validation of a scale to measure fear of pain. Pain 50:67, 1992.
74. McDonald D: Gender and ethnic stereotyping and narcotic analgesic administration. Res Nurs Health 17:45, 1994.
75. McDonald D, Bridge R: Gender stereotyping and nursing care. Res Nurs Health 14:373, 1991.
76. McGill J, Lawlis G, Selby D, et al: The relationship of MMPI profile clusters to pain behaviors. J Behav Med 6:77, 1983.
77. Melzack R: The McGill pain questionnaire: major properties and scoring methods. Pain 1:277, 1975.
78. Melzack R (ed): Pain Measurement and Assessment. New York, Raven Press, 1983.
79. Melzack R, Katz J: The McGill Pain Questionnaire: appraisal and current status. In: Turk D, Melzack R (eds): Handbook of Pain Assessment, New York, The Guilford Press, 1992, p. 152.
80. Melzack R, Katz J, Jeans M: The role of compensation in chronic pain: analysis using a new method of scoring the McGill Pain Questionnaire. Pain 23:101, 1985.
81. Mendelson G: Compensation, pain complaints, and psychological disturbance. Pain 20:169, 1984.

82. Mendelson G: Compensation and chronic pain. Pain 48:121, 1992.
83. Miller H: Accident neurosis. Br Med J 1:919, 1961.
84. Moore M, Berk S, Nypaver A: Chronic pain: inpatient treatment with small group effects. Arch Phys Med Rehabil 65:356, 1984.
85. Novy D, Nelson D, Berry L, et al: What does the Beck Depression Inventory measure in chronic pain? A reappraisal. Pain 61:261, 1995.
86. Osterhaus J, Townsend J, Gandek B, et al: Measuring the functional status and well-being of patients with migraine headaches. Headache 34:337, 1994.
87. O'Toole J (ed): Work and the Quality of Life: Resource Papers for Work in America. Cambridge, The MIT Press, 1974.
88. Parsons T: The Social System. New York, Free Press, 1951.
89. Peck C, Fordyce W, Black R: The effect of the pendency of claims for compensation upon behavior indicative of pain. Washington Law Review 53:251, 1987.
90. Polatin P, Mayer T: Quantification of function in chronic low back pain. In: Turk D, Melzack R (eds): Handbook of Pain Assessment. New York, The Guilford Press, 1992.
91. Rahe R: Subjects' recent life changes and their near-future illness susceptibility. Adv Psychosom Med 8:2, 1972.
92. Ransford A, Cairns D, Mooney V: The pain drawing as an aid to the psychologic evaluation of patients with low-back pain. Spine 1:127, 1976.
93. Richards J et al: Assessing pain behavior: the UAB pain behavior scale. Pain 14: 393, 1982.
94. Romano J, Turner J: Chronic pain and depression: does the evidence support a relationship? Psychol Bull 97:18, 1985.
95. Romano J, Syrjala K, Levy R, et al: Overt pain behaviors: relationship to patient functioning and treatment outcome. Behav Ther 19:191, 1988.
96. Rosenstiel A, Keefe F: The use of coping strategies in chronic low back pain patients: relationship to patient characteristics and current adjustment. Pain 17:33, 1983.
97. Roy R: Chronic pain and marital difficulties. Health Soc Work 10(3):199, 1985.
98. Rudy T: Multiaxial Assessment of Pain: Multidimensional Pain Inventory. Pittsburgh, Pain Evaluation and Treatment Institute, University of Pittsburgh, 1988.
99. Schwartz D, DeGood D, Shutty M: Direct assessment of beliefs and attitudes of chronic pain patients. Archives of Physical Medicine and Rehabilitation 1985; 66:806.
100. Spinhoven P, Linssen A: Behavioral treatment of chronic low back pain. I. Relation of coping strategy use to outcome. Pain 45:29, 1991.
101. Spitzer R, Williams J, Kroenke K, et al: Utility of a new procedure for diagnosing mental disorders in primary care: The PRIME-MD 1000 study. JAMA 272: 1749, 1994.
102. Spitzer R, Kroenke K, Linzer M, et al: Health-related quality of life in primary care patients with mental disorders: results from the PRIME-MD 1000 study. JAMA 274:1511, 1995.
103. Sternbach R: Psychological factors in pain. In: Bonica J, Albe-Fessard D (eds): Advances in Pain Research and Therapy. New York, Raven Press, 1976, p 293.
104. Strong J, Ashton R, Chant D: The measurement of attitudes towards and beliefs about pain. Pain 48(2):227, 1992.
105. Swanson D, Mruta T: The family's viewpoint of chronic pain. Pain 8:163, 1980.
106. Swartzman L, McDermid A: The impact of contextual cues on the interpretation of and response to physical symptoms: a vignette approach. J Behav Med 16(2):183, 1993.
107. Tait R, Chibnall J: Development of a brief version of the Survey of Pain Attitudes. Pain 70:229, 1997.
108. Tait R, Chibnall J: Observer perceptions of chronic low back pain. J Appl Soc Psychol 24:415, 1995.

109. Tait R, Chibnall J, Krause S: The Pain Disability Index: psychometric properties. Pain 40:171, 1990.
110. Tait R, Chibnall J, Margolis R: Pain extent: relations with psychological state, pain severity, pain history, and disability. Pain 41:295, 1990.
111. Tait R, Chibnall J, Richardson W: Litigation and employment status: effects on patients with chronic pain. Pain 43:37, 1990.
112. Teske K, Daut R, Cleeland C: Relationships between nurses' observations and patients' self-report of pain. Pain 16:289, 1983.
113. Todd K, Lee T, Hoffman J: The effect of ethnicity on physician estimates of pain severity in patients with isolated extremity trauma. JAMA 271:925, 1994.
114. Todd K, Samaroo N, Hoffman J: Ethnicity as a risk factor for inadequate emergency department analgesia. JAMA 269:1537, 1993.
115. Toomey T, Gover V, Jones B: Site of pain: relationship to measures of pain description, behavior and personality. Pain 17:289, 1983.
116. Toomey T, Seville J, Mann J, et al: Relationship of sexual and physical abuse to pain description, coping, psychological distress, and health-care utilization in a chronic pain sample. Clin J Pain 11:307, 1995.
117. Towery S, Fernandez E: Reclassification and rescaling of the McGill Pain Questionnaire verbal descriptors of pain sensation: a replication. Clin J Pain 12:270, 1996.
118. Turk D, Rudy T: Toward an empirically derived taxonomy of chronic pain patients: integration of psychological assessment data. J Consult Clin Psychol 56(2):233, 1988.
119. Turk D, Rudy T: The robustness of an empirically derived taxonomy of chronic pain patients. Pain 43:27, 1990.
120. Turk D, Rudy T, Stieg R: Chronic pain and depression. Pain Mgt 1:17, 1987.
121. van Dulman A, Fennis J, Mokkink H, et al: Doctors' perceptions of patients' cognitions and complaints in irritable bowel syndrome at an out-patient clinic. J Psychosom Res 38:581, 1994.
122. Vasudevan S: Impairment, disability and functional capacity assessment. In: Turk D, Melzack R (eds): Handbook of Pain Assessment. New York, The Guilford Press, 1992.
123. Vinokur A, Selzer M: Life events, stress and mental distress. Proceedings of the 81st annual convention of the American Psychological Association, 1973, p 8.
124. Waddell G, Main C: Assessment of severity in low back disorders. Spine 9:204, 1984.
125. Waddell G: A new clinical model for the treatment of low-back pain. Spine 12: 632, 1987.
126. Waddell G, Newton M, Henderson I, et al: A Fear-Avoidance Beliefs Questionnaire and the role of fear-avoidance beliefs in chronic low back pain and disability. Pain 52:157, 1993.
127. Wallis B, Lord S, Bogduk N: Resolution of psychological distress of whiplash patients following treatment by radio frequency neurotomy: a randomized, double-blind, placebo-controlled trial. Pain 73:15, 1997.
128. Ware J: The status of health assessment 1994. Annu Rev Public Health 16:327, 1995.
129. Ware J, Sherbourne C: The SF-36 health status survey. I. Conceptual framework and item selection. Med Care 30:473, 1992.
130. Weisberg J, Keefe F: Personality disorders in the chronic pain population. Pain Forum 6(1):1, 1997.
131. Williams D, Thorn B: An empirical assessment of pain beliefs. Pain 36:351, 1989.
132. Williams D, Robinson M, Geisser M: Pain beliefs: assessment and utility. Pain 59:71, 1994.

APPENDIX 6–1

Example of a Psychological Report

Reason for referral:

Identifying information and relevant history:

Age
Marital status
History of major condition
- Date of onset/span of development
- Initial treatment
- Severity of initial disability
- Additional treatments
- Future hopes and expectations

Work history
- Number of jobs
- Current job
- Job satisfaction

Additional history
- Date of birth, place of birth
- Education
- Marriage/cohabitation
- Children
- Medications, tobacco, alcohol
- History of abuse

Behavioral observations and clinical findings:

Stature
Appearance
Orthoses/Prostheses
Gait and gross motor
Speech quality and content
Mood
Affect
Cooperativeness and relatedness
Pain
- Location
- Extent
- Intensity (maximum, minimum, average)
- Variation

Understanding
Coping techniques
Pain behavior
Current living situation
Sleep patterns
Eating patterns, weight
Daily activity abilities and limitations
Family interactions
Social activities
Psychological testing
Depression
Anxiety
Coping style
Personality

Summary and recommendations:
Psychological evaluation showed the following indications:
Current emotional distress
minimal, mild, moderate, severe
Dysfunctional personality characteristics
minimal, mild, moderate, severe
Serious psychiatric disorder
minimal, mild, moderate, severe
Expression of psychosocial distress through physical symptoms
minimal, mild, moderate, severe
Potential for substance abuse
minimal, mild, moderate, severe
Generalized coping skills
poor, fair, good
Potential for gain in rehabilitation
poor, fair, good

Summary statement and recommendations:

CHAPTER 7

Physician Assessment of Working Capacity

Steven J. Scheer, MD

Half a century ago, Hanman first described the use of functional testing to assign work to those returning from World War II in accordance with the individually measured physical capacities of the workers.[23] At the time, physicians were apparently writing "light duty only" or "limited running and climbing" in pre-employment examinations without substantiating such proscriptions by appropriate testing.[30] Hanman had recommended a profile of a worker's physical abilities, describing the tolerance for numerous activities under a variety of environmental circumstances.

Fifty years later, the physician's determination of work capacity remains an important responsibility. Unfortunately, the training of physicians in the decision-making process, including information gathering, communication with representatives of the workplace, and objective measurement of employability and readiness for work return, is generally not included in medical school and residency curricula for most primary care and many specialist physicians.[43] Work-capacity determination requires a degree of experiential knowledge and significant information beyond the traditional and time-honored office physical. At one extreme, concern for patient safety and/or malpractice liability may prompt a physician to set conservative return-to-work restrictions. Alternatively, overestimation of worker capabilities, leading to premature return to regular duties, may cause reinjury. Employers too, are concerned that early work return of an injured worker will increase the liability of the company.

The purpose of this chapter is to explain a rationale and format for physicians to make work-capacity determinations. In this regard, it is understood that physicians are not always in the best position to understand the entirety of job requirements, but they are often put in a decision-making capacity regarding worker fitness nevertheless. The physician may be asked to give a general statement of physical fitness for any work, or a statement of readiness to return to specific job duties after injury or disease.

In some of the ensuing discussions, this chapter uses the example of one of the most common scenarios encountered by the physician (i.e., assessment of return-to-work capacity of a worker with a back injury). Many of the same principles apply for determination of work capacity in other circumstances. The incorporation of input from several sources—the worker, the employer, and the therapist/capacity evaluator—is described.

WORKER INPUT

An occupational history is an important inclusion in the initial workup of an injured worker. Whether the person is looking forward to returning to the original employer or to another job, the information provides a sense of transferable skills, expertise, and education. Also, inquiring about previous injury history and recovery time can be very illuminating; among industrial workers it is common to see increasingly prolonged absence during recovery after each successive injury, which is a poor prognostic sign.

Workers are often familiar with risk factors for potential injury at the workplace. Although physician evaluators need to maintain an objective and balanced view of their assessments, they should solicit the input of the evaluee regarding task difficulties and worker readiness. If available, a job analysis (JA) may lack validity or completeness. It is useful to solicit the worker's input about the accuracy of the JA. The actual poundage of material-lifting required, availability of assistance or lack thereof, awkward shifting of loads, frequency of unlisted work tasks, inaccessibility of work-saving equipment, and the supervisor's impatience over scheduled work breaks are problems that may not be reflected by the company JA. On occasion, these vaguely indicated or inexact tasks are the very problems that require special accommodation for successful work return.

It is useful to ask the worker, "What aspects of this job, as you know it, do you feel will be difficult to perform when you go back to work?" Often, it may appear that the worker's capacities and job requirements, as listed, are compatible. If additional worker input reveals there were important task variables not included on the JA, it may be possible to negotiate a more successful work return by adding a few provisos on the return-to-work prescription. For example, a plant administrative assistant with acute back pain indicated that if he went back to work soon, he could not possibly handle the frequent stair-climbing required between multiple levels of his company plant. The job description did not list stair-climbing, and there was no allowance, by precedent, for a partial-duty work return. Inquiry revealed that the climbing was necessary to transport heavy packages, and that there was an internal mail-delivery system in the plant. The "return to work at full duty" statement that the worker carried to his employer was accompanied by the words "stair climbing is limited to one flight per 2 hours; physician recheck to reassess in 2 weeks." The employer is generally more receptive to any stated work restrictions if a statement of the physician's plan for worker reassessment is included with the return-to-work statement.

In the event of a mismatch between worker capacity and the submitted JA, transitional (light-duty) work return, if available, may be indicated. The potential mismatch may be revealed by functional capacity testing, by therapist report, by a site visit performed by the physician or therapist, or by the worker. If the worker is already familiar with the proposed light duty alternative, he or she may provide useful input about how to balance the worker's functional capacity and the workplace needs. The attitude of co-workers toward a worker on light-duty should be taken into account. Resentment by co-workers may intensify if accommodation is by fiat in a union shop situation where light-duty job availability may be precluded by seniority rights.

On occasion, the injured worker reveals that he or she is not at all interested in returning to work for the previous employer. Casual questioning about job satisfaction or the date the worker expects to be ready for work return may reveal such lack of intent. Such information, if gained at an early juncture in the care, can save a great deal of time and expense for all parties.

JOB ANALYSIS

A formal job description is a legal document that outlines the duties, equipment utilized, expertise required, environmental factors, and weight limits for material handling, and is usually made available on request to the work supervisor, the medical department, or personnel department.[36] The physician is often required to read and interpret job-task data provided. At times, an engineering background would be helpful for this evaluation. More often, the job duties are easily understood, but there may be important omissions. The document may require augmentation by the worker, or site visitation by a therapist or physician. The complete JA includes a description of the following[36, 40, 56]:

1. General physical requirements (lifting and carrying, postural variations, hand/foot dexterity needs, height/weight/reach requirements, and endurance)
2. Sensory requirements (hearing, speech, sight, touch)
3. Risk-factor identification (repetitive activities, overhead work, environmental exposures, prolonged immobility)
4. Psychological stress and personality factors
5. Dexterity, skill, and intellectual requirements
6. Educational requirements

General Physical Requirements

On occasion, a job will be characterized by lifting requirements alone[22, 58] (Table 7–1, taken from the *Dictionary of Occupational Titles* [DOT]).[49–51] Smaller employers may have submitted no JA at all because a proper one has

TABLE 7–1 Definitions of the Five Degrees of Strenuousness

S	Sedentary work	Lifting 10-lb maximum and occasionally lifting or carrying articles such as dockets, ledgers, and small tools
L	Light work	Lifting 20-lb maximum and/or frequently lifting or carrying objects weighing up to 10 lb; even though the weight lifted may be only a negligible amount, a job will be in this category (1) when it requires walking or standing to a significant degree, or (2) when it requires sitting most of the time but entails pushing and pulling of arm or leg controls
M	Medium work	Lifting 50-lb maximum and/or frequently lifting or carrying objects weighing up to 25 lb
H	Heavy work	Lifting 100-lb maximum and/or frequently lifting or carrying objects weighing up to 50 lb
VH	Very heavy work	Lifting objects in excess of 100 lb and/or frequently lifting or carrying objects weighing 50 lb or more

From US Department of Labor Employment and Training Administration: Dictionary of Occupational Titles, ed 4 Suppl. Washington, DC, 1986, pp 101–102, 1986.

never been done. The choices for obtaining information then include asking the worker being evaluated or a supervisor to provide information, or utilizing the DOT. The DOT was first proposed and developed by the U.S. Department of Labor and is the most comprehensive and concise description of typical jobs, worker traits, work environments, hazards, and general lifting requirements in the U.S. labor force.[22]

When more specific job characteristics are presented to an evaluating physician, either by the employer or as inferred from the DOT, the physician may feel ill-equipped to assess the capacity of the returning worker to meet these requirements. In all such circumstances, the use of a functional capacity evaluation (FCE) is in order (see Chapter 5 and p. 125).

Sensory Requirements

Sense-organ limitations do not commonly impede the return of an impaired worker to a menial job, particularly if the worker has already shown a capability to do the job safely. In regard to new hirees with sense-organ impairments, the disability-evaluating physician should have full awareness of Public Law 101-336, the Americans with Disabilities Act (ADA).[1] The ADA was landmark legislation and pertained to protecting disabled persons seeking employment by eliminating barriers to equal opportunity. Even employers of only 15 employees are bound by the terms of the law.[1, 53]

Risk Factors Identification

Risk factors commonly encountered in the workplace include repetition, high force, prolonged posture, vibration exposure, temperature extremes, and frequent bending and twisting.[55, 56] If these maneuvers are not mentioned in the JA, the worker probably can identify them. A good example of the more common risk factors is the handling of heavy materials. Unfortunately, the NIOSH recommendations for the optimal lift of a heavy (>38 kg) object—that the object's center of gravity is only 15 cm from the body, lifted no greater than 25 cm, to a maximum height of only 75 cm, no greater than once every 5 minutes—are seldom followed by companies demanding a lot of lifting from workers.[12, 35]

There is a sizable list of potential risk factors for each body part. Tables 7–2 through 7–5 include some of these concerns, excerpted from Wells.[56] The reader is also referred to other resources for additional information about industrial risk factors.[2, 17, 27, 45, 46]

Stress, Personality Factors, and Other Requirements

Psychological stress and personality factors are real issues that relate to worker capacity and viability in a work setting, but they are seldom addressed in written form in a JA. Evidence exists that a workplace "Apgar," including questions to the worker about self-worth and co-worker appreciation, predicts the potential for future back injury, thereby attesting to the importance these psychosocial variables hold in work-capacity determinations.[5] Assessment of job skills, dexterity, intellectual prowess, and adequacy of educational attainment (at times listed in the JA) typically falls outside the realm of physician expertise.

TABLE 7–2 Assessment of Risk Factors for the Low Back

Risk factor	Look for
High trunk moment (best single predictor of a high-strain task)	Arms reaching forward; the greater the horizontal reach to handle a load, the greater the trunk moment
	Bent-over trunk posture creating large trunk moments
Sustained postures	Loss of normal (standing) curve in low back
	Lifting from below knuckle height
Time of loading: ligaments and muscles stretch, whereas discs compress or creep if loaded for long periods, which may lead to instability	Lifting immediately after prolonged immobility
	Sustained or repetitive bent or twisted torso postures
	Repeated loading of spinal tissues measured by total weight lifted

Modified from Wells R: Task analysis. In: Ranney D (ed): Chronic Musculoskeletal Injuries in the Workplace, Philadelphia, WB Saunders Co, 1997, p 53.

FUNCTIONAL CAPACITY EVALUATION

Functional assessment continues to be a valuable part of the evaluation of a previously injured worker or new employee. The ability to render a decision about work capacity based on a reasonably valid, standardized, and reproducible FCE offers the office-based physician, the workplace health-care team, and

TABLE 7–3 Assessment of Risk Factors for the Shoulder Region

Risk factor	Look for
High moments at the shoulder	Hands holding a load far from the body
	The arms held out from the body or above mid torso
Static load on the shoulder girdle; continuous low loads can be as fatiguing and injurious as infrequent high loads	The arms out from the body continuously without support
	Shoulder girdle elevation
	Tools held continuously
Awkward postures of the shoulder	Work above the shoulder level
	Work with the arm behind the trunk
No time for recovery of tissues	Continuous repetition of the same activity
	More than one third of the person's strength exerted for more than one third of the time

Modified from Wells R: Task analysis. In: Ranney D (ed): Chronic Musculoskeletal Injuries in the Workplace, Philadelphia, WB Saunders Co, 1997, p 54.

TABLE 7–4
Assessment of Risk Factors for the Hand and Forearm Region

Risk factors	Look for
High forces and highly repetitive work	Work with a cycle time of a few seconds Little "rest time" between cycles (upper limbs in constant motion) Evidence of high forces
Use of high forces	Use of a pinch grip where a power grasp is more appropriate Pressing in fasteners with a single finger Fingers forced into hyperextension Gloves (increase grip force requirements of the task)
Nonoptimal wrist postures	Sustained flexion or extension over 30 degrees Rapid, continuous wrist motions Sustained ulnar or radial deviation Jerky, flicking, or tossing motions of the wrist Sustained pronation
Static loads	Gloves (can create a "static" load on the finger flexors) Holding the wrist in extension (e.g., during typing) Continuously holding a tool or object
Power tools with high vibration, high torques, or poor torque characteristics	Evidence of "kickback," forcing the wrist rapidly into extension Vibration of the tool; can lead to callouses, nerve and blood vessel damage, or vasospasm
Sharp edges and hard surfaces	Contact with hard or sharp objects on the sides of the fingers or the base of the palm Bearing weight on the inside of the elbow or a hard surface Hammering trim or parts with the palm (striking object with the hand)
High-precision placement requirement	Holding parts stationary to fit them together Spending time in an awkward posture to thread or fit parts

Modified from Wells R: Task analysis. In: Ranney D (ed): Chronic Musculoskeletal Injuries in the Workplace, Philadelphia, WB Saunders Co, 1997, p 55.

the returning worker a greater degree of certainty about the safety of the worker's activities in the workplace. It is not failsafe as a predictor of reinjury, and assessment itself may pose some degree of risk for reinjury. Neither is it necessary for physicians to insist on formal testing of functional capacity for all work-fitness determinations. However, the physician's ability to rely on functionally based assessment appears preferable to a "fly by the seat of one's pants" approach, particularly when the job demands for material handling are significant. The greater the physical demands required, the greater the advantages of an FCE.[42]

An FCE may take one of two forms: a general FCE or a job-specific FCE.[58] The general FCE is often used to help in developing a vocational rehabilitation plan when a worker has transferable job skills and interests but is unable to return to the previous job. Generic testing is also useful when a specific JA of the work to which an injured worker is returning is not available. Aspects of the general FCE should translate directly to the generic requirements of common occupations as defined in the DOT. The general FCE may also be used to measure the progress of the recovering worker before a light-duty or full work return. The test may employ assessment of manual materials handling, aerobic capacity, posture and mobility tolerance, and anthropometric measures (size, weight, and bodily proportions).

If the specific job tasks to which a worker will return are known, a job-specific FCE can be undertaken. However, the performance of these

TABLE 7–5 Assessment of Risk Factors for Sitting and Standing

Risk factor	Look for
Sitting (better for precision tasks with low force, limited reach	Long reaches Loads over 5 kg (10 lb) Long periods of sitting (over 1 hr) without an opportunity for standing for a few minutes
Standing (better for high-force tasks)	Long periods spent standing (over 1 hr) without taking more than two steps at a time
Incorrect work-surface height	Too high a work surface, above elbow height and requiring arm abduction Too low a work surface, below elbow height and requiring the person to stoop over
Poor chair design	Inadequate knee room Seat too high or sharp edged; can lead to legs getting tired or swollen, or sore feet; a foot rest is required A bad or missing back rest; can lead to a fatigued and stiff back Lack of adjustability; makes it difficult to achieve comfort Four-legged base; more likely to tip over than five legs Arm rests that do not allow the chair to be pulled up close to the work surface

Modified from Wells R: Task analysis. In: Ranney D (ed): Chronic Musculoskeletal Injuries in the Workplace, Philadelphia, WB Saunders Co, 1997, p 56.

activities at a medical site, outside the context of the actual worksite, may ultimately and significantly limit validity of the results obtained.

There are a number of available assessment systems used to determine work capacity. The following section provides material on just a few of the available systems for which testing on reliability and/or concurrent validity assessments has been carried out.

Lifting Assessments

Lifting assessment is a form of generic testing. There are three types of lumbar strength tests: static isometric, dynamic isokinetic, and psychophysical.[3, 12, 29, 38, 48] The most studied of these is the isometric lift test,[55] performed in a leg-lift squat, torso-lift with bent back, or arm-lift upright posture. Static lift is not particularly applicable to most jobs because few tasks are performed without motion.[55, 58] However, the static strength test is safe and reliable in normal healthy workers.[13, 27] There has been some concern raised about applying the same strength assessments to chronically disabled workers.[28, 60] The original literature[13, 27] suggested that static testing was predictive of future injury, but the prospective Boeing study[3] did not show a positive correlation between results of isometric strength testing and subsequent back injury. Because of their contrived nature, static lift tests may be more useful in assessing impairment than in defining work ability.[58]

Isokinetic testing is performed to allow a determination of strength over the entire range of motion at constant speed.[32, 45] The equipment is expensive, and there are not good data showing its predictive validity. One value of such dynamic lift testing is the ability to measure consistency of effort, because maximal and submaximal effort can be compared during repeated efforts.[32]

In psychophysical testing, the worker determines the maximum weight that can be comfortably lifted. Psychophysical testing is commonly utilized in both functional capacity testing and work rehabilitation programs.[48] In all dynamometric systems of lifting assessment, the single greatest threat to validity is the subject's submaximal effort.[41]

Team-generated Work Simulation Assessments

The traditional work-capacity evaluation is a time- and personnel-intensive process, bringing together a physical therapist, an occupational therapist, and various other rehabilitation professionals (psychologist, exercise physiologist, vocational counselor, rehabilitation nurse, rehabilitation engineer, case manager, or others as the situation requires) to generate a team report about the prospects for work fitness of a returning or entering worker.[7, 11, 39] The location of the assessment is often a converted warehouse or a distinctly separate hospital-based facility. The local options may include a 4-hour, 5-day, or 2-week assessment that may range in cost between $450 and $2000, depending on personnel time, level of expertise required, and local market conditions.* Consistent opportunities to closely observe the worker for signs of fatigue, effort, pain behavior, skill, and direction-following are all advantages of a team-generated report. The ability to utilize actual equipment needed at the job site provides this FCE with a special additional advantage. However, the

*Information obtained from personal inquiries in Cincinnati; Covington, Kentucky; Tucson, Arizona.

personnel time and space needs are considerable. Inability to simulate the actual working conditions of a supervisor, co-workers, untoward working environmental conditions (e.g., slippery floors, odors, temperature alterations), and output demands could give those receiving the team-generated FCE a false sense of security about the on-site abilities of an off-site but supposedly job-exact assessment.

Systems Based on the *Dictionary of Occupational Titles*

As alluded to earlier, the DOT is a federally developed document that lists most job in the United States and categorizes them by their physical and intellectual demands. It does not, in each occupation, consider all of the job factors or working conditions and tends to focus on job titles rather than absolute job content.[22] Nevertheless, it is the most comprehensive listing and analysis of occupations available. At least three systems of work-capacity analysis have been developed and standardized after consideration of the DOT: work profiles, work samples/aptitude tests, and work simulation.

1. *Work profiles* come from the vocational counseling field, and are exemplified by the Vocational Diagnosis and Assessment of Residual Employability (VDARE)[21] developed in the 1970s. The VDARE offers a means of synthesizing work histories with current medical information and aptitudes to determine potential job options. Computerized job-matching systems have been developed as well.[8, 14, 15] Botterbusch has listed many of these systems in his text, *Vocational Assessment and Evaluation Systems: A Comparison.*[9]

2. *Work samples/aptitude tests* are exemplified by Valpar, a pioneer in establishing specific work stations evaluating 16 categories of gross movement of the trunk and extremities as the movements relate to fine manual dexterity.[52] The Valpar uses standardized work postures based on the DOT, including crouching, reaching overhead, standing, and sitting. Frustration tolerance and direction-following are also assessed.[36] Other such work sample tests include the WEST[57] and the Bennett Hand Tool Dexterity Test.[4]

3. *Work simulation assessments* can be performed by either therapist-directed standardized battery or computerized tools. Lechner et al[31] developed and tested the Physical Work Performance Evaluation (PWPE), a functional capacity tool based on the DOT. The PWPE consists of six sections: dynamic strength, fine motor skills, coordination, position tolerance, mobility, balance and endurance. The assessment takes roughly 4 hours to perform by a physical or occupational therapist. The test was designed to facilitate the objective determination of maximum lift ability and quality of movement patterns. It has been validated and tested for inter-rater reliability.

Fishbain et al[22] developed a residual functional-capacity battery for measuring injured workers after consideration of the DOT. The so-called DOT-RFC test takes roughly 3½ hours to complete and consists of 36 subtests. The authors are currently engaged in validation testing for predictive and content validity.

A work-simulation tool that was developed to give therapists immediate DOT-relevant data on work performance capacity is the ERGOS.[19, 20] The ERGOS combines static strength testing, manual-dexterity assessment, instruction following, and standardized work simulation. It uses work elements derived from industrial engineering studies. The ERGOS is similar to a battery of dynamometric tests packaged in work-like activities. A computer-generated report allows for evaluator comments of subjective effort and complaints voiced by the tested worker. Strength and endurance data generated are compared with expected capacities of competitive workers. Dusik et al[19] studied the concurrent validity of the ERGOS work simulator as compared with actual performance of formatted industrial tasks and the exercise-oriented ratings of a rehabilitation therapist over a 2-week evaluation period. There was substantial agreement among the results of the 4-hour ERGOS simulator, the 2-week therapist evaluation, and the industrial shop assessment.

Another such system is the Baltimore Therapeutic Equipment (BTE) work simulator developed in the 1980s for industrial rehabilitation programs.[16] The BTE has a passive variable resistance assembly to which tool handles are attached, allowing simulation of actual work tasks against therapist-controlled resistance levels.[36]

SITE VISITATION

Witnessing the actual working conditions to which an injured worker is going to return allows the evaluator to experience the working environment and to understand the culture, the co-worker psychodynamics, and the flow of work. The physical conditions and the environment are better appreciated in person than as passed on in a written JA. Making site visits does require advance permission from the employer and, in some cases, the union.

The value of the physician's (or a delegated therapist's) visit to the job site of an injured worker is generally considerable. Any unusual tasks that are not easily described can be more easily understood by visualizing them. The speed of work performance and the work stress, both physical and emotional, can be better appreciated. There is often value in showing the worker that the physician cares enough to take the time to understand the work situations to which the worker will be expected to return. When job-site changes are essential, advocacy for the worker is more easily defended when the physician has actually seen the problem. The major limitation to the physician in agreeing to make a site visit is the time associated with the commitment.

A checklist of the pertinent concerns to study at the job site is included in Table 7–6.[37] A limited knowledge of ergonomics will also be beneficial.

Ergonomics is concerned with human body size and anatomy, biomechanics of internal and external forces, work physiology, human behavior and decision-making, and use of equipment and tools.[44] The goal of the scientific discipline is to maximize worker capability while concurrently ensuring safety, comfort, effectiveness, and efficiency.[34] Although ergonomics is a science, it is fortunate that even untrained lay persons can at times identify obvious sources of muscle overuse or postural misuse. Table 7–6 will help focus the physician site visitor on key aspects of the analysis.

Solutions to ergonomic problems are generally either administrative interventions or engineering adaptations. Administrative solutions include preassignment capacity testing to prevent individual worker overload, incorporation of a job-task rotation to prevent prolonged exposures, and training programs to inculcate good work habits and proper use of available equipment. Engineering improvements are exemplified by tool redesign to minimize mechanical irritation or lessen worker exertion, use of special gloves to prevent vibration exposure, and purchase of wheeled dollies or carts to substitute for manual lifting.[44] Regarding ergonomic improvements for back-pain prevention, success is most likely derived from engineering/job-site adaptations; investigators have shown that workers' abilities to practice lifting precautions are usually short-lived.[47]

TABLE 7–6 Checklist of Concerns to be Considered On a Site Visit

1. General concerns
   a. Is the work performed in a fixed position or is movement at will?
   b. Can the working posture (position or static load) explain the symptoms?
   c. Is the work requiring performance at worker's maximum capacity, and if so, how much or for how long each day?
   d. Are lengthy periods of intense concentration required?
   e. Is the work satisfying, and the worker feeling appreciated?
   f. Is the work psychologically stressful?
2. For standing activities
   a. Is continuous standing (over 2 hours) repeatedly required?
   b. Is stooping frequently required?
   c. Is leaning over containers or obstacles required?
   d. Is a twisted or awkward posture required?
3. For sitting duties
   a. Is continuous sitting (over 4 hours) required?
   b. Is the seat height matched properly to leg length and working surface?
   c. Are the chair seat pan and back adjustable?
   d. For a short person, would a foot rest help; for a tall person, is a higher working surface needed?
   e. For word/data processors, is the screen easily readable without glare and visual or neck strain?
4. For repetitive* upper extremity tasks
   a. Is awkward reaching required?
   b. Are shoulders frequently elevated or arms abducted/held overhead?
   c. Is repeated forceful gripping required?
   d. Is the wrist position often flexed, extended, or abducted/adducted?
   e. Is the elbow position often pronated or supinated?
5. Lifting and handling
   a. Was training in safe lifting performed and repeated?
   b. Is lifting accompanied by frequent twisting and bending?
   c. Is worker functional lifting capacity compared to lifting tasks?
   d. Are loads distant from body, awkward, difficult to grip, bulky, shifting, or unpredictable by appearance?

*Repetitive: 1500 or more movements/hour or cycle time <30 seconds.
From Pheasant S: Ergonomics, Work and Health, Aspen Publishers Inc., Gaithersburg, Md, 1991.

Consistent with the recent trend in work reconditioning programs performed at the job site, worker capacity assessments performed on site are now also being conducted. This idea seems intuitively sensible, because the tests are conducted in the uncontrived working environment. However, there is no standardized and reproducible testing on which to base these assessments. A real advantage of on-site capacity assessments is the option of using the results to come up with proper accommodation to facilitate a disabled person's earlier return to work.

ROLE OF THE EMPLOYER

After a work injury, the return-to-work outcome is greatly affected by the relationship of the worker and the employer. The communication and show of concern, the willingness to accommodate physical limitations, and the ability to flexibly alter the job duties are all important employer variables affecting worker recovery.

1. Return to work Jan. 18, 1998 at light level of exertion: up to 20 lb of lifting occasionally, 10 lb frequently; stretch breaks each hour for 5 minutes.

2. Recheck with physician on Jan. 25, 1998. Plan to advance to medium level of exertion (up to 50 lb occasional, 25 lb frequently) during subsequent 2 weeks; continue stretch breaks every 2 hours.

3. Recheck with physician planned for week of Feb. 8 for follow-up recommendations: goal of full duty (described on job analysis as 70 lb lifting occasionally, 30 lb frequently).

FIGURE 7–1
Recommendations for return to work of Mr. Howard Jones.

The first important post-injury activity by the employer is the establishment of early and continued communication. In a survey by the Menninger Foundation,[25] only 23% of corporations contacted disabled workers within 3 days of injury, and an additional 31% made initial contact within 4 to 10 days. The physician can readily detect resentment by a disabled worker who has not heard from the employer in this timeframe, especially workers who have a long job history at that company. The trend of having third-party administrators or occupational workers' compensation case managers assigned earlier to these cases has probably helped to facilitate good communication.[24]

Availability of transitional work is the second important contribution the employer can make to protecting the future employability of injured workers. Advocacy toward this end by the occupationally involved physician may be of help. At times, the involvement of unions will prevent transitional work because of a seniority arrangement that effectively blocks light-duty options.[10] The physician may be able to finesse this problem by recommending a time-limited transitional option with step-up in physical intensity planned at each 1- or 2-week juncture (Fig. 7–1).

Since the implementation of the ADA of 1992,[1] the employer has been mandated to be more aware of possible accommodations that will facilitate work return. Accommodation can run the gamut from making light-duty job tasks available at little or no cost, to expensive job-site environmental adaptations and purchase of load-bearing equipment. Historically, employers have harbored great concern that most accommodations will be expensive, but this notion may be ill-founded. According to the Job Accommodation Network, a federally funded program for employer questions about accommodation, 80% of workplace ergonomic accommodations cost the company $1000 or less; 68% are $500 or less.[26] Regardless of company beliefs, through the ADA Title I (affecting employment practices), the disabled employee who can still perform the essential functions of a job should be accommodated by the employer for any nonessential aspects so long as to do so will not pose a significant financial hardship for the company. Unfortunately, the ADA legislation does not define what "financial hardship" means, allowing for the use of case-made law to decide precedent in this matter.[33]

PUTTING IT ALL TOGETHER

At the time of the initial physician assessment, the worker must be convinced that the physician wants to assist the worker's recovery and is willing to take the time necessary to explain the diagnosis and the likely pathomechanics of the injury. When being seen by an occupational physician, workers occasionally harbor suspicions that the physician is working for the employer. A causality dispute only adds to the intensity of the worker's concern about physician credibility.[43] The physician's emphasis on concern for the worker's recovery helps to alleviate this issue.

Once treatment is initiated, the decision regarding work capacity needs to be made. Increasingly, employers are making it easier for workers to return to the job with ongoing pain and disability to prevent development of the chronicity syndrome. That workers' compensation insurance will pay for therapy until the worker is *completely* relieved of pain has never been a mandated part of state workers' compensation laws.[43] Light-duty options are being identified as part of a "job bank" by some companies, whereby injured workers can always be utilized at the company even as they undergo therapy for their reduced physical capacity.

Assessment of work capacity requires information about the worker and the job requirements. The assessment is an active process that involves input from the worker, the employer, the physical capacity evaluator, if one is used, and at times a vocational case manager. Pain behavior and physical findings on the physician's examination have shown poor correlation with inability to work and function.[18] The need to relate a worker's physical capacities to job demands is exemplified in Figure 7–2.

In this example, a physical therapist had been permitted to perform a job analysis by visiting the job site of an ironworker who had a back injury 6 weeks earlier. The therapist determined that the job of ironworker is clearly in the "very heavy work" category (Table 7–1). After a work reconditioning program, the functional capacity evaluation of the worker shows that the only limiting factors are a balance problem on narrow support and a 93-lb lift limit. The early return to work of this ironworker will depend on the availability of work projects on the ground and the willingness of the employer to accommodate the lifting limit with equipment or a lift assist for heavier load demands.

Information obtained from functional assessment is useful in identifying ability to work, and the employer's role in relating to the injured worker's needs is important in the process of work return. One additional important ingredient is the worker's attitude about the job. Yelin et al[59] determined that disabled workers who applied for Social Security Disability Insurance differed from similarly disabled workers who did not apply in that the latter group had greater job autonomy and employers willing and able to make job modifications. Bigos et al[5] showed that psychosocial and personal factors had predictive value in picking out a group of Boeing workers more likely to have back and other musculoskeletal ailments in the subsequent period. The same research group[6] had shown in an earlier study that workers who took longer to get back to work after a back injury had poorer appraisal ratings by their supervisors than highly rated co-workers who were injured. Imminent lay-offs at the plant or a frequently injured worker's desire to take early retirement may scuttle the best work-return programs of the health-care team.

Employability is not synonymous with physical and skill-related working ability. Prediction of employability remains a difficult task. Demographic variables and psychosocial variables have both been suggested to correlate with successful rehabilitation outcome.[54] However, it is much more difficult to make predictions about an individual than a large group of individuals. Rather than attempt to use predictive tools to determine who should be rehabilitated, it is best to identify intervention strategies to maximize the chances of a successful

Functional Capacity/Job Requirement Compatibility Analysis for Journeyman Ironworker (Recovering)

Client Name: Bill Smith

Job requirement	Current level of physical capacities	Compatibility	Intervention and recommendations
Strength Very heavy work. Client is required to occasionally lift 100 lb from waist or above; frequently to push and pull up to 150 lb; frequently carry up to 50 lb	Floor to waist Occasional 93 lb Frequent 63 lb Constant 32 lb Waist to shoulder Occasional 70 lb Frequent 45 lb Constant 30 lb Shoulders or overhead Occasional 45 lb Frequent 25 lb Constant 15 lb Carry 2 hands 75 lb right or left hand 45 lb Push or pull Sled 150 lb	Moderate Moderate Moderate	Client has 93-lb maximum lift from floor to waist. For objects that weigh more than 93 lb, he will have to use a mechanical device or have assistance from another employee. His strength could improve to a lift of up to 150 lb if his employer would allow him to gradually build up to that level. He would benefit from a home program for his back strength, abdominal strength, and from further education on body mechanics.
Balance He has to maintain his balance in awkward positions on the ground and in the air on 4″ beams.	He has satisfactory balance when he has a normal or widened base of support. However, his balance is impaired moderately when he has a decreased base of support.	Satisfactory on the ground except with a narrow base of support or on 4″ beams in the air.	The deficit will prevent the client from working on small beams in the air. He has sufficient balance to work on the ground.

Frequently stoops, kneels, and crouches.	Client is able to perform these activities safely on a stable surface.	High	Client has no limitations with stooping, crouching, crawling, or kneeling.
Occasionally crawls.	Client is able to crawl normally.	High	
Climbing			
Occasionally he ascends and descends ladders, stairs, and scaffolding.	He was able to ascend and descend 100 steps safely; he could safely climb a scaffold or ladder if he had access for good upper extremity support.	Moderate	He requires a ladder or scaffold that provides good upper extremity and lower extremity support. He would not be safe climbing a beam.
Reaching			
Extending hands and arms in all directions is required.	Normal	High	No limitations with reaching.
Handling			
He is required to seize, hold, and grasp various hand tools and welding equipment.	Handgrip and finger strength is sufficient to perform his job. He appears to have no limitation in finger coordination.	High	No intervention needed.

Summary: The client has satisfactory physical capacity to substantially perform the job tasks. However, climbing onto beams above ground would be ill-advised. The client will need some additional body mechanics instruction and a home strengthening program to raise lifting capacity to 100 lb from the floor.

FIGURE 7–2

A comparison of a worker's job duties with the worker's capacities. (From Scheer S: The role of the physician in disability management. In: Shrey D, Lacerte M [eds]: Principles and Practice of Disability Management in Industry. Winter Park, Fla, GR Press Inc, 1995, pp 184–186.)

work return for all, even if some who engage in these services might be predicted to not be employable. A time may come, however, when resource limitations will not allow a casual distribution of rehabilitation dollars.

SUMMARY

The occupationally involved physician must realize the importance of communication between all of the involved parties: worker, employer, union, therapist, and vocational case worker. Being able to read and understand a job analysis allows an appreciation for worker capacity goals. Having options for work-specific rehabilitation and functional testing of the worker is important for the physician's treatment armamentarium. Input from the injured worker and the employer may suggest how a structured work return can be accomplished in workers not quite ready for full duty. Ergonomic job improvements and workplace accommodation are employer options of variable expense; their availability adds options of great flexibility for the injured worker.

ACKNOWLEDGEMENTS

The author wishes to acknowledge the assistance of John Blank, Cheryl King, Jim Keller, and Anil Mital with the development of this chapter.

REFERENCES

1. Americans with Disabilities Act of 1990. Washington, DC, US House of Representatives Conference Report 101-596, 1990. Also, Federal Register: PL 101-336, Americans with Disabilities Act, July 26, 1990, pp 327–378.
2. Armstrong T, Fine L, Goldstein S, et al: Ergonomics considerations in hand and wrist tendinitis. J Hand Surg 12A:830, 1987.
3. Battié M, Bigos S, Fisher L, et al: Isometric lifting strength as a predictor of industrial back pain reports. Spine 14:851, 1989.
4. Bennett G: Hand Tool Dexterity Test Manual. Cleveland, Harcourt, Brace, Jovanovich, 1981.
5. Bigos S, Battié M, Spengler D, et al: A prospective study of work perceptions and psychosocial factors affecting the report of back injury. Spine 16:1, 1991.
6. Bigos S, Spengler D, Martin N, et al: Back injuries in industry: a retrospective study. III. Employee-related factors. Spine 11:252, 1986.
7. Blankenship K: Industrial Rehabilitation. Macon, Ga, American Therapeutics Inc, 1988.
8. Botterbusch K: A Comparison of Computerized Job Matching Systems. Menomonie, Wis, Materials Development Center, University of Wisconsin-Stout, 1983.
9. Botterbusch K: Vocational Assessment and Evaluation Systems: A Comparison. Menomonie, Wis. Materials Development Center, University of Wisconsin-Stout, 1987.
10. Bruyere S, Shrey D: Disability management in industry: a joint labor-management process. Rehabilitation Counseling Bulletin 34:227, 1991.
11. Burke S, Harms-Constas C, Aden P: Return to work/work retention outcomes of a functional restoration program. Spine 19:1880, 1994.
12. Chaffin D, Andersson G: Occupational Biomechanics, 2nd ed. New York, Wiley and Sons, 1991.
13. Chaffin D, Herrin G, Keyserling W: Pre-employment strength testing: an updated position. J Occup Med 20:403, 1978.

14. Crewe N, Athelstan G: Functional Assessment Inventory Manual. Menomonie, Wis, Materials Development Center, University of Wisconsin-Stout, 1984.
15. Crewe N, Turner R: A functional assessment system for vocational rehabilitation. In: Halpern AS, Fuhrer MJ (eds): Functional Assessment in Rehabilitation, Baltimore, Paul H. Brookes, 1984, p 223.
16. Curtis R, Clark G, Snyder R: The work simulator. In: Hunter J, Schneider L, Macklin E, et al (eds): Rehabilitation of the Hand, St Louis, Mosby, 1984, p 905.
17. Dainoff M, Dainoff M: People & Productivity: A Manager's Guide to Ergonomics in the Electronic Office. Toronto, Holt, Rinehart and Winston of Canada, Limited, 1986.
18. Deyo R: Measuring the functional status of patients with low back pain. Arch Phys Med Rehabil 69:1044, 1988.
19. Dusik L, Menard M, Cooke C, et al: Concurrent validity of the ERGOS work simulator versus conventional functional capacity evaluation techniques in a workers' compensation population. J Occup Med 35:759, 1993.
20. ERGOS: Instruction Manual. Work Recovery, Inc, 2341 S. Friebus, Suite 14, Tucson, AZ 85713, 1991.
21. Field T, Sink J: The Vocational Diagnosis and Assessment of Residual Employability. Athens, Ga, VDARE Service Bureau, 1979.
22. Fishbain D, Abdel-Moty E, Cutler R, et al: Measuring residual functional capacity in chronic low back pain patients based on the dictionary of occupational titles. Spine 8:872, 1994.
23. Hanman B: The evaluation of physical ability. N Engl J Med 258:986, 1958.
24. Hester E: Disability and disincentives: prospective models for change. In Scheer SJ (ed): Multidisciplinary Perspectives in Vocational Assessment of Impaired Workers, Rockville, Md, Aspen Publishers, 1990, p 205.
25. Hester E, Planek T, Decellwes P, et al: Disability benefits and cost-containment practices among small, medium, large and very large employers. The Menninger Foundation, Topeka, Kan, 1990.
26. Job Accommodation Network, US Quarterly Report, President's Committee on Employment of People with Disabilities, West Virginia University, Morgantown, West Virginia, June 1995.
27. Keyserling W, Herrin G, Chaffin D: Isometric strength testing as a means of controlling medical incidents on strenuous jobs. J Occup Med 22:332, 1980.
28. Kirkeldy-Willis W, Farfan F: Instability of the lumbar spine. Clin Orthop 165: 110, 1982.
29. Kishino N, Mayer T, Gatehel R, et al: Quantification of lumbar function. IV. Isometric and isokinetic lifting simulation in normal subjects and in low-back dysfunctional patients. Spine 10:921, 1985.
30. Kuh C, Hanman B: Current development affecting the physician's role in manpower development. N Engl J Med 125:265, 1944.
31. Lechner D, Jackson J, Roth D, et al: Reliability and validity of a newly developed test of physical work performance. J Occup Med 36:997, 1994.
32. Mayer T, Barnes D, Kishino N, et al: Progressive isoinertial lifting evaluation. II. A comparison with isokinetic lifting in a disabled chronic low back pain industrial population. Spine 13:998, 1988.
33. McMahon B, Shrey D: The Americans with Disabilities Act, disability management, and the injured worker. J Workers' Comp 1:9, 1992.
34. Mital A: Ergonomics, injury prevention, and disability management. In: Shrey D, Lacerte M (eds): Principles and Practices of Disability Management in Industry, Winter Park, Fla, 1995, p 5.
35. National Institute for Occupational Safety and Health: Work Practice Guide for Manual Lifting. DHEW (NIOSH) Pub No. 81-122, 1981.
36. Osterman A, Bednar J, Skirven T, et al: Vocational capacity and physical impairment in the upper extremity. In Scheer SJ (ed): Medical Perspectives in Vocational Assessment of Impaired Workers, Gaithersburg, Md, Aspen Publishers, 1991, p 65.

37. Pheasant S: Ergonomics, Work and Health, Gaithersburg, Md, Aspen Publishers, Inc, 1991.
38. Pope M, Andersson G, Frymoyer J, Chaffin D: Occupational Low Back Pain: Assessment, Treatment and Prevention. St Louis, Mosby, 1991.
39. Pruitt W: Vocational Evaluation, 2nd ed. Menomonie, Wis, Walter Pruitt Associates Publishers, 1986.
40. Rossignol M: Establishing a prognosis for low back problems. In: Ranney D (ed): Chronic Musculoskeletal Injuries in the Workplace. Philadelphia, WB Saunders Co, 1997, p 193.
41. Rothstein J, Lamb R, Mayhew T: Clinical uses of isokinetic measurements: critical issues. Phys Ther 67:1840, 1987.
42. Scheer S: Commonalities of measuring capacity to work. In: Scheer SJ (ed): Multidisciplinary Perspectives in Vocational Assessment of Impaired Workers. Rockville, Md, 1990, p 19.
43. Scheer S: The role of the physician in disability management. In: Shrey DE, Lacerte M (eds): Principles and Practices of Disability Management in Industry, Winter Park, Fla, GR Press, Inc, 1995, p 175.
44. Scheer S, Mital A: Ergonomics. Arch Phys Med Rehabil 78:S-36, 1997.
45. Scheer S, Wickstrom R: Vocational capacity with low back pain impairment. In: Scheer SJ (ed): Medical Perspectives in Vocational Assessment of Impaired Workers, Gaithersburg, Md, Aspen Publishers, 1991, p 19.
46. Silverstein B, Fine L, Armstrong T: Hand-wrist cumulative trauma disorders in industry. Br J Indust Med 43:779, 1986.
47. Snook S, Campanelli R, Hart J: A study of three preventative approaches to low back injury. J Occup Med 20:478, 1978.
48. Troup J, Foreman T, Baxter C, Brown D: The perception of back pain and the role of psychophysical tests of lifting capacity. Spine 12:645, 1987.
49. US Department of Labor Employment and Training Administration: Dictionary of Occupational Titles, ed 4 suppl. Washington, DC, US Government Printing Office, 1986.
50. US Department of Labor Employment and Training Administration: Selected Characteristics of Occupations Defined in the Dictionary of Occupational Titles. Washington, DC, US Government Printing Office, 1981.
51. US Department of Labor Employment and Training Administration: Dictionary of Occupational Titles, ed 4. Washington, DC, US Government Printing Office, 1977.
52. Valpar Corp, 3801 East 34th St., Tucson, AZ, 1984.
53. Verville R: The Americans with Disabilities Act: an analysis. Arch Phys Med Rehabil 71:1010, 1990.
54. Walls R, Tseng M: Measurement of client outcomes in rehabilitation. In: Bolton B (ed): Handbook of Measurement and Evaluation in Rehabilitation. Baltimore, Paul H. Brookes, 1987, p 183.
55. Weinstein S, Scheer S: Industrial rehabilitation medicine. 2. Assessment of the problem, pathology, and risk factors for disability. Arch Phys Med Rehabil 73:S-360, 1992.
56. Wells R: Task analysis. In Ranney D (ed): Chronic Musculoskeletal Injuries in the Workplace, Philadelphia, WB Saunders Co, 1997, p 41.
57. Work Evaluation Systems Technology: Huntington Beach, Calif, Work Evaluation Systems Technology, 1986.
58. Wickstrom R: Functional capacity testing. In: Scheer SJ (ed): Multidisciplinary Perspectives in Vocational Assessment of Impaired Workers. Rockville, Md, Aspen Publishers, 1990, p 73.
59. Yelin E, Henke C, Epstein W: Work disability among persons with musculoskeletal conditions. Arthritis Rheum 29:1322, 1986.
60. Zeh J, Hansson T, Bigos S, et al: Isometric strength testing: recommendations based on a statistical analysis of the procedure. Spine 11:43, 1986.

SECTION III

Impairment Rating and Disability Evaluations for the Major U.S. and Canadian Disability Systems

CHAPTER 8

Impairment and Disability Under Workers' Compensation

Alan K. Novick, MD   *Robert D. Rondinelli, MD, PhD*

During the late nineteenth and early twentieth centuries injured workers had only a limited ability to recoup damages from an on-the-job injury or accident. Under tort law, a worker would have to bring civil suit against the employer for damages resulting from the work-related injury. The employee would need to prove that his employer was negligent in some fashion, resulting in the employee's direct harm. This legal process frequently was too expensive for the injured worker to pursue, and proving the employer's sole negligence was difficult. The employee or co-workers were often believed to share contributory negligence, or may have assumed the risks of injury by accepting a hazardous job. The employee claim for benefits, therefore, was frequently denied. Because of these inadequacies in the tort claims system, workers' compensation laws developed to provide medical benefits and wage replacement for injured workers with a decreased need for litigation.[14]

This chapter is intended to familiarize the health-care provider with the U.S. Workers' Compensation system, with a focus on the physician's general role and reporting requirements. In addition, a glossary of terms typically associated with workers' compensation is provided, and the varied approaches and applications of different impairment/disability rating schemes used in the system are briefly highlighted. For more detailed discussion than is possible here, a number of useful and in-depth references are cited. In addition, the reader is encouraged to review the workers' compensation laws pertaining to his or her particular jurisdiction of practice, because considerable variations exist with respect to the generalities that follow.

DEFINITIONS AND TERMINOLOGY

Within workers' compensation there are many definitions and terms of which each practitioner should have a working knowledge. These are listed in Appendix 8–1.

SYSTEM OVERVIEW

Within the United States, workers' compensation is a complex, federally mandated system of health and disability insurance that is administered at the state level. There are 53 workers' compensation jurisdictions, including the 50 states, the District of Columbia, and the U.S. territories of Puerto Rico and

TABLE 8–1 Statutory Coverage of Workers' Compensation Laws by Jurisdiction

Jurisdiction	Elective (E) or compulsory (C)	Exemption from coverage		
		Employers of fewer than:	Agricultural workers	Domestic servants
Alabama	C	5	X	Elective
Alaska	C	3	X	
Arizona	C			Elective
Arkansas	C		X	Elective
California	C			
Colorado	C			
Connecticut	C			
Delaware	C		X*	
District of Columbia	C			
Florida	C	4	X*	Elective
Georgia	C	3	X*	Elective
Hawaii	C			
Idaho	C		X	Elective
Illinois	C		X*	
Indiana	C		X	Elective
Iowa	C		X*	
Kansas	C		X	
Kentucky	C		X	
Louisiana	C			X
Maine	C		X*	Elective
Maryland	C		X*	
Massachusetts	C			
Michigan	C	3	X*	
Minnesota	C		X*	
Mississippi	C	5	X	Elective
Missouri	C	5	X*	X
Montana	C			Elective
Nebraska	C		X	Elective
Nevada	C		X	Elective
New Hampshire	C			
New Jersey	E			
New Mexico	C	3	X	Elective
New York	C		X*	
North Carolina	C	3	X*	Elective
North Dakota	C		X	Elective
Ohio	C			
Oklahoma	C		X*	
Oregon	C			Elective
Pennsylvania	C		X*	Elective
Puerto Rico	C			
Rhode Island	C	4	X	Elective
South Carolina	E	4	X	
South Dakota	C		X*	
Tennessee	C	5	X	Elective
Texas	E		X*	Elective
Utah	C		X*	

TABLE 8–1 Statutory Coverage of Workers' Compensation Laws by Jurisdiction *Continued*

Jurisdiction	Elective (E) or compulsory (C)	Exemption from coverage		
		Employers of fewer than:	Agricultural workers	Domestic servants
Vermont	C		X*	Elective
Virgin Islands	C			Elective
Virginia	C	3	X*	X
Washington	C		X*	
West Virginia	C		X*	Elective
Wisconsin	C	3	X*	Elective
Wyoming	C		X*	X

*Qualified exemptions apply.
Data from Somers H, Somers A: Workmen's Compensation: Prevention, Insurance and Rehabilitation of Occupational Disability. New York, John Wiley & Sons Inc, 1954, pp 40–43; and Brigham C, Babitsky S: Achieving Success with Workers' Compensation: Reference Manual. Falmouth, Mass, SEAK Inc, 1996. pp 17–19, 21–26.

the Virgin Islands. Recent statistics include an overall estimated 3.3 million claims filed per year for an estimated $17.9 billion in indemnities and $25.3 billion in total benefits paid. The annual operating budget excluding claims paid is estimated at $1.3 billion.[15]

Workers' compensation is compulsory in all states except Texas, New Jersey, and South Carolina (Table 8–1).[2, 14] Where applicable, all employers must pay for compensation and other benefits as defined by statute if the employee suffers an accidental injury or death arising out of employment. Individual states, however, may have special exemptions regarding workers' compensation coverage and the definition of an employee/employer relationship. For example, in Florida, "employment" does not include domestic servants in a private home, professional athletes, or seasonal agricultural labor if certain criteria are met (i.e., agricultural labor performed on a farm if the labor is completed in less than 30 days and the farmer employs less than five regular employees).[5] In addition, an independent contractor or subcontractor may not be considered an employee and may have to provide his or her own compensation insurance.[5, 8] Jurisdictional exemptions from coverage for small employers, agricultural workers, and domestic servants are summarized in Table 8–1.

Because of the multiple existing jurisdictions with varying and respective rules and regulations, it is essential that the physician be familiar with and able to apply the rules appropriate to his or her particular jurisdiction. The determination of which jurisdiction's laws apply may be difficult in certain instances. For example, a company that does business on both sides of a state line, or a business such as long-distance trucking that has employees who travel through many states could have difficulty determining which jurisdiction's laws apply when an injury occurs. Several different criteria have been applied to determine legal jurisdiction, including the principal site of employment, the location into which the contract of hire was entered, and the place where the accident occurred. Some states have legislated specific mechanisms regarding how out-of-jurisdiction injuries are handled.[5, 8]

The cost of workers' compensation benefits is financed by the employer as a recognized element of the cost of business.[14] Consequently, employers must give

TABLE 8–2 Jurisdictional Variations in Insurance Requirements, Waiting Period, and Method of Physician Selection

	Insurance requirements				
Jurisdiction	Private	State	Self-insurance	Waiting period (days) before filing	Method of physician selection
Alabama	+	–	+	3	Employer selects
Alaska	+	–	+	3	Initial choice
Arizona	+	+	+	7	Initial choice
Arkansas	+	–	+	7	Employer selects
California	+	+	+	3	Employer selects
Colorado	+	+	+	3	Employer selects
Connecticut	+	–	+	3	Employee selects (state list)
Delaware	+	–	+	3	Initial choice
District of Columbia	+	–	+	3	Employee selects (state list)
Florida	+	–	+	7	Employer selects
Georgia	+	–	+	7	Employee selects (employer list)
Hawaii	+	+	+	3	Initial choice
Idaho	+	+	+	5	Employer selects
Illinois	+	–	+	3	Initial choice
Indiana	+	–	+	7	Employer selects
Iowa	+	–	+	3	Employer selects
Kansas	+	–	+	7	Employer selects
Kentucky	+	+	+	7	Initial choice
Louisiana	+	+	+	7	Initial choice
Maine	+	+	+	7	Employer selects
Maryland	+	+	+	3	Initial choice
Massachusetts	+	–	+	5	Initial choice
Michigan	+	+	+	7	Employer selects
Minnesota	+	+	+	3	Initial choice
Mississippi	+	–	+	5	Initial choice
Missouri	+	+	+	3	Initial choice
Montana	+	+	+	6	Initial choice
Nebraska	+	–	+	7	Initial choice
Nevada	–	+	+	5	Employee selects (state list)
New Hampshire	+	–	+	3	Initial choice
New Jersey	+	–	+	7	Employer selects
New Mexico	+	–	+	7	Employer selects
New York	+	+	+	7	Employee selects (state list)
North Carolina	+	–	+	7	Employee selects
North Dakota	–	+	–	4	Initial choice
Ohio	–	+	+	7	Initial choice
Oklahoma	+	+	+	7	Initial choice
Oregon	+	+	+	3	Initial choice
Pennsylvania	+	+	+	7	Employer selects
Puerto Rico	–	+	–	3	State agency
Rhode Island	+	–	+	3	Initial choice
South Carolina	+	–	+	7	State agency

TABLE 8–2 Jurisdictional Variations in Insurance Requirements, Waiting Period, and Method of Physician Selection *Continued*

Jurisdiction	Insurance requirements: Private	State	Self-insurance	Waiting period (days) before filing	Method of physician selection
South Dakota	+	−	+	7	Initial choice
Tennessee	+	+	+	7	Employee selects (employer list)
Texas	+	+	+	7	Initial choice
Utah	+	+	+	3	Employer selects
Vermont	+	−	+	3	Employer selects
Virgin Islands	−	+	−	0	Initial choice
Virginia	+	−	+	7	Employee selects (employer list)
Washington	−	+	+	3	Initial choice
West Virginia	−	+	+	3	Initial choice
Wisconsin	+	−	+	3	Initial choice
Wyoming	−	+	−	3	Initial choice

Data from Brigham C, Babitsky S: Achieving Success with Workers' Compensation: Reference Manual. Falmouth, Mass, SEAK, Inc, 1996, pp 17, 18, 28, and 73; and Somers H, Somers A: Workmen's Compensation: Prevention, Insurance and Rehabilitation of Occupational Disability. New York, John Wiley & Sons Inc, 1954, p 94.

assurance as to their ability to meet this obligation through insurance options that vary by jurisdiction. Options include insuring through a private carrier (45 out of 53 jurisdictions), a state fund (28 out of 53 jurisdictions), or by furnishing proof of ability to carry one's own risk through a "self-insurance" fund (49 out of 53 jurisdictions) (Table 8–2).

ENTITLEMENT

When the employer and type of employment are covered by existing worker's compensation laws, an injured claimant's right to compensation is established by the following determinations:[14]

1. Is the injury compensable? Historically, the original workers' compensation statutes were intended to cover injuries that occurred by "accident" (a chance, unexpected event and one definite in time and place) in the workplace.[14] This was to be distinguished from "disease," which develops gradually over time. Because the distinction between these entities is often arbitrary and blurs in reality, and with liberalized interpretation of the original laws, extension of coverage now typically includes occupational disease, as well as death or impairment resulting from aggravation of a preexisting and underlying condition.[14]

2. Did the injury arise "out of and in the course of employment?" All workers' compensation jurisdictions share a "no-fault" concept. Unlike tort claims, under workers' compensation the employee need not prove the employer at fault for his or her injury. Instead, the determination must be made that the injury or illness arose "out of and in the course of employment" to receive benefits.

An illness or injury unrelated to employment is not intended to be covered by workers' compensation insurance. A causal relationship is established by meeting the dual requirements that the injury or illness occurred while the employee was at work and actively involved in employment activity.[14]

As can be expected, jurisdictional variations exist in the interpretation of what constitutes employment activity. For example, in Florida, an injury suffered while going to or coming from work is not considered arising out of employment, even if the employer provided transportation, unless the employee was specifically engaged in a special errand or mission for the employer. An employee, however, who is required to travel in connection with his or her job and suffers an injury while in transit is eligible for compensation. Job-related recreational and/or social activities are also not typically compensable unless the activity was a required part of the employment and provided a direct benefit to the employer.[5] For example, an employee injured at a company holiday party would not usually be covered for benefits under workers' compensation. If the employee, however, was responsible for marketing and was injured at a holiday party while entertaining potential clients, the employee then may be covered because he or she was performing specific job responsibilities.

3. **Is the resulting condition of sufficient duration to extend beyond any statutory waiting period?** In most jurisdictions, injuries are excluded from coverage for wage-loss benefits if they fail to produce disability beyond a minimum "waiting period." This exclusion is intended to minimize administrative overhead and excessive costs related to minor and inconsequential injuries.[14] Typically, this period varies from 0 to 7 days (Table 8–2). Medical benefits are provided, starting immediately at the time of injury, with no delay of care or treatment. The waiting period only applies to the wage-loss benefits.[14]

4. **Has the worker filed a claim within the specified time limits?** All jurisdictions have specified time limits from date of onset to filing a claim and notifying the employer. The range of limits is considerable, but generally an employer must be notified within 30 days of illness or injury, and a claim must be filed within 1 year for disability and 2 years for death.[14]

An employee may forfeit eligibility for medical and indemnity benefits for a work-related injury if he or she is found to be intoxicated or impaired because of substance abuse (providing the employer had maintained a drug-free workplace, including notification to the employee of the condition of employment to refrain from reporting to work or working under the influence of drugs or alcohol).[5] Furthermore, benefits may be lost or reduced if the injury was caused by refusal to use a safety appliance or observe appropriate safety rules. In Florida, for example, if an employee is warned about safety protocol before an accident and then goes on to be injured because of not following safety procedures, benefits could be reduced by 25%.[5] Benefits may also be lost if the injured worker becomes incarcerated because of criminal activities.[5] Many states will allow for continued dependent benefits and medical care but will forego wage-loss compensation if the injured worker is imprisoned. In addition, workers' compensation benefits may be in jeopardy if an employee refuses employment after he or she has been medically cleared to return to work. Even if the employee is released to work at a modified capacity, benefits are at risk if the injured employee does not return to work, assuming a job at that particular work capacity is available. The injured worker cannot collect workers' compensation benefits and an additional salary greater than their original salary at the time of injury. The worker must declare if they have become employed by anyone other than their original employer, and benefits may be reduced or eliminated based on their residual earning capacity.[5]

BENEFITS

After the work-related injury or illness, the employee has three different types of available benefits, including *survivor benefits* in cases of death, *medical and rehabilitation expenses*, and *wage-loss benefits*. In cases of severe accidents resulting in death, the employee's survivors are entitled to death benefits. Most states provide for funeral expenses and on-going compensation to the surviving spouse and/or children. In Florida, for example, funeral expenses are paid up to $5000, and survivor benefits are paid at 66⅔% of the average wage the individual was receiving at the time of death (50% to the spouse and 16⅔% to a child or children) up to a maximum value of $100,000. If the surviving spouse remarries, he or she is entitled to a lump-sum payment equal to 26 weeks of compensation at the rate of 50% of the worker's average weekly wage. The surviving children's benefits terminate at 18 years of age, or 22 years of age if the child is a full-time student, or on the child's marriage.[5]

The second type of benefit provides for medical and rehabilitative treatment of the injured worker. Most states provide for 100% of associated medical care, including but not limited to diagnostic testing, treatment, medicines, medical supplies, durable medical equipment, orthoses, prostheses, and other medically necessary apparatus.[5, 13] In addition, appropriate professional and nonprofessional attendant care is usually provided if medically necessary and under the direct orders of a physician. A variety of different health-care providers can be utilized to administer care under workers' compensation. For example, in Florida, a provider of services may include medical doctors, doctors of osteopathy, podiatrists, chiropractors, and/or optometrists. Jurisdictional laws may vary as to who controls the selection of the treating physician (Table 8–2.) Many jurisdictions will allow the employee to choose his or her own physician, whereas others allow the employer to select the treating physician. Should an injured employee seek medical care outside of the system, he or she becomes responsible for the unauthorized medical expenses thereby incurred, although several states have a set allowance for such expenses. For example, Kansas has a maximum allowance of $500 for unauthorized medical expenses.[13] Furthermore, some states have set limits for certain treatments in an attempt to contain costs. For example, in Florida, chiropractic services are limited to 18 treatments, or 8 weeks beyond the initiation of the chiropractic treatment.[5]

The third type of benefit for injured workers is cash or wage-loss compensation. This benefit provides monetary compensation because of either temporary or permanent inability to return to gainful employment. When an employee suffers an injury, this may result in impairment and/or disability. Impairment and disability are concepts that are interrelated (see Chapter 2) and are associated with wage-loss expectations under workers' compensation. Disability is typically viewed in terms relative to the individual's earning ability. For example, in Florida workers' compensation defines *disability* as an "incapacity because of the (work-related) injury to earn in the same or any other employment the wages which the employee is receiving at the time of the injury."[5]

Under workers' compensation, four separate categories of disability exist.

Disability can either be *permanent* or *temporary*. In addition, disability can be considered *total* or *partial*.[14] Permanent disability occurs when the impairment becomes static and is unlikely to change despite medical or rehabilitative treatments. During a period of temporary disability, some recovery or return of function is expected. With total disability, the injured worker is incapable of returning to any work or earning wages during a specified period after an injury. When an injured worker is able to return to work in a modified capacity but not yet to his or her full duty, a partial disability is said to exist.[6] A partially disabled worker may be considered incapable of earning his or her preinjury wages. The treating physician must give restrictions or limitations defining what the partially disabled worker is capable of performing and must indicate the anticipated duration for which those restrictions apply.

Wage-loss compensation is based on the category of disability. *Temporary total disability (TTD)* benefits are typically equal to two thirds of the average weekly wage an employee earned before the injury up to, but not exceeding, a maximum allowable cap that is set by individual statutes. TTD benefits are usually paid monthly from the time of injury until the worker reaches maximum medical improvement (MMI) or returns to a modified work status.[11] MMI identifies the point in time at which the medically determined impairment becomes stable, no further treatment is reasonably expected to improve the condition, and a permanent disability determination can therefore be made.

If an injured worker is not at MMI but is able to return to modified duty, he or she is eligible for *temporary partial disability (TPD)* benefits. TPD benefits are generally paid as two thirds of the difference between preinjury and modified-duty wages, up to a maximum allowable cap that varies by jurisdiction. Temporary disability benefits are usually paid monthly from the onset of modified duty until MMI is reached.[8]

An injured worker who is medically determined to be permanently incapable of returning to any work is considered to have a *permanent total disability (PTD)*. *PTD* is defined by statute in certain jurisdictions and for certain conditions. For example, in Florida PTD applies only to "catastrophic injury . . . in the absence of conclusive proof of substantial earning capacity"[5] where *catastrophic injury* means permanent impairment caused by conditions including spinal cord injury with paralysis, limb amputation, severe brain injury, second- or third-degree burns exceeding 5% of face and hands, total blindness, or other injuries of similar severity and incapacitation.[5] PTD benefits are payable starting at MMI, and are typically equal to two thirds of the weekly preinjury wage, up to a maximum allowable cap, which is based either on a maximum dollar value or maximum number of weeks of allowable benefits.[5, 8]

An injured worker who can no longer perform work at his or her preinjury level, but who is capable of modified duty or alternative work at MMI, is considered to have a *permanent partial disability (PPD)*. PPD benefits may be *scheduled* or *unscheduled*. Scheduled benefits are associated with impairments of certain readily identified body parts (i.e., upper limb, hand) for which predetermined and corresponding disability tables exist. Such tables specify the maximum number of weeks for which benefits must be paid at an average weekly rate based on the injured employee's wage at time of injury up to a maximum value set by each jurisdiction. PPD compensation is typically determined as the percentage of impairment (or disability) times the maximum scheduled loss for the affected body part. For example, in Kansas, the schedule for loss of an arm at the shoulder is 225 weeks at a maximum rate of $319 per week. If, however, the employee sustained an injury to the upper extremity equivalent to 20%, they would be entitled to a lump-sum payment equivalent to $14,355 ($319 per week × 225 weeks × 20%).[13] In states such as Missouri, in which impairment ratings are not recognized, a medically determined disability percentage is used instead to derive the scheduled amount.

Some injuries do not affect discrete anatomical parts but affect regions or systems instead (i.e., the spine). In such cases, unscheduled benefits provide compensation at a proportional rate to the *whole person (WP)*. Impairment or disability ratings are thus determined as a percentage, with the maximum WP loss equal to 100%. Unscheduled benefits would therefore equal a lump-sum payment at MMI equivalent to the average weekly rate up to a maximum set by individual jurisdictions paid for a period equal to the number of weeks allowed for the WP, reduced by the WP impairment percentage for that particular injury.

To better illustrate how unscheduled benefits are issued, the example of a back injury with a 5% impairment of the WP will be used. In Kansas, if the injury is to the body as a whole, an employee who is partially disabled is entitled to 415 weeks of maximal compensation. The maximum rate of disability set by state statute is $319 per week, as noted above. If the employee's preinjury wage was at or above the maximum weekly rate, then the permanent partial disability unscheduled benefit would equal $319 per week for 20.75 weeks (415 weeks per WP × 5% impairment) or a lump-sum payment of $6,619.25.[13]

A comparison of temporary and permanent benefits by jurisdiction is presented in Table 8–3. For more in-depth comparison and detailed review by jurisdiction than is possible here, the reader is referred to the U.S. Department of Labor's *State Workers' Compensation Administration Profiles,*[15] or to a summary reference manual *Achieving Success with Workers' Compensation.*[2]

SECOND INJURY FUND

Workers who have sustained a permanent partial disability often have difficulty finding employment within their new work capacity. Therefore many states have enacted a *second injury fund* to encourage the employment of individuals with preexisting disabilities by protecting the employer from excess liability for compensation and medical expenses. The criteria for recovery from the fund varies between jurisdictions. The enactment of the Americans with Disabilities Act (ADA) has reduced or eliminated the impact of the fund in many states in which workplace modifications and accommodation of the disabled are now federally mandated. For example, Kansas abolished the fund in 1994. Before that time, if employers hired an individual with preexisting work-related disability, they could recover from the fund expenses incurred for a second injury that resulted in disability or death and that would not have occurred "but for the preexisting disability." In cases in which the injury would have occurred irrespective of preexisting disability, the employer could recover any ensuing percentage of benefits apportioned to the preexisting disability.[13] Many jurisdictions, however, still utilize some form of a second injury fund. For example, in Florida, when an injury to a physically disabled worker merges with, aggravates, or accelerates a preexisting permanent physical impairment to cause a greater disability than would have resulted from the second injury alone, the employer must first pay all workers' compensation benefits, but is then eligible to receive reimbursement of 50% of all compensation expenses from the Special Disability Trust Fund.[5] No determination of apportionment is necessary. Other

TABLE 8–3 Workers' Compensation Benefits for Temporary-Total and Permanent-Total Disability*

			Time limitations on	
Jurisdiction	**Maximum % wages**	**Maximum weekly payments**	**Temporary-total disability**	**Permanent-total disability**
Alabama	66⅔	$427	DD	DD
Alaska	80% SE	$700	DD (or until medical stability)	DD
Arizona	66⅔	$323.10	DD	Life or DD
Arkansas	66⅔	$270	450 weeks	DD
California	66⅔	$406	DD	Life
Colorado	66⅔	$442.61	DD	Life
Connecticut	75% SE	$660.00	DD	DD
Delaware	66⅔	$346.17	DD	DD
District of Columbia	66⅔ (or 80% SE if less)	$701.52	DD	DD
Florida	66⅔	$453	104 weeks	DD
Georgia	66⅔	$275	400 weeks	DD
Hawaii	66⅔	$491	DD	DD
Idaho	67	$360.90 first 52 weeks; $220.55 thereafter	52 weeks; thereafter 67% of SAWW for DD	52 weeks; thereafter 67% of SAWW for DD
Illinois	66⅔	$735.41	DD	Life
Indiana	66⅔	$428.00	500 weeks (maximum $214,000)	500 weeks (maximum $214,000)
Iowa	80% SE	$817	DD	DD
Kansas	66⅔	$319	DD (maximum $100,000)	DD (maximum $125,000)
Kentucky	66⅔	$415.94	DD	DD
Louisiana	66⅔	$323	DD	DD
Maine	80% SE	$441	DD	DD
Maryland	66⅔	$525	DD	DD
Massachusetts	60	$585.66	156 weeks	DD
Michigan	80% SE	$499	DD	DD
Minnesota	66⅔	$516.60	DD (up to 90 days post-MMI)	Life
Mississippi	66⅔	$252.59	450 weeks (maximum $113,665)	450 weeks (maximum $113,665)
Missouri	66⅔	$476.28	400 weeks	DD
Montana	66⅔	$373	DD	DD
Nebraska	66⅔	$350	DD	DD
Nevada	66⅔	$432.39 (temporary total) $468.86 (permanent total)	DD	Life
New Hampshire	60	$714	DD	DD
New Jersey	70	$469	400 weeks	450 weeks

TABLE 8–3 Workers' Compensation Benefits for Temporary-Total and Permanent-Total Disability* *Continued*

			Time limitations on	
Jurisdiction	**Maximum % wages**	**Maximum weekly payments**	**Temporary-total disability**	**Permanent-total disability**
New Mexico	66⅔	$343.49	100 weeks	Life
New York	66⅔	$400	DD	DD
North Carolina	66⅔	$478	DD	DD
North Dakota	66⅔	$366	DD	DD
Ohio	72% (first 12 weeks, 66⅔% thereafter)	$493	DD	Life
Oklahoma	70	$307	300 weeks	DD
Oregon	66⅔	$489.45	DD	DD
Pennsylvania	66⅔	$509	DD	DD
Puerto Rico	66⅔	$65	312 weeks	DD
Rhode Island	75%	$474	DD	DD
South Carolina	66⅔	$422.48	500 weeks	500 weeks
South Dakota	66⅔	$349	DD	DD
Tennessee	66⅔	$382.79	400 weeks (maximum $153,116)	400 weeks, (maximum $153,116)
Texas	70%	$472	104 weeks (or MMI if sooner)	Life for statute listing (401 weeks other)
Utah	66⅔	$417 (temporary total) $354 (permanent total)	312 weeks	312 weeks (or life if rehabilitation not possible)
Vermont	66⅔	$648	DD	DD (or 330 weeks minimum)
Virgin Islands	66⅔	$298	DD	DD
Virginia	66⅔	$466	500 weeks	DD
Washington	60%–75%	$545.61	DD	Life
West Virginia	70%	$423.10	$208 weeks	Life
Wisconsin	66⅔	$479	DD	Life
Wyoming	66⅔	$421 (temporary total) $280 (permanent total)	DD	344 weeks

*As of 1995.

DD, Duration of disability; *SE,* spendable earnings; *SAWW,* state average weekly wages.

Data from Somers H, Somers A: Workmen's Compensation: Prevention, Insurance and Rehabilitation of Occupational Disability. New York, John Wiley & Sons Inc, 1954, pp 79–80, 84, 85; and Brigham C, Babitsky S: Achieving Success with Workers' Compensation: Reference Manual. Falmouth, Mass, SEAK, Inc, 1996, pp 29–34, 36–42.

jurisdictions may require the employer to pay only benefits attributed solely to the second injury, as if there had been no preexisting injury. In Missouri, the right to recover rests with the disabled employee, who may be entitled to benefits from the fund if his or her overall disability is greater than that attributable solely to the second injury. In such cases, the overall disability is first determined and an apportionment of preexisting versus subsequent disability is made. The balance due to the employee from the second injury fund would be the additive difference after the preexisting disability has been factored out.[13]

PHYSICIAN REPORTING REQUIREMENTS

The physician who practices within workers' compensation is required to complete a variety of reports and answer several specific questions throughout the treatment course. Frequently, the physician will be asked to determine causality of the specific impairment; in other words, was the worker's impairment the result of the job injury. *Causality* is defined simply as the association between a given cause and its effect. In the present context, the cause would be the work-related event and the effect would be the subsequent impairment. The determination of causality for workers' compensation injuries must be based on medical probability versus medical possibility (Appendix 8–1). For workers' compensation, the causal relationship must be established within reasonable medical probability.

The physician is also asked in each stage of the process to complete a work status report (Figure 8–1).[11] The report should identify whether the employee can return to full or modified duty, and defines the physical limitations to which the injured worker must adhere. Sitting, standing, walking, bending, stooping, climbing, crawling, squatting, kneeling, pushing, pulling, and reaching above the shoulders are all parameters that can be limited based on frequency of required versus allowed performance during the work day. In addition, lifting and carrying can be restricted by a maximum amount of allowable weight. The total number of hours an employee is allowed to work during each day may be specified. Furthermore, the work status report should identify whether the employee has reached MMI and, if not, when MMI is anticipated.

In many jurisdictions, the treating physician must issue an impairment rating for an injured worker once he or she reaches MMI. Unfortunately, not all jurisdictions use the same impairment rating systems, and some jurisdictions even use multiple rating scales depending on the date of the work-related injury. For example, Florida legislation mandates the use of the American Medical Association's *Guides to the Evaluation of Permanent Impairment, 4th Edition (AMA Guides)*[1] for injuries occurring before July 1, 1990; the *Minnesota Department of Labor and Industry's Permanent Partial Disability Schedule*[7] for injuries occurring between July 1, 1990 and October 31, 1992; and the *Florida Impairment Rating Guide*[3] for injuries occurring after October 31, 1992.[5] The most commonly used rating system nationally is the *AMA Guides*. Twenty-nine of the 53 workers' compensation jurisdictions mandate or recommend the use of the *AMA Guides*, and 11 of the 53 jurisdictions do not mandate but frequently use the *AMA Guides*. The remaining 13 of the 53 jurisdictions do not mandate or currently use the *AMA Guides*.[1] The workers' compensation physician will need to become intimately familiar with and proficient in the application of the rating guide specific to his or her particular workers' compensation jurisdiction.

PATIENT STATUS:

PATIENT NAME: ______________________ DATE OF INJURY: ______________

DIAGNOSIS: ______________________ STATUS: ☐ Improved ☐ Same ☐ Worse ☐ Resolved

WORK STATUS:

☐ RETURN TO FULL DUTY

☐ RETURN TO LIMITED DUTY NUMBER OF HOURS/DAY: _______

☐ (OFF) UNABLE TO WORK UNTIL FOLLOW-UP PROJECTED RETURN TO WORK DATE: ______________

RESTRICTIONS:

CHECK THE FREQUENCY AND NUMBER OF HOURS/DAY THE WORKER IS ABLE TO DO THE FOLLOWING ACTIVITIES:

	FREQUENCY		NUMBER OF HOURS/DAY								
Activity	**Continuous**	**Intermittent (with rest)**	**0**	**1**	**2**	**3**	**4**	**5**	**6**	**7**	**8**
Sitting											
Standing											
Walking											

	Never	**Occasionally (up to 33%)**	**Frequently (34-66%)**	**Continuously (67-100%)**
Movements:				
Bend/Stoop				
Squat				
Kneel				
Crawl				
Climb				
Pushing/Pulling				
Reach above shoulder level				
Lift:				
Up to 10 lbs				
11 - 25 lbs				
26 - 50 lbs				
> 50 lbs				
Carry:				
Up to 10 lbs				
11 - 25 lbs				
26 - 50 lbs				
> 50 lbs				

RETURN APPOINTMENT:

RETURN APPOINTMENT (DATE): ______________ TIME: __________

IS PATIENT AT MMI? ☐ YES ☐ NO IF NOT, PROJECTED MMI DATE: ______________

______________________ ______________________

Provider signature/MD Date of Exam

FIGURE 8–1

Example of a work-status report. (From Rondinelli R: Practical aspects of impairment rating and disability determination. In: Braddom R [ed]: Physical Medicine and Rehabilitation. Philadelphia, WB Saunders Co, 1996.)

MUSCULOSKELETAL IMPAIRMENT RATING

Brief Overview

Musculoskeletal impairment rating varies by jurisdiction. Three examples using the AMA *Guides, Minnesota Department of Labor and Industry's Permanent Partial Disability Schedule*, and the *Florida Impairment Rating Guide* are illustrated for comparison as follows:

The musculoskeletal chapter of the *AMA Guides* is divided into three sections: the upper extremity, the lower extremity, and the spine. Impairment ratings of the upper extremities are based on amputation, digit sensation, active range of motion, peripheral nerve injury, peripheral vascular disease, and/or certain musculotendinous impairments or bone and joint deformities. Lower-extremity impairments are determined by anatomical, functional, or diagnostic criteria. Anatomic impairments include amputations, skin loss, peripheral nerve injuries, vascular disorders, limb-length discrepancies, unilateral muscle atrophy, range-of-motion limitations, joint ankylosis, and manual muscle-strength deficits. Functional impairments include gait derangements and joint replacements, and diagnostic impairment criteria include a variety of fractures, ligamentous injuries, and surgical procedures.[1]

The *AMA Guides* allows spinal impairments to be rated based on an "injury" model or a diagnosis-related estimate (DRE) model. The DRE approach allows for specific diagnostic categories for each region of the spine to be assigned impairment ratings, thereby eliminating the need for measuring spinal motion, which is difficult to measure accurately and may not relate to disability (see Chapter 3 for a detailed discussion of this issue).

Once impairment ratings are determined for each injured body part, it is possible to express the ratings as scheduled values (for each individual body unit) or to combine these ratings as unscheduled (i.e., to the whole person) using the "combined value" chart provided at the back of the *AMA Guides*. The combined value chart is designed to ensure that cumulative scheduled ratings of regional subunits do not exceed the total value of the unit itself, and that the cumulative whole-person impairment rating does not exceed 100%. In using the combined values chart, all scheduled impairments must first be converted to whole-person equivalents using the appropriate conversion charts provided in each section of the *AMA Guides*.

Although the *AMA Guides* attempts solely to rate impairments, the application of such ratings within workers' compensation is tantamount to quantified disability ratings. Wage-loss compensation is intended to offset economic losses caused by reduction or loss of earning capacity after a work-related injury. This loss of earning ability is by definition a disability. Workers' compensation wage-loss benefits are often calculated based on an impairment rating. Functional loss, however, cannot be directly extrapolated from an impairment rating.[12] No formal functionally based disability rating scale is widely used within the workers' compensation system (see Chapter 2 for a detailed discussion of this problem and suggested alternatives).

Limitations of reliability and validity of impairment ratings are a concern when applying the *AMA Guides* (see Chapter 3). Other rating scales have been developed as alternatives to the *AMA Guides*, which may, in part, alleviate some of these shortcomings.

The *Minnesota Department of Labor and Industry's Permanent Partial Disability Schedule*[7] primarily uses diagnostic categories, with each diagnosis assigned a certain impairment percentage, thus simplifying the clinical examination and perhaps minimizing the possibility of interrater error. The *Florida Impairment Rating Guide*[3] utilizes a combination approach, with diagnostic categories for certain body regions such as the spine, and measurable determinants in other regions such as the extremities. The diagnostic categories as applied to the spine eliminate any potential error introduced because of spinal motion measurements. For example, using the Florida guide, a herniated lumbar disc treated surgically would be given an impairment rating of 7% of the whole person based on the category of "surgically treated disc lesion with or without objective neurological finding."[3, 4] Multiple operations with or without residual signs of injury would add 2% impairment per procedure.[3, 4] Unfortunately, this system does not take into account functional outcome. The patient would receive the same impairment rating whether he or she had a full recovery, with complete resolution of pain, or had persistent disabling radicular pain and weakness. The impairment rating is given only for the procedure, thus potentially encouraging patients to undergo additional procedures to increase their impairment ratings.

The Minnesota schedule[7] attempts to include functional (albeit subjective) outcomes in determining impairment ratings. For example, the same patient undergoing surgery for a lumbar herniated disc could receive an impairment rating between 9% and 15% depending on the outcome. Excellent results defined as mild low back pain, no leg pain, and no neurologic deficits would be assigned a 9% impairment rating after surgery. Average results, such as mild increase in symptoms with bending or lifting, and mild to moderate restriction of activities related to back and leg pain, would equal an 11% impairment, whereas poor surgical results as defined by persistent or increased symptoms with bending or lifting, and major restrictions of activities because of back and leg pain would equal a 13% impairment. Finally, an impairment rating of 15% is assigned when multiple operations are performed on the low back with poor surgical results, such as persisting or increased symptoms of back and leg pain.[7]

The physician disability examiner must be completely familiar with the prescribed rating system for his or her jurisdiction to meet the evaluating and reporting requirements under workers' compensation.

SUMMARY

This chapter is intended to provide a practical overview of the workers' compensation system in sufficient detail to familiarize physicians or other health-care practitioners with general jurisdictional requirements of the employer, physician, and injured worker. For a more detailed administrative account than is possible here, the reader is referred to references cited by the U.S. Department of Labor,[15] the North Carolina Industrial Commission,[10] The Minnesota Department of Labor and Industry,[8] the Florida Workers' Compensation Institute,[5, 9] and SEAK, Inc.[2] Because of the distinctive laws of each jurisdiction, medical providers who wish to practice within the workers' compensation system must familiarize themselves with the unique rules and regulations of their respective jurisdiction.

REFERENCES

1. American Medical Association: Guides to the Evaluation of Permanent Impairment, 4th ed. Chicago, American Medical Association, 1993.

2. Brigham C, Babitsky S: Achieving Success with Workers' Compensation: Reference Manual. Falmouth, Mass, SEAK, Inc, 1996.
3. Florida Workers' Compensation Institute: Florida Impairment Rating Guide. Tallahassee, Florida Workers' Compensation Institute, 1993.
4. Florida Workers' Compensation Institute: Florida Uniform Permanent Impairment Rating Schedule. Tallahassee, Florida Workers' Compensation Institute, 1996.
5. Florida Workers' Compensation Institute: Florida Workers' Compensation Reference Manual. Tallahassee, Florida Workers' Compensation Institute, 1997.
6. Meyer T: Workers' Compensation. In: Herring S, Cole A (eds): The Low Back Pain Handbook: A Practical Guide for the Primary Care Physician. Philadelphia, Hanley & Belfus, 1997.
7. Minnesota Department of Labor and Industry: Minnesota Department of Labor and Industry's Permanent Partial Disability Schedule. St Paul, Print Communication Division, Minnesota Department of Labor and Industry, 1993.
8. Minnesota Department of Labor and Industry: Minnesota Department of Labor and Industry Workers' Compensation Handbook, 1991 ed. St Paul, The Office of Revisor Statutes, 1991.
9. Nelson-Morrill C: Workers' Compensation in Florida 1935-1995: The History, People & Politics. Tallahassee, Florida Workers' Compensation Institute, 1995.
10. North Carolina Industrial Commission: North Carolina Workers' Compensation Law Annotated, 1994 ed. Charlottesville, Vir, The Michie Company, 1994.
11. Rondinelli R: Practical aspects of impairment rating and disability determination. In: Braddom R (ed): Physical Medicine & Rehabilitation. Philadelphia, WB Saunders, Co, 1996.
12. Rondinelli R, Dunn W, Hassanein K, et al: A simulation of hand impairments: effects on upper extremity function and implications toward medical impairment rating and disability determination. Arch Phys Med Rehabil 78:1358–1363, 1997.
13. Rondinelli R, Katz R, Hendler S, Eisfelder B: Disability evaluation. In: Grabois M, Garrison S, Hart K, Lemkuhl L (eds): Physical Medicine and Rehabilitation: The Complete Approach. Malden, Mass, Blackwell Science Inc, pp 311–331.
14. Somers H, Somers A: Workmen's Compensation: Prevention, Insurance, and Rehabilitation of Occupational Disability. New York, John Wiley & Sons, Inc, 1954.
15. US Department of Labor: State Workers' Compensation Administration Profiles. Washington, DC, US Department of Labor, Office of Workers' Compensation Programs, 1997.
16. World Health Organization: International Classification of Impairments, Disabilities and Handicaps: A Manual of Classification Relating to the Consequences of Disease. Geneva, WHO, 1993.

Glossary

accident An unexpected or unusual event or result that happens suddenly as a result of employment.[5] The accident produces an injury.

aggravation An ongoing effect resulting in physical worsening or accelerating of pre-existing and underlying pathology or susceptible condition.[2]

apportionment The determination of percentage of impairment directly attributable to the pre-existing versus resultant conditions related to the aggravation.[11]

causality An association between a given cause (event capable of producing an effect) and effect (a condition that can result from a specific cause) within a reasonable degree of medical probability. Causality requires a determination that:

An event took place.
The claimant experiencing the event has the condition (impairment).
The event could cause the condition (impairment).
It is medically probable that the event caused the condition (impairment).[11]

disability Any restriction or lack (resulting from impairment) of ability to perform an activity in the manner or within the range considered normal for a human being.[16]

exacerbation A temporary increase in symptoms.[2]

impairment (1) Any loss or abnormality of psychological, physiological, or anatomical structure or function.[16] (2) The loss, loss of use, or derangement of any body part, system, or function.[1]

injury Damage to a body part, or death arising out of and in the course of employment.[5]

Maximum Medical Improvement (MMI) Date after which no further significant recovery from or lasting improvement to a personal injury can reasonably be anticipated, based on reasonable medical probability.[8]

medical possibility An event is likely to occur with a probability equal to or less than 50%.[11]

medical probability An event is more likely than not to occur, with a probability exceeding 50%.[11]

occupational disease A disease peculiar to and arising out of employment, which subjects the employee to a hazard to which the public is not generally exposed.[8]

proximate causation The factor(s) that immediately or closely precede(s) the effect.[2]

ultimate causation The initial factor(s) leading to the effect.[2]

CHAPTER 9

Social Security Disability Insurance and Supplemental Security Income

James P. Robinson, MD, PhD *Claire V. Wolfe, MD*

The Social Security Administration's (SSA) disability system has evolved over time to provide benefits based on disability. There are two components to the system: (1) Social Security Disability Insurance (also known as *SSD* or *Title II*), a program for individuals who have worked, paid into the Social Security system, and subsequently become disabled and unable to work before reaching retirement age; and (2) Supplemental Security Income (also known as *SSI* or *Title XVI*), a supplemental security income program for indigent individuals who are disabled.

Qualification for either program is based on medical evidence. The physician can play an important role in assisting the patient who applies for SSA disability benefits. The purpose of this chapter is to help the reader understand the system, understand what type of objective medical evidence is needed to document disability for the purposes of the SSA, to define what other parameters may be included in assessing an individual's ability to work, and to explain the administrative options open to individuals who may have applied for and been denied benefits.

It is important to stress that both SSD and SSI are based on medically determinable impairments. The two programs differ with respect to non-medical eligibility criteria but use essentially identical definitions of disability. SSD, or Title II, provides benefits to individuals who are "insured" by virtue of their contributions through the Social Security tax on earnings, as well as to certain disabled dependents of these insured individuals. SSI, or Title XVI, provides payments to individuals, including children under age 18, who are disabled and have limited income and resources.

Persons may apply for SSD or SSI regardless of how they became disabled. Thus SSD and SSI differ from workers' compensation or Veterans Administration programs, in which eligibility depends on the circumstances under which a person was injured or became ill.

THE BASICS

The basis of the entire Social Security disability compensation system, both SSD and SSI, is the "medically determinable impairment," defined as "an impairment that results from anatomical, physiological or psychological abnormalities which can be shown by medically acceptable clinical and laboratory diagnostic techniques." A physical or mental impairment must be established by medical evidence consisting of signs, symptoms, and laboratory findings. An individual's statement of symptoms, or a physician's pronouncement that the individual is disabled without corroborating information, is insufficient for establishing disability under the Social Security programs.

Social Security Disability

Although the old-age insurance program that we know as Social Security was enacted by Congress in 1935, the disability program, SSD, was established in 1956. SSD is an insurance program. To be eligible for SSD benefits, an individual must have worked in a job covered by SSD for a minimum number of years. (The formulas for computing eligibility for SSD are complex, but in general a worker must have been in the work force for at least 5 of the 10 years before the onset of disability).

Payroll deductions for SSD are combined with payroll deductions for old-age insurance. Together, they make up the Federal Insurance Contribution Act (FICA) deduction for an employee. This contribution is matched by the employer. Employees are required to make payments into the SSD fund. Some state and federal employees may be allowed to opt out of SSD, contributing to their own retirement and disability funds. As of 1994, 96.1% of jobs in the United States were covered by SSD.

Like all SSA programs, SSD has undergone numerous modifications over the years, but the broad outlines have remained fairly constant.[21]

SSD pays monthly income support benefits to individuals under age 65 who meet the appropriate employed quarters of coverage*:

1. Whose medical condition is severely incapacitating so that they are unable "to engage in any substantial gainful activity (SGA) by reason of any medically determinable physical or mental impairment that can be expected to result in death or that has lasted or can be expected to last for a continuous period of not less than 12 months;"[21]
2. Who are widows or widowers of a covered individual and who meet the definition of disability;
3. Who are the disabled offspring (children or adult) of a covered individual.

Supplemental Security Income

The SSI program was established in 1972 as a replacement for a number of federal and/or state programs that provided income support for indigent people who were either blind, disabled, or aged (more than 65 years old). As of December 1995, 76.5% of SSI recipients were disabled, 22.2% were aged, and 1.3% were blind.[20]

SSI operates as a federal/state partnership and is funded with general tax revenues. The federal government establishes broad guidelines regarding eligibility and benefit levels, but the states have significant influence, so eligibility criteria and benefits vary widely across states. The SSI program is not an insurance program. Individuals are eligible even if they have never worked. However, SSI is a means-tested program (i.e., individuals cannot receive benefits

**Quarters of coverage* refers to those quarters worked in which the individual has earned about $500 per month. In most cases, the individual has to have worked 20 out of the last 40 quarters to be eligible for benefits. There are exceptions for younger individuals who become disabled before they have met the 40-quarter requirement.

if their assets or income are too high). In many states individuals are ineligible for SSI if they have assets of more than $2000 or an income greater than $5,808 per year.[21]

SSI eligibility includes individuals usually less than age 65:

1. With low income and assets (per individual state criteria);
2. Whose medical condition is severely incapacitating so that they are unable "to engage in any substantial gainful activity (SGA) by reason of any medically determinable physical or mental impairment that can be expected to result in death or that has lasted or can be expected to last for a continuous period of not less than 12 months;"[21]
3. Who are children less than age 18 with a "medically determinable impairment(s) that is of comparable severity" to an adult's and if it "limits the child's ability to function independently, appropriately, and effectively in an age-appropriate manner."

Similarities and differences between the two programs are summarized in Table 9–1.

THE APPLICATION PROCESS

The application process for both SSD and SSI begins when an applicant contacts a local SSA office and fills out an initial application. The SSA office then addresses non-medical eligibility issues: for SSD, whether the applicant has worked enough quarters in a job covered under Social Security; for SSI, whether

TABLE 9–1 Comparisons Between the SSD and SSI Programs

Characteristic	SSD	SSI
Purpose	Income support for disabled	Income support for disabled
Medical criteria	Inability to engage in any substantial gainful activity by reason of any medically determinable physical or mental impairment that can be expected to result in death, or that has lasted or can be expected to last for a continuous period of not less than12 months	For adult: Same as one used for SSD For child: A medically determinable physical or mental impairment that results in marked and severe functional limitations
Prior work requirement	Yes	No
Means testing	No	Yes
Average monthly payment	$682.40	$389.47
Waiting period	5 months	None
Trial work period (TWP)	Yes	Yes
Impairment-related work expenses (IRWE)	Yes	Yes
Extended period of eligibility (EPE)	Yes	No (although there is an equivalent)
Source of funding	Insurance trust fund (federal)	General revenues (federal and state)

the applicant meets the income/assets requirements. If eligibility is established, the initial application is forwarded to the state agency, the Disability Determination Service (DDS).

DDS evaluates the medical aspects of the application. The application, or case, is assigned to an adjudicator—an individual who has a college degree—who has had training in medical conditions, especially as they relate to the disability program. The adjudicator must first obtain thorough medical records on the applicant. This invariably includes obtaining records from treating and consulting physicians. The adjudicator may additionally ask the treating physician to do a report that summarizes the applicant's medical problems, documents their objective abnormalities, and identifies activity limitations.

Physicians and psychologists within the state agency are available to the adjudicator to help review the medical documentation. In about 40% of cases, the information received from treating sources is deemed insufficient, and the DDS will order a consultative examination from an independent physician, often a specialist in a field appropriate to the patient's complaints. The consultant will be asked for a history, physical, and an assessment of function based on the objective findings. The state agency may also order appropriate, noninvasive testing (e.g., ECGs, stress tests, pulmonary function studies, radiological examinations), and laboratory work.[26]

The Five-Step Process of the Application

Once the medical file is complete, the evaluating team analyzes it according to the five-step process shown in Table 9–2 and discussed here.

Step 1

Is the applicant engaged in SGA? As described earlier, this is the only step that does not consider medical evidence. If a claimant is working at a level high

TABLE 9–2 Steps In the Evaluation of SSD and SSI Applications

Step	Yes	No
1: Is applicant currently engaged in substantial gainful employment?	Application is denied, regardless of patient's medical condition	Proceed to Step 2
2: Does applicant have a medically determinable, severe impairment?	Proceed to Step 3	Application is denied; applicant can appeal denial
3: Does applicant's condition meet or equal a "listing"?	Application is accepted	Proceed to Step 4
4: Does applicant's residual functional capacity permit him/her to return to "past relevant work"?	Application is denied; applicant can appeal denial	Proceed to Step 5
5: Does applicant's residual functional capacity permit him/her to do any other kind of substantial gainful activity that exists in the national economy?	Application is denied; applicant can appeal denial	Application is accepted

enough to be "substantial gainful activity (SGA)," then regardless of the severity of the medical impairment, even if the impairment would otherwise have met all the criteria of disability for the program, the claimant cannot be found disabled.

Step 2

Does the applicant have a medically determinable severe impairment? Step 2 occurs after the medical development at the state agency. It requires that the applicant have a medically determinable "severe" impairment according to the following definition[22]:

> ...a medically determinable physical or mental impairment is an impairment that results from anatomical, physiological, or psychological abnormalities which can be shown by medically acceptable clinical and laboratory diagnostic techniques. A physical or mental impairment must be established by medical evidence consisting of signs, symptoms, and laboratory findings—not only by the individual's statement of symptoms.

Many applicants meet this test because any *documentable* impairment affecting the ability to work (e.g., even "age-appropriate" arthritis) will satisfy the requirements for step 2. However, the issue of *medically determinable* impairment has been relevant in evaluations of patients with chronic myofascial pain problems. Many of them are denied benefits at the step 2 level in the absence of documentable abnormalities.

Step 3

Does the applicant meet or equal the listings? SSA has developed a set of medical criteria, the "listings of impairments," which, if met or equaled, will result in an award of benefits without any further hearings. There are separate listings of impairments for adults and children. They are arranged by body system and set forth the medical findings deemed sufficient for an award of disability benefits. The listings are revised periodically to accommodate changes in medical diagnoses and treatment of various diseases. For example, listings involving transplants, dialysis, malignancies, and AIDS have undergone significant changes in the last few years.

A listing typically contains a diagnosis and some clinical markers of severity. For example, osteoporosis of the spine is a listed condition. If there is evidence of pain, limited back range of motion, paravertebral muscle spasm, and either a single vertebral body compression fracture with more than 50% loss of height or multiple vertebral body fractures (in the absence of a history of trauma), then the claimant will be deemed to meet the severity of the listings and benefits will be awarded regardless of age, education, or previous job history.

If a patient fails to meet the criteria for a listing, he or she may be judged to have an impairment or combination of impairments that "equals" a listing. The concept of "equals" can be applied in three different ways:

1. A patient may not have undergone the diagnostic tests described in the SSA listings but might be judged to have a listed impairment on the basis of alternative tests. For example, a patient might have received a diagnosis of osteoporosis on the basis of a bone densitometry study rather than the plain-film radiographs mentioned in the SSA listings.
2. A patient might have an impairment that is not listed but is believed to be as disabling as one that is listed by the adjudication team. For example, in the early 1980s AIDS was not a listed impairment, but would have been considered to equal a listing.
3. A patient could have a *combination* of impairments that are cumulatively as

disabling as a listed impairment, even though none of them taken in isolation is equal to a listing.

It is important that physicians be familiar with these listings; it will enable them to better assist their patients who are filing for SSD by identifying the medical documentation required by the system.*

Step 4

Can the claimant perform his or her relevant past work? Whereas steps 2 and 3 are based on strictly medical criteria, steps 4 and 5 consider medical findings, functional limitations, and vocational factors. Evaluators are asked to consider an applicant's age, educational level, past work history, and transferable skills.

As the term suggests, *residual functional capacity* (RFC) refers to the abilities that a patient still has despite his or her impairment. RFC is assessed by the DDS evaluating team on the basis of a paper review of a claimant's records. Evaluators fill out a standard form—either a Physical Residual Functional Capacity Assessment or a Mental Residual Functional Capacity Assessment—depending on the applicant's diagnosis. Treating and consulting physicians may also be asked to complete these forms, which address the physical ability of a claimant to walk, stand, sit, bend, climb, lift, and perform other physical activities. The ability of a claimant to perform various mental tasks is evaluated in any case in which a psychiatric impairment exists (including somatoform disorders). (Copies of these forms are included in Appendix 9–1; there may be slight differences among the various state agencies.)

Step 4 assesses whether a claimant with a documented impairment can return to his or her past relevant work.

Step 5

If the claimant cannot perform his or her past relevant work, can the claimant perform other work in the economy? It is here that SSD differs from most, if not all, other disability evaluations, especially the private disability arena. If a claimant can do other work, the adjudication team may determine that he or she is *not* disabled, depending on his or her age, education, literacy, ability to speak English, and past work experience. Functional restrictions are again considered at this step. An older person with little education is more likely to be found disabled under these rules than a younger person. The adjudicators determine whether the claimant's RFC, as well as age, education, and past work, allows him or her to work at any job that is available in the economy. Also considered are the numbers of jobs available locally, statewide, and nationally for each RFC. When applicants are denied at this step, the evaluating team typically identifies three different kinds of work that the applicant is judged to be capable of doing.

*See Appendix 9–2 for examples of listings of the adult impairments of musculoskeletal and neurological disorders. There are separate listings for children and additional listings for the other body systems. The handbook, *Disability Evaluation under Social Security,*[22] published by SSA, contains all the detailed listings and is available without charge from your local Social Security office, or by calling the SSA Public Information Distribution Center at 410-965-0945, or by writing to the U.S. Government Printing Office, Washington, DC, 20090, and asking for SSA Publication No. 64-039.

Outcomes of the Disability Determination Service Evaluation

The DDS team makes a determination that is forwarded to the SSA central office in Baltimore for final review. The central office does random audits, but rarely changes the decisions.

In addition to making a determination about whether disability benefits should be granted to an applicant, the DDS team may also recommend that the applicant receive vocational rehabilitation services. This recommendation can be made independent of whether the team supports a disability award for the applicant. When vocational rehabilitation is recommended, the local SSA office typically refers the patient to a state-run vocational rehabilitation agency.

Grants

When an applicant is awarded SSD benefits, there is a 5-month waiting period (benefits start 5 months after the documented onset of the disabling impairment). For SSI, the onset date is set administratively at the month of filing. For both, the evaluating team recommends how soon the patient should be re-evaluated after the benefits have been granted (the "diary"). (See p. 167 for discussion of continuing disability reviews.)

Denials

If SSD is denied on the initial evaluation by a DDS team, the claimant has several options for appeal. The sequence of appeals is as follows:

1. **Request for reconsideration:** In this situation, the applicant's file is reviewed again at the DDS office where the initial evaluation was done, and the 5-step process outlined earlier is followed. The only change in the evaluation process is that a different evaluating team is used, and the claimant may submit additional medical evidence.
2. **Request for a hearing before an administrative law judge (ALJ).** At the ALJ appeal level, the applicant is seen in person. The claimant may be accompanied by a spouse or other lay person who may testify. Also, an attorney typically represents the claimant, and may examine any witnesses present. The ALJ may seek additional medical evidence, may authorize additional examinations, and may invite consultants to the hearing to provide additional input (e.g., physicians, psychologists, and vocational rehabilitation counselors).
3. **Request for a review by the Appeals Council of the Office of Hearings and Appeals.** The evaluation at this level is a paper review, performed on appeal by the claimant of a denial by the ALJ; the emphasis is on procedural aspects of previous evaluations.
4. **The federal courts.** All of the above appeals occur within the SSA system (i.e., state agency adjudicators, ALJs, and members of the Appeals Council are all employees of the SSA). An applicant who is denied at all of the above levels can go outside the SSA system by filing an appeal in the federal courts. Appeals are submitted first to a U.S. District Court, then to the appropriate U.S. Circuit Court, and finally to the U.S. Supreme Court.

In addition to the above appeals, an applicant who has been denied benefits can file a new application for SSD or SSI at any time after a denial at the ALJ level. This starts the entire disability determination process over again.

Table 9–3 gives a flow chart of the approximate numbers of applicants who went through various appeals during 1995, and the outcomes of the appeals.

TABLE 9–3 Appeals of Disability Applications (SSD and SSI Combined—Fiscal Year 1995)

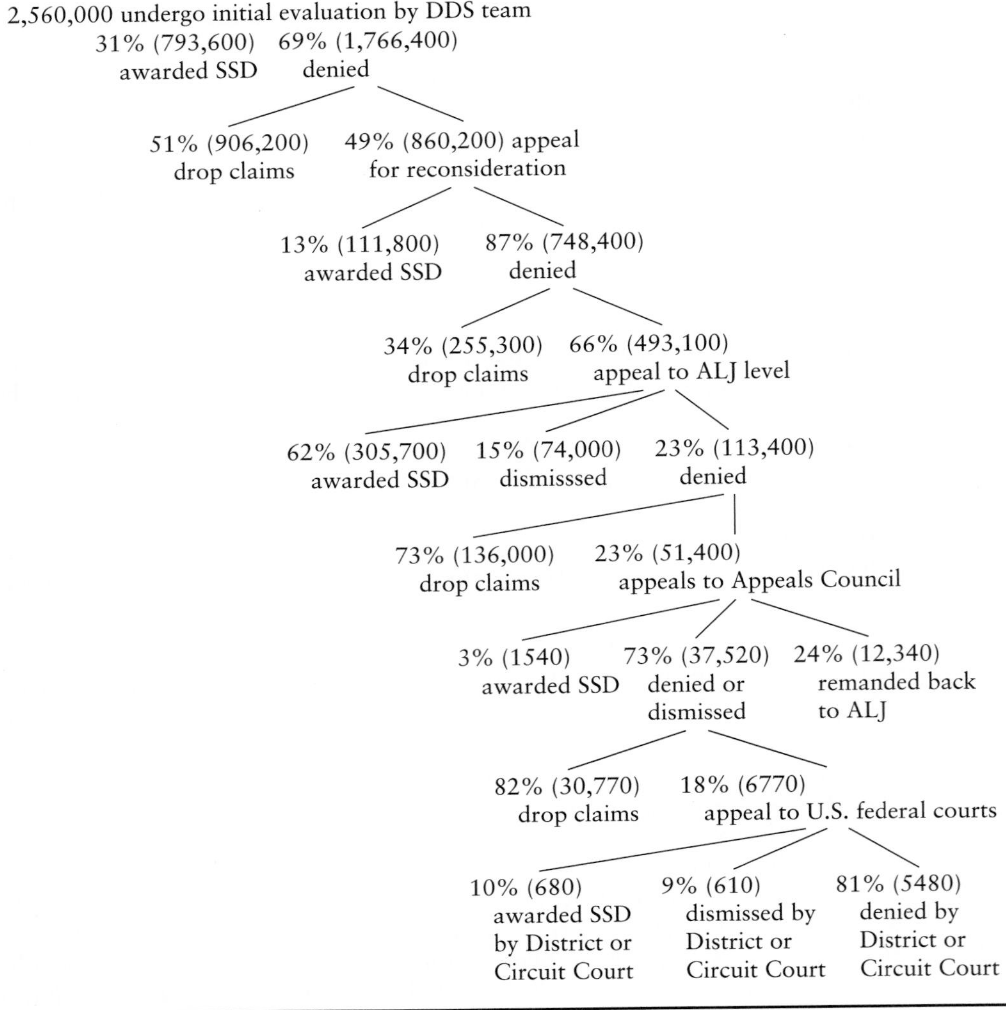

Approximately 47% of all judgments were favorable to applicants, of which 16% were awarded on appeal. Seventy-three percent of all successful appeals were awarded at the ALJ level.[4]

TERMINATION OF BENEFITS

Once a person has been granted SSD, he or she may exit the SSD system in one of four ways:

1. By death
2. By reaching the age of 65
3. By undergoing a continuing disability review (CDR) in which it is determined that he or she has shown significant medical improvement and is no longer eligible for disability
4. By returning to work

About 95% of SSD beneficiaries exit the system by routes 1 or 2: they either die or reach age 65, at which time they become eligible for old-age insurance (Social Security retirement).

Continuing disability reviews of SSD beneficiaries have been mandated by Congress. As the term suggests, the purpose of a continuing disability review (CDR) is to determine whether a beneficiary continues to be disabled enough to warrant SSD benefits. CDRs usually occur every 3 to 7 years, depending on the type of impairment; in cases in which the disability is expected to be shorter term, as with delayed fracture healing or renal transplants, the CDR may occur sooner.[17] CDRs also can be ordered if SSA staff get information that suggests a beneficiary has medically improved enough to be no longer disabled. Approximately 240,000 continuing disability reviews were performed during 1995, leading to termination of benefits for about 32,000 beneficiaries (13%).[4]

Congress and the SSA have repeatedly emphasized the importance of vocational rehabilitation for SSD and SSI beneficiaries. A recent SSA publication starts with the following:

> One of the Social Security Administration's highest priorities is to help beneficiaries with disabilities achieve a better and more independent lifestyle by helping them take advantage of employment opportunities.[18]

SSA provides the following incentives to encourage people on SSD to move out of the system by returning to gainful employment:

1. Access to vocational services. Originally, SSA paid for vocational services provided by state vocational rehabilitation departments. In recent years, regulations have changed so that SSA can also use the services of private vocational rehabilitation specialists.[4]
2. A 9-month trial work period (TWP) during which time the person receives SSD payments in addition to wages that he or she earns (see Table 9–1).
3. An extended period of eligibility (EPE) (see Table 9–1), which lasts 3 years in addition to the trial work period. During this interval, a person who has returned to work but has ceased to earn at SGA level can have SSD benefits reinstated without going through the formal application process and without the 5-month waiting period.
4. Continuation of Medicare benefits during the trial work period, the extended period of eligibility, and an additional 2 years. The overall result is that an individual is eligible for Medicare for 4 years after beginning the return-to-work process. (Patients receiving SSD benefits become eligible for Medicare in 2 years; see p. 169.)
5. Impairment-related work expenses (IRWE) (see Table 9–1). In reporting income for the purpose of determining "substantial gainful activity," individuals may deduct expenses that allow them to work despite disabilities (e.g., the cost of attendants, drugs, wheelchairs, medical devices). This applies to both SSD and SSI.

SSA is currently experimenting with new concepts designed to increase the likelihood of people who are receiving SSD or SSI returning to productivity.[7, 16] The federal budget for 1998 included funds for a pilot project in which an SSD or SSI beneficiary could choose a vocational rehabilitation provider from either the public sector (e.g., a state Department of Vocational Rehabilitation) or the private sector. If the beneficiary were successfully returned to employment, the provider would keep a share of the SSD or SSI benefits that the SSA no longer had to pay.[13]

MANAGING THE PATIENT WHO IS APPLYING FOR SOCIAL SECURITY DISABILITY

A physician who is knowledgeable about the SSD system is in a position to interact with the system in a more effective manner. Several practical points follow. These focus on the SSD application process, because this is the point at which a treating physician is most likely to be able to make an impact.

- It is important to note that the opinions of an applicant's treating physician can have a significant impact on SSA's response to the application for SSD. Federal courts have declared that the opinions of a treating physician should be given great weight in the evaluation of an applicant. Thus DDS evaluating teams will carefully consider a clear physician's statement about the ability of a patient to do work-related activities, backed by *objective* evidence of impairment. A key issue for a DDS evaluating team is whether a patient has a condition that meets an SSD listing. Criteria for listings are often stated in very specific terms, and evaluators look for these terms when they review applications. If a treating physician specifically mentions key findings, the application of the patient will more likely be approved at the DDS level.
- Applicants have the right to ask evaluators to consider information from all treating sources as well as from friends, co-workers, and relatives. This is the case even at the level of the initial DDS evaluation. Information from collateral sources can be very important in helping evaluators determine the amount of impairment associated with a medical condition.
- As noted earlier, DDS evaluators fill out a Residual Functional Capacities form for an applicant who does not have a condition that meets or equals a listing. The evaluators get information from a variety of sources when they fill out the forms. A treating physician can take a proactive step by sending information about an applicant's physical and/or psychological capacities and limitations to the local DDS office. (As noted, opinions provided by a treating physician are given special weight.)
- At the end of a DDS evaluation, the evaluating team is required to write a report that summarizes the rationale for its decision. An applicant has the right to get a copy of the report, and should request one.
- Many applicants seek the assistance of an attorney when they apply for SSD, and more do so at the appeals level. Legal aspects of SSD applications have been discussed in detail in R. C. Ruskell's book *Social Security Disability Claims, third edition.*[19]
- One crucial issue to evaluate is whether a patient's needs are likely to be well-served by SSD. First, SSD tends to be a "dead end" program in the sense that beneficiaries rarely return to competitive employment. Thus, as a practical matter, an individual who applies for SSD is, in effect, making a choice that will probably remove him or her permanently from the work force. Second, the payment levels for SSD are quite low (see Table 9–1). Thus a beneficiary may face financial hardship for the rest of his or her life. Finally, the process of seeking SSD may have adverse effects on a patient by reinforcing pain behaviors. Persons applying for SSD must convince others that they are incapacitated. There is a risk that in the course of trying to convince others, a patient may adapt to the role of a disabled person and later underestimate his or her potential for successful vocational functioning.[9, 10]

RELATIONSHIPS BETWEEN SOCIAL SECURITY DISABILITY, SUPPLEMENTAL SECURITY INCOME, MEDICARE, AND MEDICAID

Conceptually, SSD and SSI are different from Medicare and Medicaid, because the former are income-support programs whereas the latter are programs that pay for medical expenses. However, there are key links among these programs. Medicare and Medicaid were both established by Congress in 1965. Medicare was intended primarily as a health-insurance system for people age 65 or over. However, coverage is also available to individuals receiving SSD benefits. Specifically, a person who has been awarded SSD is eligible for Medicare 24 months after he or she becomes entitled to SSD.

Medicaid, like SSI itself, is a jointly financed program between the federal government and the states, and details of the program vary from state to state. It too is means-tested; individuals with assets or income above specified levels are ineligible. Federal law mandates that individuals on SSI also receive Medicaid, even though the roughly 5 million disabled people on SSI represent only a small fraction of total Medicaid beneficiaries.

Approximately 1.5 million disabled people below the age of 65 are eligible for both Medicare and Medicaid.[16] The rules for dual eligibility are complex, but, for example, a person who has been awarded SSD and also meets the means tests for Medicaid would be entitled to both types of coverage.

These links between SSD, SSI, Medicare, and Medicaid imply that an individual who meets SSA criteria for disability generally receives both income support and medical benefits.

ADEQUACY OF PAYMENTS

The SSD and SSI programs were established to protect Americans from financial devastation in the face of health problems that would render them incapable of working. Are the payments made to SSD and SSI beneficiaries adequate? From the standpoint of payment levels among beneficiaries, both the SSD and the SSI programs are fairly austere. Reno et al.[16] describe payments under the SSD program as follows:

> The modest level of DI (disability insurance) benefits can be appreciated by looking at their replacement rates (the level at which benefits replace prior earnings). Studies find that 75 to 80 percent of workers' prior earnings are needed to maintain their standard of living. DI provides much lower replacement rates than these. At average earnings and above, replacement rates range from 43 percent for a person earning $25,000 to about 26 percent for one earning $60,000. At lower earnings levels, say $15,000, benefits replace half the worker's prior earnings but are nonetheless below the poverty threshold."*

Because SSI payments average less than 60% of SSD payments, they could also be considered austere. Such statistics suggest that people do not get rich on SSD or SSI benefits, and workers take substantial cuts in income when they move from the workplace to SSD.

*From Reno VP, Mashaw JL, Gradison B (eds): Disability. Washington, DC, National Academy of Social Insurance, 1997, pp 18–19.

EPIDEMIOLOGY OF SOCIAL SECURITY DISABILITY

Trends Over Time

As of December 1995 there were 4.2 million SSD beneficiaries.[20] The average age of a beneficiary was 49.8 years. The average educational level of beneficiaries was substantially lower than that of the general population (e.g., only 16% had had some college education, compared with 45% in the general population).[4]

Data indicating trends over time need to be interpreted with caution because numbers are influenced by frequent congressional legislative directives. For example, the average age of a beneficiary dropped from about 59 years in 1958 to 50 years in 1995.[20] The interpretation of the drop is muddled, however, because before 1960 workers under the age of 50 were ineligible for SSD. Thus although there has been a real drop in the average age of beneficiaries during the past 30 years, it is much more modest than the total 9-year drop would suggest.

Overall trends in SSD applications and awards between 1970 and 1995 are shown in Table 9–4. Generally, it appears that SSD awards were made rather liberally during the 1970s, more stringently during the 1980s, and, again, with reversals in congressional directives, a return to more liberal allowances between 1991 and 1995.

The manner in which awards are granted has changed over the years in at least two respects. Between 1986 and 1993, there has been a substantial increase in the percentages of awards granted on the basis of vocational factors, as opposed to the more tightly defined medical criteria of meeting or equaling a listing.[15] Also, ALJs are playing a greater role in SSD awards. During the years from 1991 to 1995, the number of appeals was more than 50% greater than it had been from 1981 to 1985, and 70% of the decisions made by ALJs were favorable to applicants.[4]

The return-to-work record for SSD beneficiaries over the past 40 years has been dismal. Muller[12] found a recovery rate of less than 3% among a cohort followed for 10 years after receiving an SSD award. Hennessey and Dykacz[11] found lower termination rates for a cohort awarded SSD in 1985 than for a cohort awarded SSD in 1972. More recently, a report by SSA to Congress indicated that recovery rates were continuing to decline through 1994.[17]

TABLE 9–4 Trends Over Time in SSD Awards

Time period	No. of applications (in thousands)	No. of awards (in thousands)	Awards as % of applications	Awards per 1000 insured workers
1971–1975	5555	2491	45	6.3%
1976–1980	6102	2399	39	5.3%
1981–1985	5303	1719	32	3.2%
1986–1990	5298	2163	41	3.7%
1991–1995	6752	3098	46	5.0%

From Social Security Administration Office of Research, Evaluation and Statistics: Annual Statistical Supplement. Washington, DC, US Government Printing Office, 1996, p 285.

TABLE 9–5 Diagnoses of SSD Recipients—December, 1995

Diagnostic group	No. of recipients	Percentage
Infectious and parasitic diseases	85,700	2.1
Neoplasms	124,000	3.0
Endocrine, nutritional, and metabolic disease	182,000	4.4
Diseases of blood and blood-forming organs	10,700	0.3
Mental disorders (other than mental retardation)	1,069,000	25.9
Mental retardation	220,500	5.3
Diseases of		
Nervous system and sense organs	404,300	9.8
Circulatory system	553,400	12.9
Respiratory system	156,000	3.8
Digestive system	55,300	1.3
Genitourinary system	62,300	1.5
Skin and subcutaneous tissue	10,400	0.3
Musculoskeletal	879,000	21.3
Congenital anomalies	16,900	0.4
Injuries	244,100	5.9
Other	71,400	1.7
Total SSD Recipients With Diagnoses	4,125,300	100.0
Total SSD recipients	4,210,700	—

Medical Conditions Among Recipients of Social Security Disability

It is difficult to get detailed clinical information about SSD applicants or recipients. SSA uses very broad diagnostic categories that are given in Table 9–5. The table indicates that the three most common categories are mental disorders, musculoskeletal disorders, and circulatory disorders. It is impossible to determine, however, how many recipients had lumbar disk disorders or rheumatoid arthritis because individuals with either disorder would be coded as having diseases of the musculoskeletal system.

The prevalence of different kinds of medical conditions among SSD recipients varies substantially with the age of the recipients, as shown in Table 9–6. For example, 39.4% of recipients ages 30 to 39 have mental disorders, compared with 13.1% among recipients ages 60 to 64. As one would expect, musculoskeletal disorders are much more prominent among recipients ages 60 to 64 than among those ages 30 to 39.

EPIDEMIOLOGY OF SUPPLEMENTAL SECURITY INCOME

Trends Over Time

The total number of people receiving SSI for disability increased 56% from 1990 to 1995, from 3,080,982 to 4,802,709.[20] In part, the increase reflects the fact that many people receive SSI benefits when they are young, so they stay in the SSI system for many years. Because of this, the total number of beneficiaries during the 1990s reflects not only awards made during the 1990s, but also the

TABLE 9–6 Percentage Distribution of Diagnoses for SSD Recipients of Different Ages—December 1995

Diagnostic group	Percentage among all recipients	Percentage among recipients ages 30–39	Percentage among recipients ages 60–64
Infectious and parasitic diseases	2.1	4.9	0.8
Neoplasms	3.0	1.8	3.8
Endocrine, nutritional, and metabolic disease	4.4	3.4	4.4
Diseases of blood and blood-forming organs	0.3	0.5	0.1
Mental disorders (other than mental retardation)	25.9	39.4	13.1
Mental retardation	5.3	10.7	1.9
Diseases of			
Nervous system and sense organs	9.8	10.5	8.3
Circulatory system	12.9	2.8	23.8
Respiratory system	3.8	0.8	7.0
Digestive system	1.3	1.2	1.3
Genitourinary system	1.5	1.7	0.9
Skin and subcutaneous tissue	0.3	0.3	0.2
Musculoskeletal system	21.3	11.8	28.0
Congenital anomalies	0.4	0.4	0.4
Injuries	5.9	7.9	4.6
Other	1.7	1.9	1.4
Total	100.0	100.0	100.0

long-term effects of awards made during the 1970s and 1980s. A second factor is that the number of awards per year rose substantially between 1990 and 1995. Among adults, there was a 22% increase in the number of awards per year. Among children, the increase was 116%,[20] in large part the result of legislative liberalization of definitions for learning and behavior disorders.

Medical Conditions Among Recipients of Supplemental Security Income

Much of the difference in diagnostic profiles between SSI and SSD recipients can be attributed to the fact that SSI recipients are younger than SSD recipients. The average age for disabled SSI recipients in 1995 was 34.9 years, compared with 49.8 years for SSD recipients.

The most striking feature of the profile of diagnoses among disabled SSI recipients is that mental disorders dominate, with 59% of recipients having either mental retardation or a mental disorder other than mental retardation (Table 9–7). For example, approximately 10% of SSI recipients carry a diagnosis of schizophrenia. (People with chemical dependency are also included in the mental disorders group, although congressional amendments in 1996 preclude disability awards based solely on impairment from chemical dependency.)

As with SSD recipients, the diagnostic profile of SSI patients varies substantially with age (Table 9–8). In fact, comparison between Tables 9–4 and 9–6 indicates that at least among people in the 60 to 64 age group, SSD and SSI recipients are similar with respect to the frequency with which various groups of conditions occur.

STRAINS AND CONFLICTS WITH SOCIAL SECURITY DISABILITY AND SUPPLEMENTAL SECURITY INCOME

The SSA is in a difficult position as it attempts to administer the SSD and SSI programs. Decisions about who is sufficiently disabled to deserve societal aid are complex. The SSA must walk a fine line between those people who may be exaggerating disability and those who genuinely need help. Additionally, SSA must deal with the whims of the political process; the executive, legislative, and judicial branches of the federal government; and its own bureaucracy and lack of consistency.

These conflicts raise several ongoing issues:

- How can the SSA convert the vague mandates provided by Congress into

TABLE 9–7 Diagnoses Among People Receiving SSI Benefits—December 1995

Diagnostic group	No. of recipients	Percentage
Infectious and parasitic diseases	58,000	1.7
Neoplasms	47,700	1.4
Endocrine, nutritional, and metabolic disease	139,800	4.1
Diseases of blood and blood-forming organs	20,500	0.6
Mental disorders (other than mental retardation)	1,063,500	31.2
Mental retardation	937,400	27.5
Diseases of		
Nervous system and sense organs	313,600	9.2
Circulatory system	163,600	4.8
Respiratory system	88,600	2.6
Digestive system	23,900	0.7
Genitourinary system	30,700	0.9
Skin and subcutaneous tissue	6,800	0.2
Musculoskeletal system	225,000	6.6
Congenital anomalies	64,800	1.9
Injuries	85,200	2.5
Other	139,800	4.1
Total disabled SSI recipients with diagnoses	3,408,600	100.0
Total disabled SSI recipients	4,220,100	—

TABLE 9–8 Percentage Distribution of Diagnoses for SSI Recipients of Different Ages—December 1995

Diagnostic group	Percentage among all recipients	Percentage among recipients ages 30–39	Percentage among recipients ages 60–64
Infectious and parasitic diseases	1.7	3.4	1.0
Neoplasms	1.4	0.8	2.4
Endocrine, nutritional, and metabolic disease	4.1	3.2	8.0
Diseases of blood and blood-forming organs	0.6	0.6	0.1
Mental disorders (other than mental retardation)	31.2	39.4	20.0
Mental retardation	27.5	31.2	6.8
Diseases of			
Nervous system and sense organs	9.2	8.6	6.0
Circulatory system	4.8	1.6	18.8
Respiratory system	2.6	0.5	6.8
Digestive system	0.7	0.5	1.1
Genitourinary system	0.9	1.0	0.9
Skin and subcutaneous tissue	0.2	0.3	0.1
Musculoskeletal system	6.6	3.6	23.7
Congenital anomalies	1.9	0.9	0.3
Injuries	2.5	3.3	2.2
Other	4.1	1.1	1.7
Total	100.0	100.0	100.0

regulations and policies that can be administered uniformly throughout the country?

- How independent of the overall SSA system can administrative law judges be? Should they be conceptualized as administrators of SSA policy or as independent judges within the SSA system?
- How can SSA maintain uniformity and consistency in its policies in the face of rulings in federal district courts that apply to only some parts of the country?
- Is the SSA subservient to the federal courts, or can it be selective in accepting and implementing court rulings? These issues crop up repeatedly. For example, in late 1997 the SSA was involved in a controversy about SSI benefits for disabled children. It had interpreted the 1996 welfare reform act (The Personal Responsibility and Work Opportunity Reconciliation Act of 1996) as tightening the criteria for SSI eligibility for children, and had cut some 142,000 children from the SSI roles. By November of 1997, it was faced with criticism from children's advocates and a 57% reversal rate of its decisions among appealed cases.[5, 6] In response, the SSA agreed to reexamine the files of 60,000 children who had been denied benefits and to give new opportunities for appeal to 80,000 other families.

FINAL THOUGHTS

Experience during the past century has shown that disability programs are difficult to administer.[1] In common with other disability programs such as the workers' compensation programs, SSD and SSI could be faulted for being bureaucratic and for failing to distinguish clearly between disabled and non-disabled applicants. However, it is important to note some of the strengths of the SSD and SSI programs in comparison with workers' compensation programs and disability programs administered by private insurance companies.

A major strength is that some of the most difficult questions surrounding disability have been debated openly in relation to the SSA programs, whereas the same issues have not been given the same open, fair hearings in, for example, workers' compensation cases. Assessment of pain is an excellent example. The SSA has commissioned two detailed examinations of the role of pain in disability.[14, 17] Moreover, federal court decisions have contributed to a dialog about how pain should be considered in the evaluation of an SSD applicant. Interactions between the SSA and the courts lead to *Rulings and Acquiescences,* which is published periodically by the SSA.[24, 25] Ultimately, these rulings become codified in SSA regulations.[3]

A second strength of the SSD and SSI programs is that the SSA has given serious attention to the issues of reliability and validity of disability ratings with internal reviews of determinations at the initial and reconsideration levels. This is in contrast to other programs in which impairment or disability is assessed, such as workers' compensation systems, where no internal checks of reliability exist.

Finally, the SSA has gone further than other disability systems in supporting research on its beneficiaries. A steady stream of research is published in the *Social Security Bulletin*. A few of the workers' compensation systems have done outcome-based research on disabled workers,[2, 8] but their research is dwarfed by the efforts of the SSA.

The relative openness of the SSA, along with its attention to reliability of decisions and outcome-based research, creates the framework for a system that is self-correcting and responsive to the perceptions and preferences of Americans. Even the most ardent supporters of SSA would not argue that the agency has "solved" the problem of how to determine disability, but it has set up an infrastructure that makes improvement possible and measurable.

ACKNOWLEDGEMENTS

Hon. Susan Blaney, Administrative Law Judge, Kansas City, Kansas, reviewed the 5-step application process and provided helpful clarification to same.

REFERENCES

1. Berkowitz ED: Disability insurance and the social security tradition. In: Nash GD, Pugach NH, Tomasson RF (eds): Social Security: The First Half-Century. Albuquerque, University of New Mexico Press, 1988.
2. Cheadle A, Franklin G, Wolfhagen C, et al: Factors influencing the duration of work-related disability: A population-based study of Washington State workers' compensation. Am J Public Health 84(2):190–196, 1994.

3. Code of Federal Regulations, Title 20. Parts 400 to 499; paragraph 404, 1529. Washington, DC, US Government Printing Office, 1997.
4. Committee on Ways and Means, US House of Representatives: 1996 Green Book. Washington, DC, US Government Printing Office, 1996.
5. Disabled Children Denied Aid to Get New Chance, US Says. New York Times, Dec. 18, 1997.
6. Disabled Youths Are Wrongly Cut From Aid Program. New York Times, November 16, 1997.
7. Ferrell D: Director of Public Affairs, Seattle Regional Office, Social Security Administration. Personal Communication, November, 1997.
8. Franklin GM, Haug J, Heyer NJ, et al: Outcome of lumbar fusion in Washington State workers' compensation. Spine 19(17):1897–1904, 1994.
9. Hadler NM: Disability determination and the social conscience. Arthritis Care Res 9:163–169, 1996.
10. Hadler NM: If you have to prove you are ill, you can't get well: The object lesson of fibromyalgia. Spine 21:2397–2400, 1996.
11. Hennessey JC, Dykacz JM: A comparison of the recovery termination rates of disabled-worker beneficiaries entitled in 1972 and 1985. Soc Secur Bull 56(2): 58–69, 1993.
12. Muller LS: Disability beneficiaries who work and their experience under program work incentives. Soc Secur Bull 55(2):2–19, 1992.
13. Office of Management and Budget: Budget of the United States Government: Fiscal Year 1998. Washington, DC, US Government Printing Office, 1997.
14. Osterweis M, Kleinman A, Mechanic D (eds): Pain and Disability. Washington, DC, National Academy Press, 1987.
15. Quadagno J: Incentives to disability in federal disability insurance and supplemental security income. Clin Orthop Rel Res 336:11, 1997.
16. Reno VP, Mashaw JL, Gradison B (eds): Disability. Washington, DC, National Academy of Social Insurance, 1997.
17. Report to Congress on rising cost of Social Security Disability Insurance Benefits. Soc Secur Bull 59(1):67, 1996.
18. Rupp K, Scott CG: Length of stay on the Supplemental Security Income Disability Program. Soc Secur Bull 58(1):29–47, 1995.
19. Ruskell RC: Social Security Disability Claims, 3rd ed. Norcross, Ga, The Harrison Company, 1993.
20. Social Security Administration Office of Research, Evaluation and Statistics: Annual Statistical Supplement. Washington, DC, US Government Printing Office, 1996.
21. Social Security Administration Office of Research, Evaluation and Statistics. Social Security Programs in the United States (SSA Pub No. 13-11758). Washington, DC, US Government Printing Office, 1997.
22. Social Security Administration: Disability Evaluation Under Social Security (SSA Pub No. 64-039). Washington, DC, US Government Printing Office, 1994.
23. Social Security Administration: Report of the Commission on the Evaluation of Pain. (SSA Pub No. 64-031). Washington, DC, US Government Printing Office, 1987.
24. Social Security Administration: Social Security Ruling 96-3p. 61 Federal Register, #128 (2 July 1996), p 34468–34470.
25. Social Security Administration: Social Security Ruling 96-7p. 61 Federal Register, #128 (2 July 1996). p 34483–34488.
26. Stine F: Director, Renton Office, Division of Disability Determination Services. Personal communication, November, 1997.

APPENDIX 9-1

Examples of Forms Used for Physical and Mental Capacity Assessments

MEDICAL ASSESSMENT OF ABILITY TO DO WORK-RELATED ACTIVITIES (PHYSICAL)

____

Name of Individual | Social Security Number

____

(Please Print or Type)

To determine this individual's ability to do work-related activities on a day-to-day basis in a regular work setting, please give us an assessment--BASED ON YOUR EXAMINATION--of how the individual's physical capabilities are affected by the impairments(s). Consider the medical history, the chronicity of findings (or lack thereof), and the expected duration of any work-related limitations, but not the individual's age, sex, or work experience.

For each activity shown below:

(1) Check the appropriate block

(2) Respond to the questions concerning the individual's ability to perform the activity; and

(3) Identify the particular medical findings (i.e., physical exam findings, x-ray findings, laboratory test results, history, symptoms (including pain), etc.) which support your assessment of any limitations.

IT IS IMPORTANT THAT YOU RELATE PARTICULAR MEDICAL FINDINGS TO ANY ASSESSED REDUCTION IN CAPACITY. tHE USEFULNESS OF YOUR ASSESSMENT DEPENDS ON THE EXTENT TO WHICH YOU DO THIS.

I. Are LIFTING/CARRYING affected by impairment?

What are the medical findings that support this assessment?

( ) No
( ) Yes

If "yes" how many pounds can the individual lift and/or carry?

Maximum Occasionally (from very little up to 1/3 of an 8-hour day) ______________

Maximum Frequently (from 1/3 to 2/3 of an 8-hour day) ______________

II. Are STANDING/WALKING affected by impairment?

What are the medical findings that support this assessment?

( ) No
( ) Yes

If "yes," how many hours in an 8-hour workday can the individual stand and/or walk: total? ______________

without interruption? ______________

Form SSA-1151 (4/84) TEST (OVER)

III. Is SITTING affected by impairment?

( ) No
( ) Yes

If "yes," how many hours in an 8-hour workday can the individual sit: total? ____________

without interruption? ____________

What are the medical findings that support this assessment?

IV. How often can the individual perform the following POSTURAL ACTIVITIES?

	Frequently	*Occasionally	*Never
Climb			
Balance			
Stoop			
Crouch			
Kneel			
Crawl			

What are the medical findings that support this assessment?

*Frequently: from 1/3 to 2/3 of an 8-hour day.
*Occassionally: from very little up to 1/3 of an 8-hour day.

V. Are the following PHYSICAL FUNCTIONS affected by the impairment?

	No	Yes
Reaching		
Handling		
Feeling		
Pushing/Pulling		
Seeing		
Hearing		
Speaking		

A. How are these physical functions affected?

B. What are the medical findings that support this assessment?

VI. Are there ENVIRONMENTAL RESTRICTIONS caused by the impairment?

	No	Yes
Heights		
Moving Machinery		
Temperature Extremes		
Chemicals		
Dust		
Noise		
Fumes		
Humidity		
Vibration		
Other		

A. How do the checked restrictions affect the individual's activities?

B. What are the medical findings that support this assessment?

Continued on following page

VII. State any other work-related activities which are affected by the impairment, and indicate how the activities are affected. What are the medical findings that support this assessment?

____
(Signature)

____
(Title/Medical Specialty)

____
(Date)

FORM APPROVED
OMB NO. 0960-0431

MENTAL RESIDUAL FUNCTIONAL CAPACITY ASSESSMENT

NAME

SOCIAL SECURITY NUMBER

CATEGORIES *(From IB of the PRTF)*

ASSESSMENT IS FOR:

☐ Current Evaluation

☐ 12 Months After Onset: ______ *(Date)*

☐ Date Last Insured: ______ *(Date)*

☐ Other: ______ *(Date)* to ______ *(Date)*

I. SUMMARY CONCLUSIONS

This section is for recording summary conclusions derived from the evidence in file. Each mental activity is to be evaluated within the context of the individual's capacity to sustain that activity over a normal workday and workweek, on an ongoing basis. Detailed explanation of the degree of limitation for each category (A through D), as well as any other assessment information you deem appropriate, is to be recorded in Section III (Functional Capacity Assessment).

If rating category 5 is checked for any of the following items, you MUST specify in Section II the evidence that is needed to make the assessment. If you conclude that the record is so inadequately documented that no accurate functional capacity assessment can be made, indicate in Section II what development is necessary, but DO NOT COMPLETE SECTION III.

	Not Significantly Limited	Moderately Limited	Markedly Limited	No Evidence of Limitation in this Category	Not Ratable on Available Evidence
A. UNDERSTANDING AND MEMORY					
1. The ability to remember locations and work-like procedures.	1. ☐	2. ☐	3. ☐	4. ☐	5. ☐
2. The ability to understand and remember very short and simple instructions.	1. ☐	2. ☐	3. ☐	4. ☐	5. ☐
3. The ability to understand and remember detailed instructions.	1. ☐	2. ☐	3. ☐	4. ☐	5. ☐
B. SUSTAINED CONCENTRATION AND PERSISTENCE					
4. The ability to carry out very short and simple instructions.	1. ☐	2. ☐	3. ☐	4. ☐	5. ☐
5. The ability to carry out detailed instructions.	1. ☐	2. ☐	3. ☐	4. ☐	5. ☐
6. The ability to maintain attention and concentration for extended periods.	1. ☐	2. ☐	3. ☐	4. ☐	5. ☐
7. The ability to perform activities within a schedule, maintain regular attendance, and be punctual within customary tolerances.	1. ☐	2. ☐	3. ☐	4. ☐	5. ☐
8. The ability to sustain an ordinary routine without special supervision.	1. ☐	2. ☐	3. ☐	4. ☐	5. ☐
9. The ability to work in coordination with or proximity to others without being distracted by them.	1. ☐	2. ☐	3. ☐	4. ☐	5. ☐
10. The ability to make simple work-related decisions.	1. ☐	2. ☐	3. ☐	4. ☐	5. ☐

Continued on following page

	Not Significantly Limited	Moderately Limited	Markedly Limited	No Evidence of Limitation in this Category	Not Ratable on Available Evidence
Continued—SUSTAINED CONCENTRATION AND PERSISTENCE					
11. The ability to complete a normal work-day and workweek without interruptions from psychologically based symptoms and to perform at a consistent pace without an unreasonable number and length of rest periods.	1. ☐	2. ☐	3. ☐	4. ☐	5. ☐
C. SOCIAL INTERACTION					
12. The ability to interact appropriately with the general public.	1. ☐	2. ☐	3. ☐	4. ☐	5. ☐
13. The ability to ask simple questions or request assistance.	1. ☐	2. ☐	3. ☐	4. ☐	5. ☐
14. The ability to accept instructions and respond appropriately to criticism from supervisors.	1. ☐	2. ☐	3. ☐	4. ☐	5. ☐
15. The ability to get along with coworkers or peers without distracting them or exhibiting behavioral extremes.	1. ☐	2. ☐	3. ☐	4. ☐	5. ☐
16. The ability to maintain socially appropriate behavior and to adhere to basic standards of neatness and cleanliness.	1. ☐	2. ☐	3. ☐	4. ☐	5. ☐
D. ADAPTATION					
17. The ability to respond appropriately to changes in the work setting.	1. ☐	2. ☐	3. ☐	4. ☐	5. ☐
18. The ability to be aware of normal hazards and take appropriate precautions.	1. ☐	2. ☐	3. ☐	4. ☐	5. ☐
19. The ability to travel in unfamiliar places or use public transportation.	1. ☐	2. ☐	3. ☐	4. ☐	5. ☐
20. The ability to set realistic goals or make plans independently of others.	1. ☐	2. ☐	3. ☐	4. ☐	5. ☐

II. REMARKS: If you checked box 5 for any of the preceding items or if any other documentation deficiencies were identified, you MUST specify what additional documentation is needed. Cite the item number(s), as well as any other specific deficiency, and indicate the development to be undertaken.

☐ Continued on Page 3

☐ Continued on Page 4

III. FUNCTIONAL CAPACITY ASSESSMENT

Record in this section the elaborations on the preceding capacities. Complete this section ONLY after the SUMMARY CONCLUSIONS section has been completed. Explain your summary conclusions in narrative form. Include any information which clarifies limitation or function. Be especially careful to explain conclusions that differ from those of treating medical sources or from the individual's allegations.

☐ Continued on Page 4

MEDICAL CONSULTANT'S SIGNATURE	DATE

Continued on following page

Continuation Sheet—Indicate section(s) being continued.

Paperwork/Privacy Act Notice: The information requested on this form is authorized by Section 223 and Section 1633 of the Social Security Act. The information provided will be used in making a decision on this claim. Failure to complete this form may result in a delay in processing the claim. Information furnished on this form may be disclosed by the Social Security Administration to another person or governmental agency only with respect to Social Security programs and to comply with federal laws requiring the exchange of information between Social Security and other agencies.

TIME IT TAKES TO COMPLETE THIS FORM: We estimate that it will take you about 20 minutes to complete this form. This includes the time it will take to read the instructions, gather the necessary facts and fill out the form. If you have comments or suggestions on how long it takes to complete this form or on any other aspect of this form, write to the Social Security Administration, ATTN: Reports Clearance Officer, 1-A-21 Operations Bldg., Baltimore, MD 21235, and to the Office of Management and Budget, Paperwork Reduction Project (0960-0431), Washington, D.C. 20503.

APPENDIX 9–2

Examples of Listings of Adult Impairments of Musculoskeletal and Neurological Disorders

LISTING OF IMPAIRMENTS*

Part A (applicable to individuals age 18 and over and to children under age 18 where criteria are appropriate)

Sec 1.00	MUSCULOSKELETAL SYSTEM†
1.01	CATEGORY OF IMPAIRMENTS, MUSCULOSKELETAL
1.02	*Active rheumatoid arthritis and other inflammatory arthritis*
1.03	*Arthritis of a major weight-bearing joint (due to any cause)*
1.04	*Arthritis of one major joint in each of the upper extremities (due to any cause)*
1.05	*Disorders of the spine*
1.08	*Osteomyelitis or septic arthritis (established by X-ray)*
1.09	*Amputation or anatomical deformity*
1.10	*Amputation of one lower extremity (at or above the tarsal region)*
1.11	*Fracture of the femur, tibia, tarsal bone, or pelvis*
1.12	*Fracture of an upper extremity*
1.13	*Soft tissue injury of an upper or lower extremity*
Sec 11.00	NEUROLOGICAL‡
11.01	CATEGORY OF IMPAIRMENTS, NEUROLOGICAL
11.02	*Epilepsy: major motor seizures (grand mal or psychomotor), documented by EEG and by detailed description of a typical seizure pattern, including all associated phenomena; occurring more frequently than once a month, in spite of at least 3 months of prescribed treatment*
11.03	*Epilepsy: minor motor seizures (petit mal, psychomotor, or focal), documented by EEG and by detailed description of a typical seizure pattern, including all associated phenomena; occurring more frequently than once weekly in spite of at least 3 months of prescribed treatment*
11.04	*Central nervous system vascular accident*

*For each italicized listing, specific criteria are provided (not listed here) whereby the condition of disability can be met. The reader is referred to the complete listings for further information.

†Social Security Administration: Disability Evaluation Under Social Security (SSA Pub No. 64-039). Washington, DC, US Government Printing Office, 1994, p 16–20.

‡Op cit. pp 62–67.

11.05 *Brain tumors*
11.06 *Parkinsonian syndrome*
11.07 *Cerebral palsy*
11.08 *Spinal cord or nerve root lesions, due to any cause*
11.09 *Multiple sclerosis*
11.10 *Amyotrophic lateral sclerosis*
11.11 *Anterior poliomyelitis*
11.12 *Myasthenia gravis*
11.13 *Muscular dystrophy*
11.14 *Peripheral neuropathies*
11.15 *Tabes dorsalis*
11.16 *Subacute combined cord degeneration (pernicious anemia) with disorganization of motor function . . . not significantly improved by prescribed treatment*
11.17 *Degenerative diseases not listed elsewhere, such as Huntington's chorea, Friedreich's ataxia, and spino-cerebellar degeneration*
11.18 *Cerebral trauma*
11.19 *Syringomyelia*

CHAPTER 10

Disability Evaluation Under the Department of Veterans Affairs

Steven Oboler, MD

The Department of Veterans Affairs (VA) was established in 1930 as the Veterans Administration, when Congress authorized President Herbert Hoover to "consolidate and coordinate government activities affecting war veterans." In 1946 the Department of Medicine and Surgery (now the Veterans Health Administration [VHA]) was established to provide health-care services to eligible veterans. In 1953 the Department of Veterans Benefits (now the Veterans Benefits Administration [VBA]) was created to administer the GI Bill and the VA's compensation and pension programs. On March 15, 1989 the Veterans Administration became the Department of Veterans Affairs, the fourteenth department in the president's cabinet.

By 1996 the VHA operated 173 medical centers, more than 375 outpatient clinics, 134 nursing homes, and 39 domiciliaries, which are located in all 50 states, the Philippines, and Puerto Rico. The VHA is responsible for conducting examinations required for the adjudication of claims for VA benefits.[37] The VBA operates 58 regional offices, with at least one in every state, and is responsible for administering a wide variety of Congressionally authorized benefits programs, including disability compensation and pension (the focus of this chapter), burial assistance, rehabilitation assistance, education and training assistance, home-loan guarantees, life-insurance coverage, and special benefits for homeless veterans.[41]

Total compensation and pension expenditures for the Department of Veterans Affairs for 1996 were estimated to be $18,152,769,000.[40] In 1997 there were an estimated 25,422,900 veterans, of whom 2,256,700 (8.9%) were receiving service-connected benefits. Assuming there are no wars, these figures are estimated to be 17,930,200 veterans and 1,818,830 receiving service-connected benefits by the year 2015.[74] The number of veterans receiving compensation (actual and projected) by period of military service between 1990 and 2015 is shown in Fig. 10–1; in 1996, Vietnam veterans exceeded World War II veterans as the largest group receiving compensation benefits.[72]

Unlike Social Security, insurance, and workers' compensation benefit programs, there is no "finality" to the VA disability claims adjudication process. As long as certain limited criteria are met, veterans can file and refile, with claims for survivor benefits often extending the process for years after a veteran's death. Repeat claims, which outnumber original claims by an almost three to one margin, dominate the VA adjudication and appeals system. The 1996 *Report to Congress* by the Veterans' Claims Adjudication Commission projected that even if the VA received no new compensation claims for the next 20 years, the volume of repeat claims in 2015 would be at least 55% of the 1995 level.[73] During

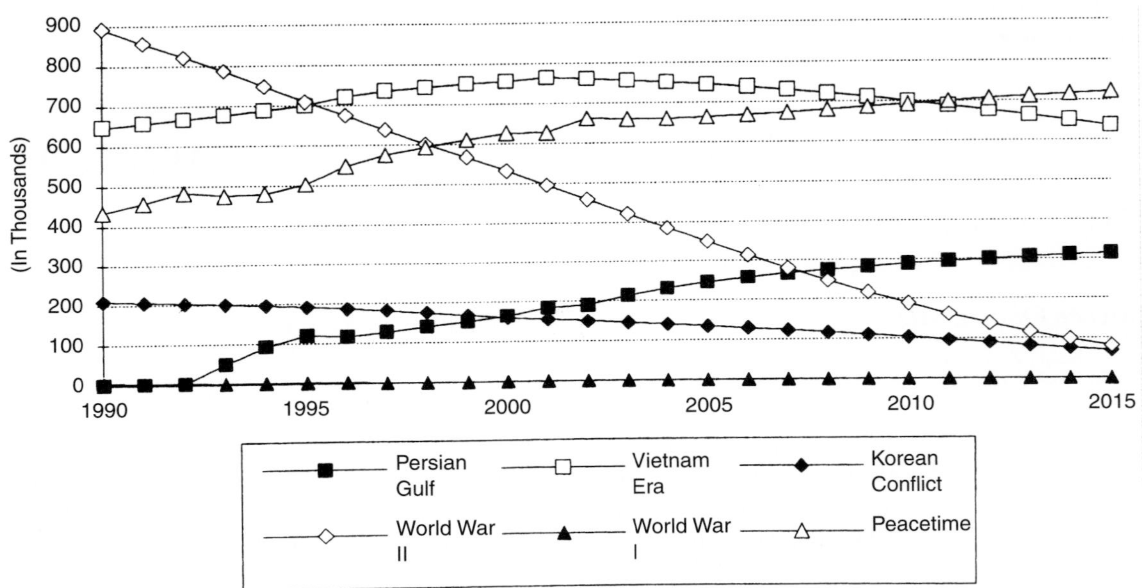

FIGURE 10–1
Numbers of veterans receiving compensation (actual and projected) by period of service from 1990 to 2015. (From Veterans Claims Adjudication Commission: Report to Congress, December 1996. Pub No. 1997-516-422/83512, Washington, DC, US Government Printing Office, 1997, p 39.)

1996, there were a total of 266,938 visits to VA facilities specifically for compensation and pension (C&P) examinations.[60] As the VA reorganizes, more and more C&P examinations are being done under fee-base, contract, and other off-site arrangements with community practitioners.

WHO IS ELIGIBLE?

VA benefit eligibility, including disability, is based on discharge from active military service under other than dishonorable conditions. *Active service* means full-time service as a member of the Army, Navy, Air Force, Marines, or Coast Guard, or as a commissioned officer of the Public Health Service, the Environmental Services Administration, or the National Oceanic and Atmospheric Administration. *Honorable* and *general* discharges qualify a veteran for VA benefits, whereas *dishonorable* and *bad-conduct* discharges issued by general court-martial bar VA benefits. Veterans in prisons and parolees may be eligible for some VA benefits.[5]

Disability Compensation

Disability compensation is monthly monetary benefits paid to veterans who are disabled by injury or disease incurred or aggravated during active military service. Compensation may also be paid for diseases or injuries suffered as a result of VA hospitalization, medical or surgical treatment, or vocational rehabilitation training.[15] Decisions on entitlement to compensation are determined by the Adjudication Division of the Compensation and Pension Service of the VBA. Veterans with residuals of conditions determined by adjudication to be related to injuries or diseases incurred or aggravated while on active duty or as a result of VA care are referred to as *service connected;* illnesses and injuries determined not to have been incurred or aggravated while on active duty are referred to as being *non-service connected.* The amount of monetary benefits a veteran receives depends on the amount of impairment caused by an injury or disease, with the rating percentages representing the "average impairment in earning capacity resulting from such disease and injuries and their residual conditions in civil[ian] occupations."[16] Disability compensation is not subject to state or federal income tax, is adjusted by Congress to reflect changes in cost of living, and varies with the number of dependents. Compensation rates effective December 1, 1998,[71] for a single veteran without dependents, are shown in Table 10–1.

Disability Pensions

Veterans with low incomes may be eligible for monthly monetary support if they have 90 days or more of active military service, 1 day of which was during a period of war. The veteran must be *permanently and totally disabled.* Non-service–connected pensions are not payable to those who have assets that can be used to provide adequate maintenance[6]; Table 10–2 shows pension rates effective December 1, 1998 for a variety of situations. Payments shown are reduced by the amount of countable income of the veteran and the income of any spouse or dependent children.[70]

Presumptive Service Connection

A number of chronic diseases (e.g., hypertension, diabetes mellitus, peptic ulcer disease, arthritis) and tropical diseases (e.g., malaria, amebiasis, dysentery) are eligible for presumptive service connection if the diseases become manifest to a degree of 10% or more within 1 year of discharge from active duty, even if there is no record of the condition during service (3 years for leprosy and tuberculosis and 7 years for multiple sclerosis).[7] In addition, ongoing research involving

TABLE 10–1 1999 VA Disability Compensation Rates

Disability (%)	Monthly rate ($)
10	96
20	184
30	282
40	404
50	576
60	726
70	916
80	1062
90	1196
100	1989

From Federal Benefits for Veterans and Dependents, 1999 ed. VA pamphlet 80-99-1. Washington, DC, Dept of Veterans Affairs, 1999, p 59.

TABLE 10–2 1999 VA Disability Pension Rates

Status	Maximum annual rate ($)
Veteran without dependent spouse or child	8778
Veteran with one dependent spouse or child	11,497
Veteran permanently housebound with no dependents	10,729
Veteran permanently housebound with one dependent	13,448
Veteran in need of aid and attendance with no dependents	14,647
Veteran in need of aid and attendance with one dependent	17,365
Increase for each additional dependent child	1496

From Federal Benefits for Veterans and Dependents, 1999 ed. VA pamphlet 80-99-1. Washington, DC, Dept of Veterans Affairs, 1999, p 59.

several groups of veterans, including former prisoners of war, Vietnam veterans exposed to toxic herbicides (Agent Orange), and veterans exposed to ionizing radiation, has identified a number of long-term medical and psychiatric conditions that occur more frequently in these groups, for which presumptive service connection is available.

Former Prisoners of War

The VA has long recognized the special hardships associated with prisoner-of-war (POW) confinement, and has conducted longitudinal studies of the health status of former POWs after World War II and the Korean conflict.[3] As a result of these and other studies from the United States and abroad, the list of presumptively service-connected conditions continues to expand. For example, severely malnourished POWs, with a history of localized edema (possibly related to thiamine deficiency [beriberi]) were found to have an increased risk for the subsequent development of ischemic heart disease.[62, 63] Recent Congressional legislation now provides former POWs who had at least 30 days of captivity presumptive service-connection for ischemic heart disease, even though this condition usually does not develop until many years after the veteran leaves military service. The list of presumptively service-connected conditions for former POWs follows[8]:

Avitaminosis
Any anxiety disorder (including posttraumatic stress disorder)
Beriberi (including ischemic heart disease in former POWs with a history of localized edema during captivity)
Chronic dysentery
Cold injuries
Dysthymic disorder (or any depressive disorder)
Helminthiasis
Irritable bowel syndrome
Malnutrition (including optic atrophy)

Pellagra
Peptic ulcer disease
Peripheral neuropathies
Posttraumatic arthritis
Psychosis

Agent Orange

Between 1962 and 1971, U.S. military forces sprayed nearly 19 million gallons of herbicides in Vietnam. The preparation known as *Agent Orange*—named for the orange identification band on storage drums—accounted for approximately 11.2 million gallons. Herbicides were used to defoliate the jungle canopy that concealed enemy troops, to destroy enemy crops, and to clear vegetation around U.S. bases. Spraying with Agent Orange was suspended in 1970 after a report that one of the primary herbicide components—2,4,5-trichlorophenoxyacetic acid—could cause birth defects in laboratory animals. Use of other herbicides, including picloram and cacodylic acid, was stopped in 1971. By the time the United States withdrew its last troops in May 1975, some 3 million U.S. men and women had served in Vietnam. Over the past 25 years research studies from around the world have identified a number of medical conditions that occur more frequently in those exposed to the herbicides used in Vietnam. Although the VA recognized several conditions as being presumptively service connected in the years after the end of the Vietnam War, this list was greatly expanded after a 1994 report by the Institute of Medicine of the National Academy of Sciences, which found *statistically sufficient associations* between herbicide exposures and the subsequent development of soft-tissue sarcomas, non-Hodgkin's lymphomas, Hodgkin's disease, chloracne, and porphyria cutanea tarda. In addition, the Institute of Medicine reported *limited/suggestive evidence of an association* between herbicide exposure and the development of respiratory cancers (lung, larynx, and trachea), prostate cancer, and multiple myeloma.[31] Because of the government's inability to determine an accepted "exposure index" for U.S. forces possibly exposed to herbicides, the VA currently grants presumptive service connection to any eligible veteran with documented land, air, or naval (including offshore waters) service in Vietnam between January 9, 1962 and May 7, 1975. At present, the VA recognizes 12 conditions as being presumptively service connected for veterans who served in Vietnam[10]:

Acute and subacute peripheral neuropathy*
Chloracne (or other acneform disease consistent with chloracne)*
Hodgkin's disease
Multiple myeloma
Non-Hodgkin's lymphomas
Porphyria cutanea tarda*
Prostate cancer
Respiratory cancers (cancer of the lung, bronchus, larynx, or trachea)†
Soft-tissue sarcomas (other than osteosarcoma, chondrosarcoma, Kaposi's sarcoma, or mesothelioma)

*Must be diagnosed within 1 year of last service in Vietnam.
†Must be diagnosed within 30 years of last service in Vietnam.

Ionizing Radiation

From the first atomic explosion in July 1945 at White Sands, New Mexico until the Nuclear Test Ban Treaty went into effect in August 1963, the United States conducted over 230 atmospheric and underwater nuclear explosions, involving at least 210,000 military participants. Despite the awesome destructive power of nuclear weapons and the increased morbidity and mortality among survivors of Hiroshima and Nagasaki, there were no long-term efforts to monitor the health status of U.S. military personnel exposed to low levels of ionizing radiation until the 1980s.[69] Anecdotal reports of increases in thyroid abnormalities, leukemia, and other malignancies in the late 1970s resulted in a number of reports in the early 1980s on the health status of both military and civilian populations exposed to ionizing radiation, many with conflicting conclusions.[4, 54, 55, 58] Congressional legislation authorized the VA to treat veterans exposed to ionizing radiation, and compensation benefits were authorized in the late 1980s. Currently veterans exposed to ionizing radiation as a result of participation in atmospheric or underwater detonation of nuclear devices between 1945 and 1962, and those who were stationed in Hiroshima or Nagasaki, Japan between August 1945 and July 1946 or were interned near these cities as POWs, may be presumptively service connected for the following conditions[9]:

Leukemia (other than chronic lymphocytic leukemia)
Breast cancer
Cancer of the gallbladder or bile ducts
Cancer of the small intestine
Cancer of the urinary tract
Esophageal cancer
Lymphoma (except Hodgkin's disease)
Multiple myeloma
Pancreatic cancer
Pharyngeal cancer
Primary liver cancer (except if cirrhosis or hepatitis B is indicated)
Salivary gland cancer
Stomach cancer
Thyroid cancer

Claims for service connection for other conditions claimed by the veteran to be related to ionizing radiation exposure will also be considered by the VA, but such claims must be reviewed in terms of the likelihood that the size and nature of the radiation exposure caused the claimed condition, rather than approved on simple presumption.[11]

Mustard Gas

Although they were never used, during World War II both sides produced millions of tons of chemical weapons. The United States established secret research programs to develop both better chemical weapons and better methods of protection against these weapons. Some of this research focused on the development of protective clothing and skin ointments, which could prevent or lessen the severe blistering effects of mustard agents (sulfur and nitrogen mustard) and Lewisite (an arsenic-containing compound). By the end of World War II, an estimated 60,000 U.S. servicemen had been used as human subjects in this chemical-defense research program. At least 4000 of these subjects were exposed to high concentrations of mustard agents or Lewisite in gas chambers or in field exercises over contaminated ground. Participants were given little or no information about the nature or possible long-term effects; record-keeping was minimal to nonexistent. Public attention was finally drawn to these experiments when some of the exposed veterans began to seek compensation from the VA for health problems they believed were caused by exposure to mustard gas or Lewisite. In 1991 the VA requested the Institute of Medicine of the National Academy of Sciences to convene a committee to survey the scientific and medical literature regarding the long-term health effects of these agents. The committee's findings were released in 1993,[64] and the VA now awards presumptive service connection for the following conditions related to blistering agent–exposure while on active duty[12]:

Chronic conjunctivitis
Acute nonlymphocytic leukemia
Asthma
Chronic bronchitis
Chronic laryngitis
Chronic obstructive pulmonary disease
Corneal opacities
Emphysema
Keratitis
Laryngeal cancer
Lung cancer (except mesothelioma)
Nasopharyngeal cancer
Scar formation
Squamous cell cancer of the skin

Gulf War Veterans

Between August 1990 and March 1991, the United States deployed 697,000 troops to the Persian Gulf region in response to Iraq's invasion of Kuwait. Many troops were exposed to a variety of potentially adverse substances, including oil-well fires, fumes and smoke from military operations, toxic paints, depleted uranium, chemoprophylactic agents, and multiple immunizations. In addition, some troops, possibly over 100,000, were potentially exposed to unknown quantities of chemical and possibly biological warfare agents released from Iraqi production and storage facilities destroyed by coalition forces. Although fewer than 150 Americans died during the 6-week war and most troops left the Gulf area by May 1991, there have been persistent reports of adverse health effects among both U.S. and other coalition forces. The most commonly reported symptoms have been fatigue, headaches, joint pains, skin rashes, shortness of breath, sleep disturbances, difficulty concentrating, and forgetfulness. These symptoms have not been localized to any one organ system, and there have been no consistent physical or laboratory abnormalities pointing toward a single specific disease or syndrome.[56, 65] Although there are no chronic medical conditions that have been found to occur with increased frequency among veterans who served in southwest Asia during the Gulf War, in November 1994 Congress passed legislation authorizing the VA to compensate Gulf War veterans with disabling undiagnosed illnesses.[66] To qualify for compensation, the chronic disability resulting from an undiagnosed illness must have persisted for at least 6 months, must have appeared during active duty in the southwest Asia theater of operations during the Persian Gulf War, or to a degree of 10% or more not later than December 31, 2001. Signs or symptoms that may be manifestations of undiagnosed illness include, but are not limited to the following:

Fatigue
Abnormal weight loss
Cardiovascular signs or symptoms
Gastrointestinal signs or symptoms
Headaches
Joint pain
Menstrual disorders
Muscle pain
Neurological signs or symptoms
Neuropsychological signs or symptoms
Signs or symptoms involving the skin
Signs or symptoms involving the upper or lower respiratory tract
Sleep disturbances

Benefits based on undiagnosed signs and symptoms, which over time progress or evolve to the point at which a diagnosis of a recognized pathologic condition can be made, may result in discontinuation of benefit payments if proof of service connection cannot be continued under any other regulation.[13] In addition to compensation benefits, Gulf War veterans are entitled to free VA health care for conditions that may be related to exposure to toxic substances or environmental hazards encountered while serving in southwest Asia. In 1992 a "Persian Gulf Registry Program" was established by the VA for concerned veterans "to identify possible diseases which may result from service in . . . southwest Asia"[45] (see also Gulf War "undiagnosed illness," p. 201).

PROCESS OF DISABILITY DETERMINATION

When a veteran submits a claim for benefits, the VBA and VHA have a shared set of responsibilities to ensure that the veteran is moved through the claims process as quickly as possible. The VBA is primarily responsible for rating decisions, and the VHA's primary focus is performing necessary evaluations. However, recent years have witnessed a blurring of these formerly sharp distinctions, primarily because of precedent-setting decisions from the Court of Veterans Appeals. Although there are many different benefit programs available to veterans, there are four basic steps in the process of determining whether benefits will be granted: applying for benefits, initial claims review, disability examinations, and claims adjudication.

Step 1: Applying for Benefits

To request the necessary application forms (e.g., disability compensation, non-service–connected pension, insurance, specially adapted housing), veterans may contact a veterans benefits counselor at the nearest VA regional office in person or by calling a nationwide, toll-free number, 1-800-827-1000. Information and applications can also be obtained from VA medical facilities and from veterans service organizations (e.g., American Legion, Disabled American

Veterans, Veterans of Foreign Wars). Completed applications are then submitted to the nearest VA regional office for processing.

A recently discharged veteran applying for compensation for injuries or illnesses incurred or aggravated while in military service, or any first-time applicants for VA compensation or pension benefits, must submit a *Veteran's Application for Compensation or Pension* form (VA Form No. 21–526). Claimants who wish to reopen a claim may send a letter detailing the issues or use a *Statement in Support of Claim* (VA Form No. 21–4138). Those applying for pension benefits must complete a detailed financial questionnaire; this information is not required for compensation claims. The claimant may also submit medical and/or other records in support of the claim with the application form.

Step 2: Initial Claims Review

The veteran's application for benefits will be reviewed by benefits personnel in the Adjudication Division at one of 58 VA regional offices. For first-time applicants, a claims folder will be established and documentation of dates and character of military service (e.g., honorable discharge, general discharge, or dishonorable discharge) will be verified using a national computerized data bank or by inquiry to the Department of Defense. Obtaining service medical records (SMRs) often requires considerable effort on the part of the VA because the records may be sent to a number of different repositories, depending on the date of discharge, branch of service, reserve obligation, and length of service. Obtaining SMRs can often be the single greatest cause for delay in processing original claims for VA compensation. Once all evidence is available, adjudication personnel will then determine whether the veteran is eligible for the claimed benefit. For original or new compensation claims, this involves reviewing SMRs to document the presence of an illness or injury that could reasonably be associated with a current chronic problem, and (if not already available) requesting that the veteran submit records documenting ongoing problems related to the active military service illness or injury. For recently discharged military personnel, it is generally sufficient to list all conditions he or she wishes to have considered for service connection. Adjudication personnel will then request a complete general medical examination to identify any chronic residuals of the claimed in-service illnesses or injuries. Depending on the nature of the claim and the availability of supporting medical documentation, the VA may also require an evaluation at a VHA facility.

Step 3: VA Disability Examinations

Requests for examinations

VA regional offices request disability examinations at VHA facilities utilizing the Automated Medical Information Exchange (AMIE) data processing system, which allows electronic transfer of information between VA regional offices and VHA medical facilities. The AMIE system also allows tracking of case load, pending examinations, average time to complete an examination, and the number of examinations returned to each VHA facility for additional information because they are "insufficient" or "inadequate" for rating purposes. Although most disability examinations are performed at VHA facilities (often with fee-base or contract examiners), depending on availability of resources examinations can also be done in non-VA facilities at VA expense[47] (see Appendix 10–A).

Examination procedures

Disability examinations in the VA are to be conducted in accordance with guidelines set forth on AMIE Disability Examination Worksheets and in the *Physician's Guide for Disability Evaluation Examinations*.[59]

Worksheets. When a C&P examination request is initiated by the adjudication team through the AMIE system, one or more "worksheets" will be identified that may be used by the examiner to obtain the information required for rating purposes (see Appendix 10–1). Examination worksheets are "living" documents that are continuously being revised and updated to cover all issues required for rating each body system, as well as guidelines for conducting special examinations, such as POW and Cold Injury protocols. At present, in addition to a General Medical Examination worksheet, there are 53 worksheets. Although their use is not mandatory, examination reports must be complete and cover all issues required for rating. Examiners can obtain copies of these worksheets from VHA administrative personnel responsible for C&P programs (see Appendix 10–2).

Physician's guide. Up until 1994, a hard copy of *Physician's Guide for Disability Evaluation Examinations* was available for use by VA disability examiners. In 1994 the guide was extensively revised by a joint VBA/VHA task force and made available in electronic format only through the VA's computer system. The revised guide was indexed to the diagnostic codes used by the adjudication team in its *Schedule for Rating Disabilities*[24] and contained very specific guidelines as to information needed for rating. Unfortunately, the lack of a hard copy and incomplete indexing of the electronic guide makes this a very underutilized resource. At present, VHA and VBA are discussing whether to reissue an updated hard copy of the guide or simply expand the AMIE worksheets to include an introductory section and additional information on examination techniques. The most recent hard copy of the guide was published in 1985 and provides helpful background information on VA C&P examinations, but many sections are outdated and in general should not be used as a reference to what is currently required for rating purposes.[34]

Schedule for rating disabilities

Because the 54 disability examination worksheets do not cover all medical and psychiatric conditions for which veterans may claim benefits, and an up-to-date *Physician's Guide* is not currently available, it is extremely important that anyone performing VA disability examinations obtain a copy of the VA's *Schedule for Rating Disabilities,* which is published as Part 4 of *Title 38 Code of Federal Regulations*.[17] The issues that need to be addressed on VA C&P examinations are determined by the factors that are used in deciding the various levels (percentage) of disability that can be awarded. Review of the *Schedule for Rating Disabilities* will give the VA C&P examiner valuable insight as to what historical information needs to be documented, what examinations need to be performed, and what studies need to be ordered. Current copies of the *Title 38 Code of Federal Regulations* are located in most VA medical facility libraries, at all VA regional offices, or may be purchased from the U.S. Government Printing Office (202-512-1800), which operates bookstores in major metropolitan areas throughout the United States.

Who can do examinations?

VA C&P examination regulations have been recently revised to allow examinations by "any qualified clinical personnel." Thus, unless a specialist is specifically required as part of the AMIE request, VA C&P examinations may be done by physicians, nurse practitioners, physician assistants, psychologists, optometrists, audiologists, as well as other "qualified" clinical personnel. VHA is responsible for ensuring that C&P examiners are adequately qualified, and all examination reports must be signed by physicians or psychologists.[42]

Specialist examinations

In general, unless specifically requested by the adjudication team, VA C&P examinations do *not* need to be performed by specialists. Requests for specialty examinations are made only when there are special circumstances, such as conflicting diagnoses, or if required by a Board of Veterans' Appeals (BVA) remand. VHA examiners can also request specialist examinations if a diagnosis is not well established; any additional evaluations should be completed before the examination report is returned to the VA regional office for rating consideration.[43]

Medical records

Availability of medical records at the time of a VA disability examination is sometimes problematic. Medical records to be considered for VA disability examinations (including SMRs) are usually contained in the veteran's claims folder (also referred to as a *C-file*). The claims folder also contains records of benefit activity (e.g., applications for benefits, correspondence, rating decisions, and award letters). Because these files are often needed for other benefit activity, such as home and educational loans, and may contain records accumulated over many decades, VA regional offices strictly control access and movement of claims folders. For original claims for service-connection benefits, the SMRs may not have been received by the VA regional office and the claims folder will not be forwarded for the C&P examiner's review. In addition, for routine C&P review examinations or examinations related to claims for increase of established conditions, the claims folder is generally not forwarded. Examinations for which the claims folder will routinely be made available include claims involving former POWs, BVA remands, and cases requiring opinions. In addition, if necessary, the examiner may request the claims folder at the time of the examination. As the records contained in the claims folder are largely irreplaceable, these files should be stored in a secure location and nothing should ever be removed from the claims folders. Veterans should not be allowed to handle, transport, or in any way alter the contents of claims folders. Veterans can request copies of claims folder records by contacting a veteran benefits counselor at 1-800-827-1000. Veterans may bring medical records with them at the time of their C&P examinations, and these records should be associated with the current claim and returned with the completed examination report to the VA regional office. C&P examiners should document in the report whether the claims folder (or other medical records) was reviewed at the time of the examination.[48]

Examination techniques

The 54 C&P worksheets give specific details regarding information required for VA rating purposes (see Appendix 10–2). Because disabilities related to impairment of joint function are the most common awards under the VA disability program, accurate assessment of joint range of motion (ROM) is extremely important. Figs. 10–2 and 10–3 provide a standardized description of joint-motion measurement.[27] Examiners are instructed to use a goniometer to measure both passive and active ROM, including movement against gravity and strong resistance. ROM should be indicated in degrees; it is not acceptable simply to note that ROM is "normal," or "within normal limits." It is good practice to include ROM measurements of the contralateral joint whenever possible. This is particularly true if a joint ROM is believed to be "normal," but the measured ROM in degrees is different from the average normal ROM as shown in Figs. 10–2 and 10–3.

Impairment ratings and examination requirements for the spine are currently

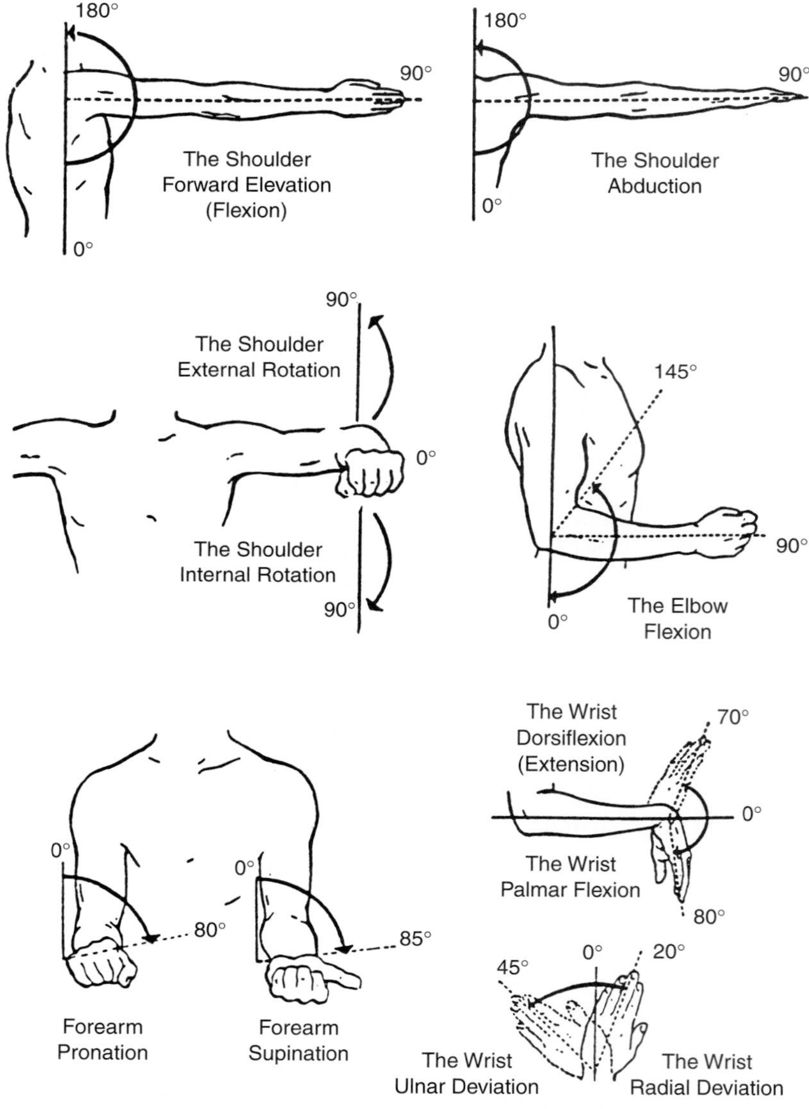

FIGURE 10–2
Normal ranges of motion in joints of upper extremities. (From 38 CFR. Part 4.71. Measurement of ankylosis and joint motion. Washington, DC, U.S. Government Printing Office, 1997, pp 352–353.)

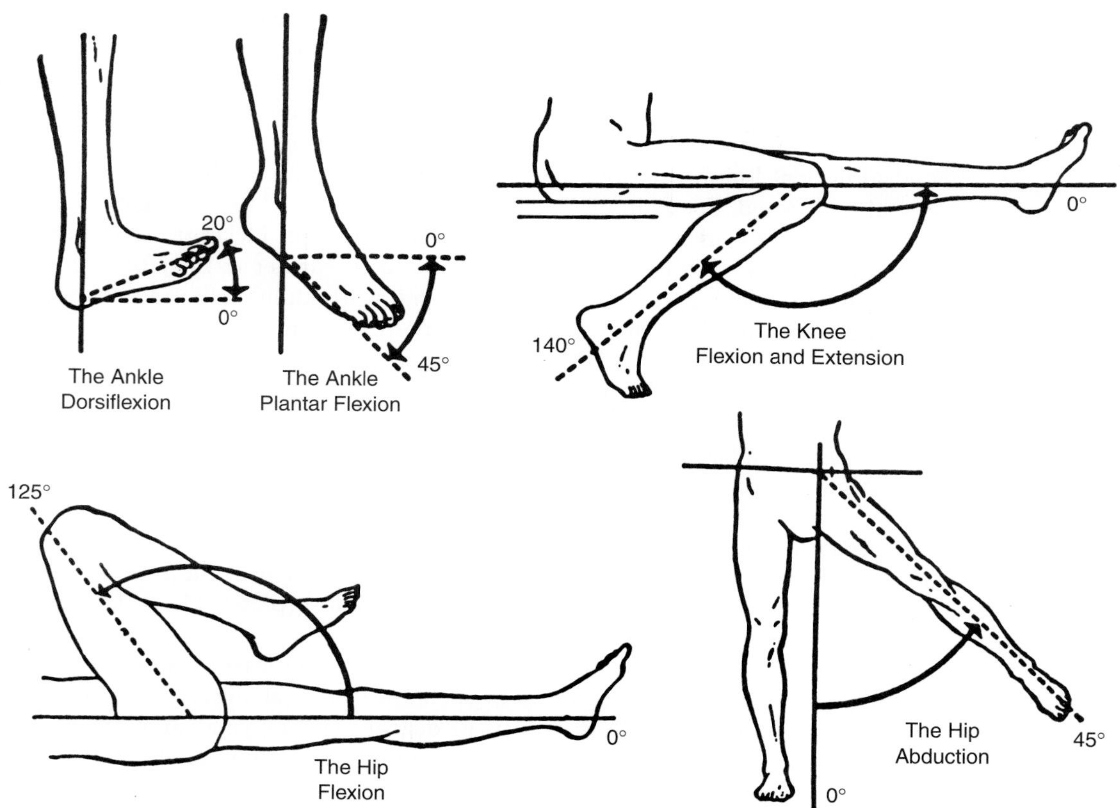

FIGURE 10–3
Normal ranges of motion in joints of lower extremities. (From 38 CFR. Part 4.71. Measurement of ankylosis and joint motion. Washington, DC, U.S. Government Printing Office, 1997, pp 352–353.)

under review, and no average normal ROM measurements for the spine are included in the current Spine worksheet. Measurement of spine ROM should be made with a goniometer (not inclinometer). Average normal ROM measurements from the 1994 computerized *Physician's Guide for Disability Evaluation* are as follows:

Cervical spine
- Forward flexion = 0° to 65°
- Backward extension = 0° to 50°
- Left and right lateral flexion = 0° to 40°
- Left and right rotation = 0° to 55°

Lumbosacral spine
- Forward flexion = 0° to 95°
- Backward extension = 0° to 35°
- Left and right lateral flexion = 0° to 40°
- Left and right rotation = 0° to 35°

Functional assessment of joints. Recent landmark Court of Veterans Appeals' decisions[33, 52] found that the traditional VA method of assessing joint disabilities for rating purposes—one-time measurement of active and passive ROM—was inadequate because functional impairment may be underestimated. Additional factors that now must be considered include (1) pain with joint movement, (2) weakened movement against varying resistance, (3) excess fatigability with use, (4) incoordination, and (5) the effects of episodic exacerbations (flare-ups) on functional ability.[18, 23, 25] Each of these issues should be assessed, and the amount of limited motion (if any) resulting from one or more of these factors should, if feasible, be reported in degrees of additional loss of motion. The absence of any or all of these factors should also be noted. For example, if shoulder abduction is 0° to 180° against gravity but there is evidence of pain (e.g., verbal complaint, facial grimace) between 120° and 180°, this should be documented. If further testing for endurance against resistance (e.g., 10 repetitions using a 5-lb dumbbell) reduces shoulder abduction to 90°, this should be reported. If more than one factor is contributing to loss of ROM, the examiner should state, if possible, which has the major functional impact. This can be done as a comment. For the above example, this might read: "Comment: Although shoulder abduction against gravity is full, 0° to 180°, because of the combined effects of pain and lack of endurance, the veteran's functional ROM is best estimated to be 0° to 90°." At present, there are no guidelines as to which tests should be used to determine strength and endurance for the various joints. These tests should be individualized, keeping in mind patient safety and that the results must, if possible, be reported in terms of additional loss of ROM *in degrees* (see Appendixes 10–2 and 10–3).

Imaging studies. In general, the least invasive and least expensive means of objectively documenting pathology such as arthritic changes and/or structural defects is preferred. The diagnosis of degenerative or posttraumatic arthritis of a joint requires radiological confirmation. However, once the diagnosis of arthritis has been confirmed in a joint, further imaging studies of that joint are generally not required because benefits are determined by the amount of functional impairment and not by the severity of radiological or other imaging-study findings. For example, if the AMIE request specifies a veteran's left knee for examination, and the request notes that the veteran is service connected for "left knee degenerative arthritis," then additional radiographs are not required. On the other hand, if the veteran is only claiming service connection for left knee degenerative arthritis and is not yet service connected and no past imaging reports are available documenting arthritic changes, then appropriate radiological studies should be obtained and the results included with the final examination report.[36]

Psychiatric examinations. Diagnoses of psychiatric conditions for VA benefit purposes must be made in accordance with the criteria contained in the American Psychiatric Association's *Diagnostic and Statistical Manual of Mental Disorders, fourth edition (DSM-IV)*.[1] Occasionally a VA regional office may require evaluations under *DSM-III-R* criteria; this will always be noted at the time of the examination request. The complete multi-axial format as specified by *DSM-IV* may be required as part of BVA remands or specifically requested by a VA regional office. If so, the examiner should include a Global Assessment of Function (GAF) score and note whether it refers to current functioning or functioning over some specific period of time.[2] If multiple Axis I and/or Axis II diagnoses exist, the examiner should attempt, to the extent possible, to separate and/or differentiate the symptomatology among the various disorders; if it is not possible to differentiate symptoms, an explanation should be provided. In addition to final diagnoses conforming to the *DSM-IV* format, psychiatric evaluations should include a statement regarding the veteran's competency. For VA benefit payments, "a mentally incompetent person is one who because of injury or disease lacks the mental capacity to contract or to manage his or her own affairs, including disbursement of funds without limitation."[14]

Employability

In considering the issue of unemployability caused by service-connected conditions, the examiner should bear in mind that age, individual preferences, and non-service–connected conditions should not, to the extent possible, influence the examiner's professional opinion as to whether employment is feasible. For VA rating purposes, total disability is considered to exist when there is impairment of mind or body sufficient to make it impossible for the average person to follow a substantially gainful occupation.[20] Total disability may be permanent and is generally not assigned for temporary exacerbations or acute infectious diseases. Although the adjudication team is ultimately responsible for determining if a veteran meets the criteria for a "total disability rating" based on "unemployability,"[21] examiners are frequently asked to comment on the combined effects of service-connected conditions on employability. For service-connected medical conditions, a useful way to consider whether minimum employability criteria can be met is to ask the question: Is sedentary employment feasible? For service-connected psychiatric conditions, minimum employability criteria may be met if employment would be feasible in a loosely supervised situation requiring little interaction with the public.

Change in diagnosis or etiology

Once it has been established that a disease, injury, or residual disability is attributable to military service (i.e., service connected for VA compensation purposes), any change in the diagnosis or etiology can have serious rating repercussions. If after careful review of all evidence (including the SMR or other records on which the original diagnosis was made), a change in diagnosis or etiology involving a service-connected condition is necessary, the examiner should certify that the previous diagnosis or attributed etiology on which the service connection was originally granted was "in error." This certification should be placed at the end of the report and should summarize the facts, findings, and reasons supporting the conclusion.[19] On the other hand, if the change in diagnosis is the result of maturation of the disability into another, or the change merely reflects a change in nomenclature related to more updated classification, this should be clearly documented.[28]

Suspected malingering or misrepresentation of the facts

If malingering is detected or suspected, the examiner should so state, together with a complete description of the observed behavior that lead the examiner to suspect malingering. However, the possible serious consequences should be carefully considered by the examiner before arriving at such an opinion. Any evidence of evasion or misrepresentation of facts that can be substantiated by findings should also be reported in detail. If the veteran refuses or obstructs the examination, the examiner should document the specific actions by which the veteran obstructed the examination or failed to cooperate.[35] Claimants are not entitled to use a recording device or have their attorney present during the examination.[61]

Gulf War "undiagnosed illness"

The concept of "undiagnosed illness" has proved problematic for VA clinicians. To qualify for these benefits, a Gulf War veteran must have objective indications of an undiagnosed chronic illness. For VA compensation purposes, "objective indications" means signs, symptoms, and other indicators of illness. *Signs* in the medical sense are objective findings perceptible to an examining clinician (e.g., unexplained fever, tachycardia, abnormal weight loss, laboratory abnormalities) that cannot be attributed to a known pathological process. *Symptoms* can be either objectively measured indicators (e.g., an elevated blood pressure with a headache, or lack of energy in someone with unexplained weight loss) or subjective indicators, (e.g., complaint of pain, fatigue, or dizziness). *Non-medical indicators* of unexplained illness can include time lost from work, evidence that a veteran has sought medical treatment, or statements from laypersons documenting changes in appearance, physical abilities, or mental or emotional attitude.[44] For VA compensation evaluations, examiners must do everything reasonable to evaluate a Gulf War veteran's symptoms.[46] If a diagnosis of a chronic medical condition can be made, compensation benefits will be awarded if there is evidence that the condition was incurred or aggravated during active military service. If no diagnosis of an accepted pathological (including psychiatric) condition can be made, the examiner should make a final diagnosis that (1) identifies the claimed symptom(s)/findings, (2) includes any objective abnormalities found and states these are of unknown etiology, and (3) states that no diagnosis of any chronic pathological condition can be made. Example: "Chronic abdominal pain with occasional nausea, abdominal pain and tenderness on examination of unknown etiology, with insufficient clinical evidence at present to warrant a diagnosis of any chronic pathological disorder." Conversely, if there are no objective abnormalities on examination, the final diagnosis should reflect this fact. Example: "Racing heart, with normal cardiac examination, normal heart rate and rhythm, normal electrocardiogram, and insufficient clinical evidence at present to warrant a diagnosis of any chronic pathological disorder." Benefits might be awarded under the provisions of "undiagnosed illness" in the first example, but probably not for the second.

Report format

The scope of VA C&P examinations varies considerably depending on a number of factors, including the type of examination (e.g., a claim for increase in compensation for a single joint versus a claim for original service connection for multiple illnesses and injuries incurred over a 20-year period in a recently discharged veteran) and length of time since discharge (i.e., a veteran discharged within the last 12 months usually undergoes a complete general medical examination regardless of duration of military service, whereas a veteran discharged 2 or more years previously will generally be examined only for specific issues noted on the AMIE request).

All C&P reports should include the following: complete name and Social Security number; date of examination; name, professional credentials (e.g., MD, DO, PA [physician's assistant], NP [nurse practitioner], etc.), and signature of the examiner; whether the claims folder and/or other medical records were reviewed; date of most recent VA disability examination (date of discharge from active duty for recently discharged veterans); interim history (since most recent disability examination: hospitalizations, surgeries, significant outpatient treatment, current medications [name, dose, frequency, condition for which prescribed, compliance, and side effects]); occupational history (current employment status; if unemployed, the date last employed, type of work, and reason for termination; medical absenteeism past 12 months [number of days and medical reason for absence]). In addition, for each condition listed under "General Remarks" on the AMIE request, the examiner should include a separate, problem-oriented discussion, including the history since last evaluated for VA claims purposes, current symptoms, limitations, and current treatment. The examiner should consult the relevant worksheet to be sure that all historical issues needed for rating have been addressed. The worksheet will also identify what is required on physical examination and if any specific laboratory, radiological, or other studies are required.

Final diagnoses

After review of any requested studies, the examiner should include a final diagnosis for each condition, complaint, or symptom listed on the AMIE request, or—if a complete general medical examination was requested—all complaints noted at the time of the examination. To alert the adjudication team that all issues listed on the AMIE request have been addressed, symptoms or conditions for which no acute or chronic pathological disorder can be diagnosed should also be listed in the "Final Diagnoses" section, and the fact that no pathological condition was identified should be noted. For example, if "Pneumonia" was listed on the AMIE request, but the current history shows no chronic sequelae and the current evaluation (physical examination, chest radiograph, and spirometry) are normal, the final diagnosis would be: "Pneumonia, treated and resolved, with insufficient clinical evidence at present to warrant a diagnosis of any chronic pathological disorder." For VA rating purposes, final diagnoses should not be expressed in ambiguous or equivocal terms. Avoid qualifiers such as "possible," "may be due to," or "rule out." Be sure that the final diagnoses are supported by the diagnostic studies. For example, if the lumbosacral spine radiograph does not show degenerative changes, a final diagnosis of "degenerative arthritis" is not acceptable. Also, the examiner should be sure that the final diagnosis identifies a pathological process. Thus "lumbosacral pain" is *not* acceptable, whereas "lumbosacral strain" is an acceptable final diagnosis. Other examples of unacceptable final diagnoses would include arthralgia (versus arthritis confirmed by radiograph or laboratory studies) and elevated blood pressure (versus hypertension).

Comments

In general, the examiner should avoid "Comments" after the "Final Diagnoses" section. Any comments should not raise questions about the certainty and/or correctness of the final diagnosis and should not suggest additional studies or examinations that have not been included as part of the final examination package.

Example: Final Diagnosis: (1) Posttraumatic headaches.

Comment: Although the veteran may have postconcussive headaches, some of his symptoms may be related to atypical seizures, and an EEG would be helpful.

Note how the comment undermines the final diagnosis of posttraumatic headaches and suggests another possible diagnosis for the veteran's symptoms. If a seizure disorder is really a likely possibility, the examiner should order an EEG. On the other hand, if this is merely speculation, this comment should not be included in the examination report because it is confusing to the adjudication team, and the case will have to be returned to the examining facility for clarification.

Opinions

Unless specifically requested on a BVA remand or AMIE request, examiners should avoid giving opinions. If an opinion is requested, examiners should include as much of their reasoning as possible, including specific references (including page number) to any medical literature that may have been used to support their conclusions.

Example: A veteran is service connected for a left leg fracture with leg shortening. He is now claiming service connection for right hip degenerative arthritis, and the AMIE request asks for an opinion. An acceptable response might be as follows:

Opinion: Because of the service-connected left tibia/fibula fracture, there is angulation and significant shortening of the left lower extremity. Despite lifts and other orthotics, over the years the veteran has had an abnormal gait, which has caused wear-and-tear on the right lower extremity. This is evidenced by asymmetric arthritic changes, worse on the right. Therefore it is my professional opinion that the veteran's service-connected left-leg condition caused his current right-hip arthritis.

In weighing the evidence for and against a claimed relationship, a useful way to consider the issues is in terms of probability. For VA rating purposes, the three levels of probability are as follows: (1) it is likely that condition x caused condition y, (2) it is as likely as not that condition x caused condition y, and (3) it is not likely that condition x caused condition y. In general, the veteran will receive benefits if it is likely or as likely as not that condition x caused condition y.

Final report

The completed report should be reviewed by a VHA clinician familiar with VA regional office rating requirements to be sure that all AMIE issues have been adequately addressed, that all diagnostic studies are available and support the final diagnoses, and to ensure that non-physician reports are reviewed and co-signed by a physician (see Appendix 10–3).

There are several important issues examiners should keep in mind when performing VA disability examinations. These examinations are for evaluative purposes only. The examiner should not discuss treatment options or provide treatment. If unexpected abnormalities that require follow-up are identified, the veteran should be referred to the nearest VA medical facility for appropriate treatment and follow-up. These referrals should be documented in the examination report. The examiner should not discuss possible rating outcomes with the claimant. Unlike examinations performed using the American Medical Association's *Guides to the Evaluation of Permanent Impairment*,[50] VA C&P examination reports should never include statements regarding the magnitude of impairment in terms of percent disability; this is an adjudicative function reserved for VA regional office rating specialists.

Timeliness of examinations

C&P examinations have one of the highest priorities among all VHA activities.[49] After receipt of an electronic AMIE request, VHA examining facilities must complete all examinations, including any necessary studies, and return the completed report to a VA regional office in an average of 35 days or less.[57]

Common problems

VA rating guidelines require C&P examinations that are "inadequate as a basis for the required consideration of service connection and evaluation" to be returned to the examining facility for corrective action.[26] Increasing judicial scrutiny of VA C&P examinations over the past decade has underscored the issue of "inadequate" reports. VA C&P examiners must clearly understand the differences between adequate clinical reports for treatment purposes and C&P examination reports that are adequate for VA rating purposes. For clinical examinations, reports must meet the community and/or facility standard of care. For VA rating purposes, completed reports must contain sufficient detail and documentation to address the issues required by the VA's *Schedule for Rating Disabilities*.[42] Attention to necessary examination procedures and/or requirements has the obvious benefits of reducing both the number of appeals and the time required for appellate review by minimizing the number of claims returned for re-examination and/or clarification. The magnitude of these "inadequate" (also referred to as *insufficient*) examinations cannot be ignored, as evidenced by the fact that 71.5% of 12,834 BVA remands returned during 1996 included instructions to conduct a medical examination.[39] Table 10–3 shows the 15 most common reasons for "insufficient" C&P examinations in a 1996 review by VBA of

TABLE 10–3 15 Most Common Reasons for Insufficient VA Compensation & Pension Examinations

Frequency (%)	Reason insufficient
10.8	All claimed/noted disabilities not examined
9.4	Final diagnosis not supported by exam findings
7.3	Functional impairment not adequately described
7.2	Failed to provide requested medical opinion
6.7	Complaints described, but no final diagnosis
6.6	Joint exam: range of motion in degrees not given
5.8	Orthopedic exam: radiographs not provided
5.3	Required specialty exam(s) not conducted
5.2	Final diagnosis not meaningful (e.g., history of hand injury)
5.1	Laboratory studies, radiographs, other studies requested by examiner not conducted or provided
4.3	Joint exam: presence/absence of pain not shown
3.6	Chronic disability or disease not ruled out
3.4	Failed to comply with BVA remand instructions
2.9	Restrictions of activities, occupational impairment not adequately described
2.1	Exam did not distinguish manifestations between coexisting service-connected and non-service–connected conditions
14.3	Other reasons (each less than 2.0%)

From Veterans Claims Adjudication Commission: Report to Congress, December 1996. Pub No. 1997–516–422/83512, Washington, DC, US Government Printing Office, 1997, p 39.

21,600 C&P examinations, of which 2600 (12%) were found to be "inadequate for rating purposes."[71]

Step 4: Claims Adjudication

Information received from the veteran, community, and VA medical treatment records, and the completed C&P examination are all reviewed by rating personnel in the Adjudication Division of the VA regional office. The *Schedule for Rating Disabilities*[42] is used by rating personnel to convert a claimant's clinical findings to standard diagnostic codes and evaluations for purposes of authorizing monthly monetary benefits to claimants based on average loss of earning capacity in civilian occupations as a result of specific diseases or injuries. The *Schedule* provides for evaluating disabilities in multiples of 10%, from zero to 100% (see Table 10–1). The total percent disability for a veteran with more than one service-connected condition is not necessarily the additive sum of each percent disability assigned to the various conditions, but is determined from a "Combined Ratings Table."[22] Illnesses or residuals of injuries that are determined to be less than 10% disabling may still be service-connected at the "zero percent" level, which entitles the veteran to free treatment for that condition at a VA medical facility, but no monetary compensation. Compensation in addition to the standard zero to 100% schedule may be awarded for a variety of conditions, including the need for specially adapted housing and clothing and automobile allowances. Veterans are notified by letter from the VA regional office as to the results of rating action, as well as their appeal rights if they are dissatisfied with the decision.

Appeals process

As previously noted, the VA benefits system is different from Social Security, insurance, and workers' compensation claims programs because there is no "finality" to the VA disability claims adjudication process. Repeat claims, including appeals of decisions on claims for benefits issued by a VA regional office, outnumber original claims by an almost three to one margin.[73] However, unlike most other U.S. benefits programs, clinicians involved in examining veterans for C&P purposes are not called on or required to testify in person as part of the appeals process involving VA benefits. If adjudication personnel at a local VA regional office, the BVA, or the Court of Veterans Appeals require additional clarification, opinions, examinations, or studies, written requests outlining what is needed will be submitted to the examining facility for further action.

Claimants may appeal benefit decisions and have 1 year from the date of notification of a VA decision to file an appeal. The first step in the appeals process is for the claimant, or someone authorized to act on the claimant's behalf, to file a written statement that the claimant disagrees with the VA's decision ("Notice of Disagreement"). After receipt of the notice, the VA regional office will furnish the claimant with a "Statement of the Case," which describes the facts, laws, and regulations that were used in deciding the case. If the claimant decides to pursue the appeal, a "Substantive Appeal" must be filed within 60 days of the mailing of the Statement of the Case, or within 1 year from the date the VA regional office mailed its rating decision, whichever period ends later. Claimants also have the right to representation and personal hearings to discuss the merits of their cases before the local rating board and BVA.[30]

Board of Veterans' Appeals

The BVA is a VA organization located in Washington, D.C. that makes final decisions on benefits on behalf of the Secretary of Veterans Affairs in cases in which the claimant disagrees with the decision of a VA regional office or medical center.[29] Any decision issued by a VA regional office on a claim for benefits, and some decisions issued by VA medical centers (such as eligibility for medical treatment), can be appealed to the BVA. Most commonly, veterans appeal either a denial of a claim or the level of the benefits granted. For example, if a veteran who is service connected for a knee disability is dissatisfied with the 10% disability award made by the local VA regional office, this decision can be appealed to the BVA. Claimants are usually represented by a veterans service organization (e.g., American Legion, Disabled American Veterans) or attorneys. The BVA is composed of "Members of the Board," and attorneys experienced in veterans' law and who are assisted by staff attorneys. During 1996 the BVA issued 33,944 appellate decisions, with almost 45% of the compensation claim decisions involving "remands" back to local VA regional offices for further development, often requiring additional examinations at VA C&P units. Despite recent streamlining of BVA appellate procedures, there were over 60,000 BVA appeals pending in 1996, with the average BVA decision requiring 595 days (down from 781 days in 1994).[38]

U.S. Court of Veterans Appeals

Although the United States has been providing pensions and medical care to its veterans since the Revolutionary War, up until 1988 these activities were largely insulated from both the courts and attorneys. In 1933, only 3 years after the VA's inception, Congress barred federal court review of individual VA benefit determinations, and attorney representation was rare because an 1864 law prohibited attorneys from charging more than $10 for prosecuting a claim for VA benefits. The VA's "splendid isolation" from judicial oversight and attorney involvement ended on November 18, 1988, with the enactment of "The Veterans' Judicial Review Act"[67, 68] which had five major provisions[53]:

1. Retained the BVA as the VA's final administrative body
2. Repealed the law precluding judicial review of individual benefit issues
3. Established a new court, the U.S. Court of Veterans Appeals, separate from the VA, to which adverse final decisions of the BVA could be appealed by individual veterans
4. Abolished the $10 cap for attorney fees, allowing attorneys and others authorized to practice before the Court of Veterans Appeals to charge a "reasonable fee" for representation
5. Created another level of judicial review so that under certain circumstances appeals of Court of Veterans Appeals decisions could be taken to the U.S. Court of Appeals for the Federal Circuit, and in some cases to the U.S. Supreme Court

Only claimants may seek review by the Court of Veterans Appeals; the VA may not appeal BVA decisions. The Court of Veterans Appeals is empowered to affirm, modify, reverse, or remand decisions of the BVA, and to establish binding precedents with regard to the VA's administration of the law. To appeal to the Court of Veterans Appeals, a claimant must have filed a "Notice of Disagreement" on or after November 18, 1988. The appeal must be filed with the Court of Veterans Appeals within 120 days after the BVA mails its final decision. The

Court of Veterans Appeals does not hold trials or receive new evidence, but rather reviews the record that was considered by the BVA. Both the VA and appellants may appeal decisions of the Court of Veterans Appeals to the U.S. Court of Appeals for the Federal Circuit and to the Supreme Court of the United States. Appellants may represent themselves or have lawyers or approved agents as representatives before the Court of Veterans Appeals.[51]

Over the past decade, the impact of The Veterans' Judicial Review Act and Court of Veterans Appeals' decisions on the conduct of VA C&P examinations has been enormous. Although more than 90% of the 30,000 to 40,000 cases appealed to the BVA each year involve medical issues, physician involvement at the VA regional office and BVA levels has been sharply curtailed because medical experts and consultants involved in rating decisions can no longer render opinions based simply on their medical experience.[32] This has resulted in increased importance of the findings of the clinicians actually examining the veterans, reviewing the claims folder, and providing supporting "reasons and bases" for any medical opinions. A number of areas that were formerly the near exclusive purview of VA regional offices rating specialists have now been returned, at least in part, to the examining clinicians for input and comment, including issues relating to employability, causality, aggravation, and severity of impairment.

Court of Veterans Appeals decisions are published in *West's Veterans Appeals Reporter* in the WESTLAW and LEXIS online services, and in the Court of Veterans Appeals' electronic bulletin board. For information about the Court of Veterans Appeals' rules and procedures, contact the Clerk of the Court at 625 Indiana Avenue NW, Suite 900, Washington, DC 20004, or call 1-800-869-8654. Additional information can be viewed on the Internet at *www.vetapp.uscourts.gov.*

ACKNOWLEDGEMENTS

I am indebted to Ms. Jan Herrera for preparing drafts of the manuscript and to Drs. Sandra Baker, Thomas Meyer, and Sylvia K. Oboler for their encouragement, reviews, and comments.

REFERENCES

1. American Psychiatric Association: Diagnostic and Statistical Manual of Mental Disorders, 4th ed. Washington, DC, American Psychiatric Association, 1994.
2. Op. cit. p 32.
3. Beebe GW: Follow-up studies of World War II and Korean War prisoners. II. Morbidity, disability, and maladjustments. Am J Epidemiol 101:400–422, 1975.
4. Caldwell GG, Kelley D, Zack M, et al: Mortality and cancer frequency among military nuclear (Smoky) participants, 1957 through 1979. JAMA 250:620–624, 1983.
5. 38 CFR. Part 3.1–3.100: Pension, compensation, and dependency and indemnity compensation. Washington, DC, U.S. Government Printing Office, 1997, pp 137–320.
6. 38 CFR. Part 3.3. Pension. Washington, DC, U.S. Government Printing Office, 1997, pp 140–142.
7. 38 CFR. Part 3.307. Presumptive service connection for chronic, tropical or prisoner-of-war related disease, or disease associated with exposure to certain her-

bicide agents; wartime and service on or after January 1, 1947. Washington, DC, U.S. Government Printing Office, 1997, pp 217–223.
8. 38 CFR. Part 3.309(c). Diseases specific as to former prisoners of war. Washington, DC, U.S. Government Printing Office, 1997, pp 220–221.
9. 38 CFR. Part 3.309(d). Diseases specific to radiation-exposed veterans. Washington, DC, U.S. Government Printing Office, 1997, pp 221–222.
10. 38 CFR. Part 3.309(e). Diseases associated with exposure to certain herbicide agents. Washington, DC, U.S. Government Printing Office, 1997, pp 222–223.
11. 38 CFR. Part 3.311. Claims based on exposure to ionizing radiation. Washington, DC, U.S. Government Printing Office, 1997, pp 223–226.
12. 38 CFR. Part 3.316. Claims based on chronic effects of exposure to mustard gas. Washington, DC, U.S. Government Printing Office, 1997, pp 229–230.
13. 38 CFR. Part 3.317. Compensation for certain disabilities due to undiagnosed illness. Washington, DC, U.S. Government Printing Office, 1997, pp 230–231.
14. 38 CFR. Part 3.353. Determination of incompetency and competency. Washington, DC, U.S. Government Printing Office, 1997, pp 247–248.
15. 38 CFR. Part 3.358. Determinations for disability or death from hospitalization, medical or surgical treatment, examinations or vocational rehabilitation training. Washington, DC, U.S. Government Printing Office, 1997, pp 250–251.
16. 38 CFR. Part 4.1. Essentials of evaluative rating. Washington, DC, U.S. Government Printing Office, 1997, p 331.
17. 38 CFR. Part 4.1–4.150. Schedule for Rating Disabilities. Washington, DC, U.S. Government Printing Office, 1997, pp 329–434.
18. 38 CFR . Part 4.10. Functional impairment. Washington, DC, U.S. Government Printing Office, 1997, p 332.
19. 38 CFR. Part 4.13. Effect of change of diagnosis. Washington, DC, U.S. Government Printing Office, 1997, pp 332–333.
20. 38 CFR. Part 4.15. Total disability ratings. Washington, DC, U.S. Government Printing Office, 1997, p 333.
21. 38 CFR. Part 4.16. Total disability ratings for compensation based on unemployability of the individual. Washington, DC, U.S. Government Printing Office, 1997, pp 333–334.
22. 38 CFR. Part 4.25. Combined rating table. Washington, DC, U.S. Government Printing Office, 1997, pp 336–338.
23. 38 CFR. Part 4.40. Functional loss. Washington, DC, U.S. Government Printing Office, 1997, p 341.
24. 38 CFR. Part 4.40–4.150. Disability Ratings. Washington, DC, U.S. Government Printing Office, 1997, pp 341–419.
25. 38 CFR. Part 4.45. The joints. Washington, DC, U.S. Government Printing Office, 1997, p 342.
26. 38 CFR. Part 4.70. Inadequate examinations. Washington, DC, U.S. Government Printing Office, 1997, pp 350–351.
27. 38 CFR. Part 4.71. Measurement of ankylosis and joint motion. Washington, DC, U.S. Government Printing Office, 1997, pp 352–353.
28. 38 CFR. Part 4.125. Diagnosis of mental disorders. Washington, DC, U.S. Government Printing Office, 1997, p 416.
29. 38 CFR. Part 19.1–19.14. Operation of the Board of Veterans' Appeals. Washington, DC, U.S. Government Printing Office, 1997, pp 60–62.
30. 38 CFR. Part 19.25–19.38. Appeals processing by the agency of original jurisdiction. Washington, DC, U.S. Government Printing Office, 1997, pp 62–65.
31. Committee to Review the Health Effects in Vietnam Veterans of Exposure to Herbicides: Veterans and Agent Orange: Health Effects of Herbicides Used in Vietnam. Washington, DC, National Academy Press, 1994, p 6.
32. Cragin CL: A time of transition at the Board of Veterans' Appeals: The changing role of the physician. Fed Bar News J 38:500–504, 1991.
33. DeLuca v. Brown, 8 Vet. App. 202 (1995).

34. Department of Medicine and Surgery: Physician's Guide for Disability Evaluation Examinations. Pub no. 19850-461-890/24994;Washington, DC, US Government Printing Office, March 1, 1985.
35. Op. cit. Chapter 1, paragraph 1.16: Suspected malingering or misrepresentation of facts; and paragraph 1.17: Refusal or obstruction of examination.
36. Op. cit. Paragraph 1.20: Overexposure to x-ray.
37. Department of Veterans Affairs: Annual Report of the Secretary of Veterans Affairs, Fiscal Year 1996. Washington, DC, Department of Veterans Affairs, 1997, p ix.
38. Op. cit. pp 43–46.
39. Op. cit. p 44.
40. Op. cit. p 148.
41. Department of Veterans Affairs: Federal Benefits for Veterans and Dependents, 1999 ed. VA pamphlet 80-99-1. Washington, DC, Department of Veterans Affairs, 1999.
42. Department of Veterans Affairs: Medical examiner's signature. In: Veterans Benefits Administration Manual M21-1. Part VI. Rating board procedures, subparagraph 1.07d. Washington, DC, Department of Veterans Affairs, May 19, 1997.
43. Op. cit. Subparagraph 1.02b: Specialist examinations.
44. Op. cit. Subparagraph 7.22: Compensation for undiagnosed illnesses of Persian Gulf veterans.
45. Department of Veterans Affairs: Persian Gulf Program. In: Veterans Health Administration Manual M-10. Part III. Environmental Agents Service. Washington, DC, Department of Veterans Affairs, August 8, 1995.
46. Op cit. Chapter 3. Phase II: Persian Gulf Uniform Case Assessment Protocol.
47. Department of Veterans Affairs: Requests for examinations. In: Veterans Health Administration Manual, M-1. Operations. Part I. Medical administration activities; Chapter 20. Examinations: C&P/Other federal agencies; paragraph 20.03. Washington, DC, Department of Veterans Affairs, July 6, 1993.
48. Op. cit. Paragraph 20.05. Request for claims folders.
49. Op. cit. Chapter 16. Paragraph 16.31. Priority sequence.
50. Doege TC, Houston TP (eds): Guides to the Evaluation of Permanent Impairment, 4th ed. Chicago, American Medical Association, 1993, pp 1–6.
51. Farley JJ III: The new kid on the block of veterans' law: the United States Court of Veterans Appeals. Fed Bar News J 38:488–492, 1991.
52. Floyd v. Brown, 9 Vet. App. 88 (1996).
53. Fox WF Jr: The US Court of Veterans Appeals: A Comprehensive Analysis of the Jurisprudence, Organization and Operation of the Newest Article I Court. Washington, DC, Paralyzed Veterans of America, 1994.
54. Johnson CJ: Cancer incidence in an area of radioactive fallout downwind from the Nevada test site. JAMA 251:230–236, 1984.
55. Johnson JC, Thaul S, Page WF, et al: Mortality of Veteran Participants in the CROSSROADS Nuclear Test. Washington, DC, National Academy Press, 1996.
56. Joseph SC: A comprehensive clinical evaluation of 20,000 Persian Gulf veterans. Mil Med 162:149–155, 1997.
57. Kizer KW: Memorandum of Understanding Between Veterans Benefits Administration and Veterans Health Administration on Processing Examination Requests. Veterans Health Administration directive 10-95-023, Washington, DC, Department of Veterans Affairs, March 3, 1995.
58. Larsen PR, Conrad RA, Knudsen KD, et al: Thyroid hypofunction after exposure to fallout from a hydrogen bomb explosion. JAMA 247:1572–1576, 1982.
59. Lemons SL, Kizer KW: Examination Worksheets for Disability Claims. Washington, DC, Department of Veterans Affairs, September 14, 1997, Memorandum.
60. National Center for Veteran Analysis and Statistics: Summary of Medical Programs, October 1, 1995 through September 30, 1996. Washington, DC, Department of Veterans Affairs, 1997, p 104.

61. Office of General Counsel: Failure to Submit to Medical Examination: Insistence on the Presence of an Attorney and Use of a Recording Device. OGC Precedent Opinion 4-91. Washington, DC, Department of Veterans Affairs, February 13, 1991.
62. Page WF: The Health Status of Former Prisoners of War. Washington, DC, National Academy Press, 1992, p 113.
63. Page WF, Ostfeld AM: Malnutrition and subsequent ischemic heart disease in former prisoners of war of World War II and the Korean Conflict. J Clin Epidemiol 47:1437–1441, 1994.
64. Pechura CM, Rall DP (eds): Veterans at Risk: The Health Effects of Mustard Gas and Lewisite. Washington, DC, National Academy Press, 1993.
65. Persian Gulf Veterans Coordinating Board: Unexplained illnesses among Desert Storm veterans: a search for causes, treatment and cooperation. Arch Intern Med 155:262–268, 1995.
66. Public Law 103–446. Persian Gulf War Veterans' Benefits Act. In: Veterans' Benefits Improvement Act of 1994.
67. Public Law 100–687, 102 Stat. 4105 (1988).
68. Stichman BF: The Veterans' Judicial Review Act of 1988: Congress introduces courts and attorneys to veterans' benefits proceedings. Admin Law Rev 41:365–397, 1989.
69. Titus AC: Governmental responsibility for victims of atomic testing: a chronicle of the politics of compensation. J Health Polit Policy Law 8:277–292, 1983.
70. Veterans Benefits Administration, Compensation and Pension Service: 12/1/97 Legislative Adjustment. Fast Letter (97-146). Washington, DC, Department of Veterans Affairs, November 20, 1997.
71. Veterans Benefits Administration, Compensation and Pension Service: White paper: Study of VA Examination Report Adequacy. Washington, DC, Department of Veterans Affairs; December 17, 1996.
72. Veterans' Claims Adjudication Commission: Report to Congress, December 1996. Pub No. 1997-516-422/83512, Washington, DC, US Government Printing Office, 1997, p 39.
73. Op. cit. p 5.
74. Veterans' Claims Adjudication Commission: Report to Congress: Appendices, December 1996. Pub No. 1997-516-423/83513, Washington, DC, US Government Printing Office, 1997, p A–2.

Sample AMIE VA C&P Examination Request

Date: Oct. 30, 1998 COMPENSATION AND PENSION EXAM REQUEST
For Denver VAMC Medical Center Division at DENVER
Requested by DENVER, CO-RO

Date Requested: Oct. 29, 1998@8:35:40

Name: DOE, JOHN J. **SSN:** 123 45 6789
C-Number: 21098765
DOB: JUL 30, 1947
Address: 123 Anywhere St
City, State, Zip: Denver, Colorado 80220 **Res Phone:** 303-555-1212
Bus Phone: 303-555-2222
Entered active service: DEC 27, 1967
Released active service: DEC 24, 1969

** **Priority of exam:** Increase

Selected exams: Shoulder, Elbow, Wrist, Knee, and Ankle

Current Rated Disabilities:

Rated Disability	Percent	SC?	Dx Code
Arm, limitation of motion	0%	Yes	5201

Other Disabilities:

General Remarks:

Examine SC: Right Shoulder, Degenerative Arthritis

Remarks: Examiner is to furnish an opinion as to the number of additional degrees of range-of-motion loss caused by pain on use, weakened movement, excess fatigability, incoordination and/or during flare-ups.

VA Form 21-2507

APPENDIX 10–2

Sample VA Examination Worksheet*

JOINTS (SHOULDER, ELBOW, WRIST, HIP, KNEE, AND ANKLE)

Name: **SSN:**
Date of Exam: **C-number:**
Place of Exam:

A. Review of Medical Records:

B. Medical History (Subjective Complaints)

Comment on:

1. Pain, weakness, stiffness, swelling, heat and redness, instability or giving way, "locking," fatigability, lack of endurance, etc.
2. Treatment: Type, dose, frequency, response, side effects
3. If there are periods of flare-up of joint disease:
   a. State their severity, frequency, and duration
   b. Name the precipitating and alleviating factors
   c. Estimate to what extent, if any, they result in additional limitation of motion or functional impairment during the flare-up
4. Describe whether crutches, brace, cane, corrective shoes, etc., are needed
5. Describe details of any surgery or injury
6. Describe any episodes of dislocation or recurrent subluxation
7. For inflammatory arthritis, describe any constitutional symptoms
8. Describe the effects of the condition on the veteran's usual occupation and daily activities
9. For upper extremity, state which is dominant and means used to identify dominant extremity
10. If there is a prosthesis, provide date of prosthetic implant and describe any complaint of pain, weakness, or limitation of motion. State whether crutches, brace, etc., are needed.

C. Physical Examination (Objective Findings):

Address each of the following as appropriate to the condition being examined and fully describe current findings: *A detailed assessment of each affected joint is required, including joints with prostheses.*

1. Using a goniometer, measure the *passive* and *active* range of motion, including movement against gravity and against strong resistance. Provide range of motion in degrees.
2. If the joint is painful on motion, state at which point in the range of motion pain begins and ends.
3. State to what extent (if any) and in which degrees (if possible) the range

*From Lemons SL, Kizer KW: Examination Worksheets for Disability Claims. Washington, DC, Department of Veterans Affairs, September 14, 1997. Memorandum.

of motion or joint function is *additionally limited* by pain, fatigue, weakness, or lack of endurance after repetitive use or during flare-ups. If more than one of these is present, state, if possible, which has the major functional impact.

4. Describe objective evidence of painful motion, edema, effusion, instability, weakness, tenderness, redness, heat, abnormal movement, guarding of movement, etc.

5. For weight-bearing joints (hip, knee, ankle), describe gait and functional limitations on standing and walking. Describe any callosities, breakdown, or unusual shoe wear pattern that would indicate abnormal weight bearing.

6. If ankylosis is present, describe the position of the bones of the joint in relationship to one another (in degrees of flexion, external rotation, etc.), and state whether the ankylosis is stable and pain free.

7. If indicated, measure the leg length from the anterior superior iliac spine to the medial malleolus.

8. For *inflammatory arthritis*, describe any constitutional signs.

9. Describe range of motion with prosthesis in same detail as described above for nonprosthetic joints.

D. Normal Range of Motion: All joint Range of Motion measurements must be made using a *goniometer*. Show each measured range of motion separately rather than as a continuum. For example, if the veteran lacks 10° of full knee extension and has normal flexion, show the range of motion as extension to –10° (or lacks 10° of extension) and flexion 0° to 140°.

(**Note:** Elbow, wrist, hip, knee, and ankle ranges of motion not included here.)

4. Shoulder, elbow, forearm, and wrist range of motion:
   a. Normal range of motion is measured with zero° the anatomical position *except* for 2 situations:
      (1). Supination and pronation of the forearm is measured with the arm against the body, the elbow flexed to 90°, and the forearm in mid position (zero°) between supination and pronation.
      (2). Shoulder rotation is measured with the arm abducted to 90°, the elbow flexed to 90°, and the forearm reflecting the midpoint (zero°) between internal and external rotation of the shoulder.
   b. Shoulder forward flexion = 0° to 180°
   c. Shoulder abduction = 0° to 180°
   d. Shoulder external rotation = 0° to 90°
   e. Shoulder internal rotation = 0° to 90°

E. Diagnostic and Clinical Tests:

1. As indicated: Radiological examinations, including special views or weight-bearing films, MRI, arthrogram, diagnostic arthroscopy.

2. Include results of all diagnostic and clinical tests in the examination report.

Note: The diagnosis of degenerative arthritis or posttraumatic arthritis of a joint requires radiographic confirmation. Once the diagnosis has been confirmed in a joint, further radiographs of that joint are not required.

F. Diagnosis

Signature: Date:

APPENDIX 10-3

Sample VA C&P Examination Report

Compensation & Pension Examination
November 15, 1997

This veteran is a 50-year-old right-handed male, who is appointed for disability evaluation per AMIE request. The veteran was last evaluated for claims purposes in October 1990. The veteran's claims folder was reviewed at the time of this examination. For pertinent past medical history and findings of record, please see the claims folder.

Interim History: Since the veteran's 1990 disability evaluation, he has not been hospitalized or undergone any surgical procedures.

Current Medications: (1) Ibuprofen, 800 mg tid, for shoulder pain; (2) atenolol, 50 mg qd, for hypertension; and (3) acetaminophen with codeine (½ gr), 2 to 3 per week for severe shoulder pain. The veteran states he is compliant with his prescribed medications, although he sometimes gets an upset stomach from the ibuprofen. The veteran is currently followed on a regular basis by his general practitioner, Dr. Maxwell Smart, in Denver and was last seen 3 weeks ago.

Occupational History: Works full-time (40 hr/wk) as a checker and stocker at a local supermarket × 18 years. Has missed 2 weeks work in the past year because of "right shoulder pain."

Present Status: Right Shoulder Arthritis: As documented in the veteran's claims folder, he was originally injured in Vietnam in 1968, when he was "blown out of a jeep," landing on his right shoulder. Radiographs at that time showed no fractures, and he was treated conservatively with a sling "for a couple of weeks" and then returned to full combat duty. He continued to seek medical care because of pain with lifting, and at the time of discharge in 1969, was diagnosed as having "right shoulder bursitis." In 1970, he was service connected at 0% for "bursitis" and this rating was continued at the 0% level when he was last evaluated for VA claims purposes in 1990.

The veteran denies any further injuries to his right shoulder since the jeep accident in 1968, but states that over the past 2 to 3 years he has had increasing difficulty doing the full range of duty at work and is afraid he might lose his job. Specifically, the veteran relates that when he arrives at work at 5 AM to begin stocking shelves he's "fine for about an hour." At the end of that time he describes a constant "ache" in the right shoulder, which intensifies to a "sharp" pain if he continues to work or works above shoulder level. He uses a step-stool as much as possible. He also notes decreased endurance and weakness, but admits that this really may be more related to increasing pain. He denies incoordination, but does describe two episodes in recent months where he was "laid up on a heating pad" for 2 to 3 days, both instances after he worked overtime to help stock shelves. The "sharp" discomfort gradually subsides over a period of several hours when he goes home or keeps his arm below shoulder level. The ibuprofen is helpful, but he is "never" pain-free while working, and is taking increasing amounts of acetaminophen with codeine (2 to 3/week) for sleep. He avoids any non-work activities that require work above shoulder level, including painting and baseball. He saw an orthopedic specialist about a year ago, who diagnosed "impingement" and "posttraumatic degenerative arthritis" (report in claims file). Short-term physical therapy "was a waste of money," but he continues to do range-of-motion exercises. The veteran denies any numbness or tingling in his right arm or hand.

Physical Examination: Per AMIE-2507 request, the examination was confined to the right upper extremity. The veteran presented as a WDWN muscular adult male. Wt = 206 lb; Height = 5′11″. Veteran was cooperative and appeared to give full effort throughout the interview and examination.

On observation, the shoulders were symmetrical without obvious atrophy, scars, or deformity. Mid-biceps circumference was 36.7 cm on the right (dominant) and 36.0 cm on the left. On palpation there was no muscle spasm detected over the upper back and neck, but there was mild tenderness with direct palpation over the rotator cuff on the right. Both active and passive range of motion (ROM) of both upper extremities was tested and the results were consistent. The veteran had full left shoulder ROM, including abduction (= 0–180°); forward flexion (= 0–180°); internal and external rotation (= 0–90°). Right shoulder range of motion was abnormal, with abduction free of pain only from 0–80°. The veteran was able to abduct the right shoulder to 165°, with pain and hesitation from 80–165°. Moderate crepitus was noted with passive ROM. Forward flexion was also abnormal, with a pain-free arc from 0–85° and pain and hesitation from 85–160°. Right shoulder external rotation was 0–65° with only mild discomfort, but internal rotation was limited to 0–45° because of pain. Strength of the LUE was normal, 5/5, for all muscle groups. Right shoulder muscle strength was 4+/5 because of pain. Grip strength was normal in both hands. Neurologic testing in both upper extremities was normal, including 2+ and symmetrical reflexes, normal sensation, coordination and fine movements (buttoning and unbuttoning his shirt).

Functional testing was assessed using standard 5-lb dumbbells. With the veteran's left arm, he was easily able to perform 10 repetitions, 0–135°, of shoulder forward flexion and abduction, simulating the motion he commonly uses to stock shelves at the supermarket. On functional testing of the right shoulder there was marked abnormality. Amplitude progressively decreased because of pain, so that after only 4 repetitions the veteran was only able to bring the dumbbell to 75° of abduction and stopped after the sixth repetition because of pain.

Diagnostic Studies: Outside x-ray films of the right shoulder, dated 11/14/95, were reviewed by our radiologist and were interpreted as showing mild to moderate degenerative changes in the glenohumeral joint, as well as calcification within the rotator cuff complex, consistent with calcific tendinitis.

Final Diagnosis:

Right Shoulder: Posttraumatic degenerative arthritis and calcific tendinitis, with limitation of motion, function, and discomfort, as described.

Comment: Although active and passive right-shoulder ROM is only slightly restricted, 0–165° (normal abduction and forward flexion = 0–180°), the veteran has marked functional limitations that are consistent with his objective pathology. While working, the veteran's right shoulder functional range of motion is estimated to be 0–75°, for an additional loss of abduction and forward flexion of 80° (difference between 75° and 165°). Although this additional loss of ROM is primarily caused by pain and decreased endurance, it also takes into account weakened movement. There was no demonstrable incoordination, and any estimate of further loss of ROM because of episodic flares is not feasible.

[**Rating Decision:** The completed report and claims folder were returned to the VA Regional Office Adjudication Division for rating consideration. After review of the C&P examination report and all other information related to the claim, the veteran's right shoulder condition was rated under Diagnostic Code 5201, "Arm, limitation of motion of," and given a disability rating of 20% (= arm motion limited to shoulder level). This 20% rating translates to a payment (in 1999) of $184 per month.]

CHAPTER 11

The Canadian Disability System

Michel Lacerte, MDCM, MSc

When Canada became a nation in 1867, the British North America (BNA) Act—now the Constitution (Act)—outlined the areas of jurisdiction for which the federal government had responsibility and those that were under the control of the provincial governments. At that time, health and welfare issues were not seen as key governmental concerns (people were expected to look after themselves) and, by default, were assumed to fall under provincial jurisdiction.[6]

As health and welfare issues became more salient, the provincial governments were not financially able to provide the required services and programs. As a result, advances in social welfare legislation had to wait for one of the following three developments[7]:

> . . . a provincial government's willingness and ability to finance needed measures; an amendment to the B.N.A. Act to permit federal entry into an area of jurisdiction otherwise assigned to the provinces; or the development of stratagems to secure federal financial help without appearing to violate the provisions of the B.N.A. Act.

All three developments have occurred—although legislation continues to evolve—with the result that both levels of government now have important roles in providing public health and income-security programs.

Some key federal programs include Old Age Security, the Guaranteed Income Supplement, the Canada Pension Plan, Employment Insurance (formerly Unemployment Insurance), and the Child Tax Benefit. The provinces are in charge of such areas as health care, social assistance, and workers' compensation. Through the Canada Health and Social Transfer, the federal government also contributes toward the cost of certain provincial/territorial programs.

For individuals with a disability, programs are provided by both levels of government. It is important to note, however, that Canada has no overall framework for social justice for persons with disabilities and, unlike for seniors or the unemployed, has never aspired to build one.[2] Nevertheless, there are five major programs designed to assist those who are disabled and who qualify: provincial workers' compensation programs, the Canada Pension Plan, Veterans Affairs Disability Pensions, provincial social assistance programs, and the federal Disability Tax Credit. The administration of private disability insurance in Canada is very similar to that in the United States.

WORKERS' COMPENSATION

Like the United States and Australia, Canada is one of only three countries that has a non-nationwide workers' compensation system.[27] Instead, each of Canada's 10 provinces and two territories has a Workers' Compensation Board

(WCB) (or equivalent) that is set up either as a statutory agency (equivalent to a Crown corporation) or as part of a ministry of labor.[3] Each WCB is governed by provincial or territorial legislation. The federal government has no meaningful operational role in workers' compensation.

Canadian WCBs were designed to ensure that a public insurance fund was available to compensate workers who became injured or ill because of work-related activities. In the case of a worker's death, families are compensated. Compensation programs are premised on a no-fault principle. Employees, therefore, cannot sue their employers, and an injured worker is guaranteed limited compensation regardless of whether the employer has been negligent or not.[22]

As is the case for other policy areas that fall under provincial jurisdiction, such as education, medical care, and natural resources, workers' compensation programs vary throughout the country. Bogyo explains[4]:

> A bank clerk must be covered for workers' compensation in Quebec but not in Manitoba; a worker in British Columbia can receive a benefit that is 50 percent higher than the maximum in Newfoundland; a restaurant owner will have to pay twice as much for coverage in Ontario as in British Columbia. This variety of benefits, coverage, and services reflects the political, social, and economic environment present in each province.

Nevertheless, Canadian workers' compensation programs do share similar characteristics in terms of administration, financing, and benefits.[23]

Administration

As previously noted, WCBs in Canada are governed by guidelines set out in provincial or territorial legislation. Board members are appointed by their respective provincial or territorial government. Daily operations are carried out by a chief administrative officer and accompanying public service staff. WCBs establish their own policies and procedures, adjudication rules, decisions and orders, and assessment (insurance premium) schedules and manage their own funds, anticipate future liabilities, and create reserves out of current earnings to fund these future liabilities.[12]

Workers' compensation claims can be initiated either by the injured worker, the employer, or the examining physician.[23] Workers wishing to appeal a WCB decision do so first through a somewhat informal internal review process. The next, and final, level of appeal is done through a hearing with an appeals body or tribunal, which in most provinces is independent of the WCB. Except for judicial review cases involving a violation of process under the Workers' Compensation Act or a decision that was arbitrary and patently unreasonable, decisions of appeal bodies are not subject to review in court.[13]

Financing and Costs

Workers' compensation is directly funded by compulsory contributions made by employers through an employer's payroll tax. Assessment (tax) rates are calculated in terms of amounts for each one hundred dollars of payroll, and vary depending on the amount of risk involved. To determine rates, rating groups (or classes) and experience-rating programs (also known as *merit* or *merit/demerit* programs) are used.

With rating groups, employers are stratified by industrial sectors, with each group paying a potentially different rate that reflects (more or less, depending on the province) the costs incurred by that group.[24] The more hazardous a group, the higher the rate companies or employers must pay.[23] The number of rating groups used by WCBs varies from province to province, as do the rates assessed for each group.

Experience-rating programs determine a specific company's actual WCB payroll tax based on its past injury and illness record or history. If the company's injury or accident record is higher than the average for its rating group, then it pays more. Conversely, if its record is better than average, it pays less. As such, employers have a financial incentive to reduce both accidents and potentially dangerous working conditions. Experience ratings are intended to encourage rehabilitation and re-employment of injured workers because these result in lower claims costs, which are then reflected in the calculation of the experience rating.[20]

In recent years, employers of the same industrial sector have started to create "safety groups" or "pools" to minimize their exposure by adopting actuarial and disability management principles. As well, many occupational health and safety departments have developed return-to-work programs and in-house treatment facilities.

Benefits

Workers receive different kinds of benefits depending on the nature of their injury or impairment. They can receive vocational and physical rehabilitation services, cash payments (based on a percentage of lost wages), their medical costs (wherein the provincial/territorial health-care system is reimbursed by WCBs), and a pension if the injury is permanently disabling or results in a permanent loss of earnings.[14] The definition of accident, injury, disability, and scope of entitlement, as well as the percentage of reimbursable earnings, varies according to province. Benefits are not taxed.

Until recently, WCBs based the amount of a disability pension for permanently disabled workers on the degree of their medical impairment. Such pensions were not affected by future employment prospects, so it led to situations in which some workers received a WCB lifetime pension even though they had returned to work with little or no earnings loss.[21]

Now, however, most Canadian WCBs, including Quebec, Alberta, and Ontario, have moved to a dual award system for permanently disabled workers. Workers are compensated for both future economic losses, or loss of earnings, and the presence of a permanent physical or psychological impairment (also referred to as a *non-economic loss*). Awards for loss of earning capacity make up a portion of the difference between a worker's pre-accident earning level and what he or she is currently earning or is deemed capable of earning. Consequently, one worker may be able to maintain earnings capacity despite a major medical impairment, particularly in jobs that are sedentary or professional in nature, whereas others may experience earnings loss with a relatively minor medical impairment, particularly in jobs that require manual dexterity or special skills.[14]

Awards for permanent impairment (non-economic loss) reflect the extent of the worker's impairment and are determined by the WCBs in accordance with prescribed rating schedules. Some provinces use recent editions of the American Medical Association's *Guides to the Evaluation of Permanent Impairment*,[1] some have developed their own tables, and some use a combination of the two. Impairment evaluations are generally performed by a WCB roster of physicians.

After registering with a WCB and obtaining a billing number, physicians can bill for services that are permitted under each Board's health professional fees schedule. Fees schedules, which are determined by each jurisdiction, are generally comparable to those of the respective provincial or territorial health insurance plan.

Research

Canadian WCBs fund and conduct research on compensation-related matters. For example, the Quebec WCB funded the Institute for Workers' Health and Safety of Quebec, which, in turn, funded the Quebec Task Force on Spinal Disorders. The resulting manuscript, *A Scientific Approach to the Assessment and Management of Activity-related Spinal Disorders,* was published in *Spine* in 1987.[16]

CANADA PENSION PLAN

The Canada Pension Plan (CPP) and the Quebec Pension Plan (QPP) were introduced in 1966 primarily in an attempt to provide all Canadians with a wage-related retirement pension system. The two plans are similar in terms of contributions and benefits; CPP is administered by Human Resources Development Canada, QPP by the Quebec provincial government. Entitlement and benefit credits are transferable, and together the two plans can be seen as making up a nationwide system.[11] In addition to a retirement pension, the plans provide survivor benefits (which include a death benefit, a children's benefit, and a surviving spouse's pension) and disability benefits.

For practical purposes, CPP is "a pay-as-you-go program," which means that current benefits are financed by current contributions.[19] Contributions are mandatory and are paid equally by the employer and employee. Self-employed workers pay both portions. Yearly contributions are determined on the basis of earnings—more specifically, on a percentage of earned income between a prescribed minimum and maximum figure. (Other sources of income, such as investment earnings, are not included.) Assuming they earn more than the minimum amount, all Canadian workers over the age of 18 contribute to CPP and do so until they turn 70 or retire (qualified individuals can retire and receive the Canada Pension at age 60). As of 1998, the maximum yearly contribution for both employees and employers was $1068.80; for self-employed workers it was $2137.60.

Disability Benefits

Workers who suffer a severe and prolonged physical or psychological impairment may be eligible to receive disability benefits. Benefits include a monthly pension to qualified workers and monthly benefit payments for their dependent children. According to the Canada Pension Plan[5]:

> A disability is **severe** only if by reason thereof the person in respect of whom the determination is made is incapable regularly of pursuing any substantially gainful occupation, and a disability is **prolonged** only if it is determined in prescribed manner that the disability is likely to be long continued and of indefinite duration or is likely to result in death.

To qualify for disability benefits, however, workers must also be under 65 and have contributed to CPP for 4 of the last 6 years. Further, earnings for each of those 4 years have to have reached at least 10% of that year's given maximum earnings figure. At age 65, the disability pension is switched over to a CPP retirement pension.

The disability pension consists of two parts, a flat-rate component, which is the same for all workers, and an earnings-related component, which varies depending on contributions made and years worked. In 1998 the flat-rate portion was $336.77 a month; the maximum monthly earnings-related amount was $558.59. Like all CPP benefits, disability pensions are considered taxable income and are fully indexed to the consumer price index.

As mentioned, the CPP also provides a monthly benefit payment for the dependent children of a disabled contributor. A "dependent child" is considered the natural or adopted child of the contributor, or a child in the care and control of the contributor, and who is either under age 18 or between the ages of 18 and 25 and in full-time attendance at a recognized institution.[8] The monthly benefit payment in 1998 for dependent children was $169.80.

Application Procedure

Contributors must apply for disability benefits in writing using a government application kit, which can either be picked up at a local client service center or mailed directly to the applicant. Kits contain instructions, application and consent forms, a questionnaire about employment history and medical situation, and a medical report. The medical report (Fig. 11–1) is usually filled out by the applicant's family physician or by the specialist most knowledgeable about the disabling medical condition.

As specified in CPP legislation, depending on the circumstances an application for the children's benefit may be made by the claimant parent, by the child, or by a provincial agency or other adult in charge of the child. Similarly, payments may go to the parent, another adult, an agency, or to the child.

After an application for a disability pension is approved by CPP adjudicators (most of whom are nurses), the claimant must wait for a period of 4 months before payments begin. It is incumbent on beneficiaries to inform CPP in writing if: their medical condition improves; they return to any job full-time, part-time, temporarily, or on a seasonal basis; they go to work on a trial basis; or they successfully complete a school, college, university, upgrading, or retraining program.[9] Once notified of such changes, CPP initiates a review of the claimant's file, which can result in benefits being cancelled if eligibility criteria are no longer being met. A claimant who fails to inform CPP about changes in his or her work or medical status and is later deemed to have received unwarranted benefits will be responsible for paying them back.

CPP Disability Vocational Rehabilitation Program

CPP recently introduced a Disability Vocational Rehabilitation Program predicated on the idea that advances in technology, medicine, and training techniques now make it possible to make some disabled workers employable. The voluntary program, established specifically to assist CPP disability pension recipients in rejoining the workforce, was approved after an evaluation of CPP's National Vocational Rehabilitation Project, which was started in 1993.

CPP reviews an individual's situation to determine his or her suitability for the program. An attempt is made to determine if a person has the motivation

Text continued on page 228

Government of Canada | Gouvernement du Canada
Income Security Programs | Programmes de la sécurité du revenu
Canada Pension Plan | Régime de pensions du Canada

Personal Information Bank
HWC PPU 146
Fichier de renseignements personnels
SBSC PPU 146

MEDICAL REPORT - RAPPORT MÉDICAL

Protected "B" When Completed
Protégé "B" une fois rempli

SECTION A To be completed by Applicant - Doit être remplie par le demandeur

First Name - Prénom	Initial - Initiale	Last Name - Nom de famille	
Home Address (No., Street, Apt., or R.R.) Adresse du domicile (numéro, rue, app., ou route rurale)		City - Ville	Province / Territory Province / territoire
Postal Code Code postal	Telephone No. - N° de téléphone ( )	Date of Birth Date de naissance D/J M Y/A	**Social Insurance Number** **Numéro d'assurance sociale**

SECTION B To be completed by Physician - Doit être remplie par le médecin

Please provide factual objective opinions - Veuillez donner une opinion factuelle objective

1 Height - Taille Weight - Poids	2 a) How long have you known the patient? Depuis quand connaissez-vous le patient?	b) When did you start treating the patient for the main medical condition? Quand avez-vous commencé à traiter le patient pour son état pathologique principal? M Y/A	c) Date of the last visit Date de la dernière visite D/J M Y/A

3 Diagnosis (es) - Diagnostic(s) :

4 Relevant/significant medical history relating to the main medical condition:
Antécédents médicaux pertinents/importants reliés à l'état pathologique principal :

ISP 2519 (06-94)

Printed on recycled paper  Imprimé sur du papier recyclé

Canada

FIGURE 11–1
Medical report form. (Courtesy Canada Pension Plan.)

Social Insurance Number
Numéro d'assurance sociale

5 **Over the past two years, has the patient been admitted to a hospital/institution?**
Au cours des deux dernières années, le patient a-t-il été admis à l'hôpital ou dans une institution?

○ Yes / Oui **If yes**, please list:
Dans l'affirmative, veuillez indiquer :

○ No / Non

Name of the Hospital(s)/Institution(s) - Nom de(s) l'hôpital(aux) ou de(s) l'institution (institutions)

The date(s) of admission La (les) date(s) d'admission	The reason(s) for admission La (les) raison(s) de l'admission

6 **Is there supporting evidence for the main medical condition?**
Y a-t-il des preuves à l'appui de l'état pathologique principal du patient?

Laboratory reports Rapports de laboratoire	○ Yes / Oui	○ No / Non
X-rays reports Radiographies	○ Yes / Oui	○ No / Non
Consultants' opinions Opinions de consultants	○ Yes / Oui	○ No / Non
Other Autre	○ Yes / Oui	○ No / Non
Documentation attached Documents ci-joints	○ Yes / Oui	○ No / Non
Documentation to be returned Documents devant être retournés	○ Yes / Oui	○ No / Non

Please describe relevant physical findings and functional limitations **or** attach supporting documentation.
Veuillez décrire les observations physiques et les limitations fonctionnelles pertinentes **ou** joindre les documents à l'appui.

FIGURE 11–1 *Continued*

Illustration continued on following page

Social Insurance Number
Numéro d'assurance sociale

7 **Are further consultations or medical investigations planned relating to the main medical condition?**
Prévoyez-vous effectuer d'autres consultations ou évaluations médicales en rapport avec son état pathologique principal?

○ Yes / Oui — **If yes**, please specify:
Dans l'affirmative, veuillez préciser :

○ No / Non

8 **Is the patient currently on medication(s) as a result of the main medical condition?**
Le patient prend-il présentement des médicaments en raison de son état pathologique principal?

○ Yes / Oui — **If yes**, please indicate dosage and frequency.
Dans l'affirmative, veuillez indiquer la dose et la fréquence.

○ No / Non

9 **Treatment:** List type and response.
Traitement : Indiquez le genre et la réaction.

FIGURE 11–1 *Continued*

Social Insurance Number
Numéro d'assurance sociale

10 **Prognosis of the main medical condition of this patient - Pronostic au sujet de l'état pathologique principal du patient :**

FIGURE 11–1 *Continued*

Illustration continued on following page

Social Insurance Number Numéro d'assurance sociale

11 Additional Information - Renseignements supplémentaires

SIGNATURE (Please print or use a stamp - Veuillez écrire en lettres moulées ou estampiller)		
Physician's Full Name - Nom du médecin au complet		
Address - Adresse Postal Code Code postal	○ Family Physician Médecin de famille ○ Specialty Spécialité ______	
Signature X	D/J M Y/A	Telephone No. - N° de téléphone ( )

FOR OFFICE USE ONLY - À L'USAGE EXCLUSIF DU BUREAU		
☐ A.C. - C.V.	Initials - Initiales	D/J M Y/A

FIGURE 11–1 *Continued*

and capability to go through work-related rehabilitation, a medical condition that allows it, a likelihood of actually returning to work, and a family physician who approves it. Some of the services that can be available through the program include skills enhancement, educational upgrading, retraining, guidance, and job-search training. Private-sector companies are contracted to provide the services. Participants continue to receive their full CPP disability benefits throughout the time they are involved in the program and during the period they spend looking for work. After obtaining employment, a claimant's benefits remain intact for 3 months.

Appeals

CPP contributors and beneficiaries may appeal any decision regarding benefits and eligibility. Appeals must be made in writing and within 90 days after receiving the disputed decision. There is a three-stage appeal process, starting with an appeal to the minister of human resources development. At this stage, an adjudicator unfamiliar with the initial decision reviews the claimant's file. If still dissatisfied, the claimant may appeal to a Review Tribunal, a three-member committee chaired by a lawyer and usually including at least one health-care professional. Hearings are informal, closed to the public, and usually held in or near the appellant's community.[10] If requested by the claimant, the third stage involves a hearing by the Pension Appeals Board. Made up of government-appointed judges, its decisions are final.

For the purpose of appeals, CPP does request independent medical evaluations from specialists. The referral letter to the specialist provides an outline of the components of the evaluation report to determine if the disabling condition(s) is prolonged and severe.

VETERANS AFFAIRS DISABILITY PENSIONS

Veterans Affairs Canada (VAC) provides a service-related disability pension to former, current, and reserve members (and their survivors) of the Canadian Armed Forces. Among those included are veterans of the two world wars and the Korean war, as well as Allied veterans and civilians who, during wartime, worked in organizations affiliated with the Canadian military. In 1998, disability pensions were provided to approximately 151,000 veterans and their survivors. Pensions are awarded for service-incurred disabilities/conditions, including aggravation of pre-enlistment conditions arising from or attributable to military service, either in peacetime or time of war.[26] Survivor pensions are also awarded for a death related to military duty.

The applicant for a VAC disability pension must provide personal information, as well as information about his or her service record and the current status of the medical condition in question (Fig. 11–2). They must also submit a completed physician's statement (Fig. 11–3).

Approval of an application involves two steps. First, using a claimant's application form, service record documents, and medical records, a VAC adjudicator (many of whom are nurses) must determine that the medical problem is connected to military service. Next, the degree of the disability must be assessed by a VAC or a VAC-contract physician who reviews the applicant's VAC files and medical reports and, in some cases, conducts a medical examination.[15] The doctor's recommended assessment is then sent to the VAC main office for approval.

The degree of disability (which is determined using VAC's Table of Disability) is then checked with VAC's rate table to establish the amount of the pension. A disability assessed from 1% to 4% results in a single, lump-sum payment. A disability assessed at 5% or greater results in the payment of a monthly pension.[25] Pension payments are increased for each 5% increment in assessed disability.

In 1998 the minimum monthly pension for a single veteran was $85.81; the maximum monthly benefit for 100% disability was $1716.20. Pensioners with a spouse (including a common-law spouse) and/or dependant children, parents,

B - APPLICANT'S STATEMENT **Protected information when completed.**

Disability being claimed

To what period of service is the claimed condition related? How is the claimed condition related to service (give details of any relevant events during service, including any medical treatment provided during service)? For a hearing loss claim, indicate the types of noise exposure (guns, artillery, etc.).

Describe how you have coped with the claimed condition since discharge. Have you had any medical attention for this condition since discharge? When and where was this medical attention received?

What effect has this claimed condition had on your everyday activities?

Name and address of physician from whom current information on the claimed condition can be obtained.

Name and address of physician(s)/consultant(s) seen for this condition in the past, if different from above.

Page 3 of 4

FIGURE 11–2
Applicant's statement from Application for Disability Pension. (Courtesy Veterans Affairs Canada.)

Veterans Affairs Canada / Anciens Combattants Canada

Protected information when completed.

HO file No.	Service No.(s)

PHYSICIAN'S STATEMENT

RE ______________________________

Patient's family name	Patient's given name(s)	Date of birth (y-m-d)

Specific medical diagnosis

X-rays / other tests / consultations Yes ☐ No ☐ Pending ☐ If **yes**, include a copy of the results. If **pending**, expected date of receipt. Year Month Day

Complaints/symptoms

Physical findings, i.e. limitation in movement

Duration and type of treatment/medication/surgery/recent hospitalization

Effects on everyday activities

Physician's name (printed)	Telephone No. Area code	Physician's signature	Date

PEN 819 (95-05)

Français au verso.

Canada

FIGURE 11–3
Physician's statement. (Courtesy Veterans Affairs Canada.)

or siblings can receive an additional pension. The 1998 maximum monthly married rate was $2145.25. Pensions are not taxable and are indexed for inflation.

Pensioners also receive treatment benefits, which must be related to their pensionable medical condition. Such benefits can include medical treatment when outside of Canada and expenses not covered by provincial health plans, such as for prescription drugs, wheelchairs, hearing aids, and hearing aid batteries. Some pensioners may also be eligible for a wider array of medical and related benefits under the Veteran's Independence Program (which is also available to eligible veterans who do not receive a disability pension).

In addition to their regular disability pension, veterans who are severely disabled (but not from their pensionable disability) may be eligible to receive either an attendants' allowance (if they need help with personal care) or an exceptional incapacity allowance. Pensioners who require orthotic or prosthetic devices secondary to their pensioned conditions may receive a clothing allowance.

For the first year after the death of a disability pensioner, the surviving spouse receives a pension equivalent to the original amount, which is usually reduced thereafter. Dependant children, as well as parents and/or siblings supported by a deceased pensioner, may also qualify for survivor benefits.

VAC disability claimants dissatisfied with a decision can appeal and, if they have new supportive medical information, can ask for a review of their case. In such situations, VAC may call in a specialist to do an independent medical evaluation to determine if the claim is, indeed, supported by new medical evidence.

PROVINCIAL SOCIAL ASSISTANCE PROGRAMS

A non-working person in Ontario (as an example) who believes he or she is disabled may apply to the local municipality for social assistance (general welfare assistance [GWA]). The person goes to the appropriate municipal office and makes an appointment to see a counselor. If the applicant claims disability, he or she is sent a province-wide medical report form to be completed by his or her physician.

If the physician states that the worker is temporarily unemployable because of disability, eligible applicants may collect GWA. If the physician states that the applicant is permanently unemployable because of a medical impairment and unlikely to resume remunerative employment, the applicant's file is sent to the province, which administers Family Benefits Assistance (FBA). FBA provides a client with more robust benefits than does GWA.

Recently, the Ontario government set up a separate income-support system for the disabled. The Ontario Disability Support Program takes people with disabilities off social assistance and is designed to be more responsive to their overall needs.

THE DISABILITY TAX CREDIT

The nonrefundable Disability Tax Credit lowers the amount of income tax paid by persons with a disability or by those individuals who support them. The credit is based on the realization that severely disabled persons have an elevated

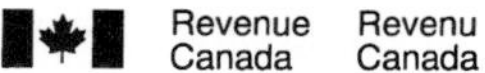
Revenue Canada / Revenu Canada

DISABILITY TAX CREDIT CERTIFICATE

Please read the attached information sheet carefully. It is important that you understand the eligibility requirements, and that you complete this form correctly.

Revenue Canada or one of our medical advisors may ask for more information about this claim.

Any medical fees related to this credit are the responsibility of the applicant or representative. Provincial medicare plans do not cover these fees.

Part A – To be completed by the applicant or representative

Complete this part before taking the form to your medical doctor, optometrist, or audiologist for completion of part B of the form.

Name of person making this claim	Social insurance number of person making this claim	6730 Relationship of person with disability to person making this claim: 1. ☐ Self 2. ☐ Spouse 3. ☐ Other (indicate relationship)	
6732 Date of birth of person with disability: Year / Month / Day	Maiden name of person with disability (if applicable)	Name of dependant with disability	6734 Social insurance number of dependant with disability

If you are claiming the credit for a dependant, does the dependant reside with you? **Yes** ☐ **No** ☐ If no, indicate the dependant's address.

Please provide the name, address, and telephone number of medical doctors, optometrists, or audiologists who know about the individual's disabling condition(s). Attach a separate sheet if you need more space.

Name	Address	Telephone number

I authorize any medical doctor, optometrist, or audiologist having medical records to disclose the information contained in these records to Revenue Canada for the purpose of determining whether the person with a disability meets the eligibility requirements for the disability tax credit.

Signature of person with disability or person with Power of Attorney — Telephone number — Date

Part B – To be completed by a medical doctor, optometrist, or audiologist

Complete the boxes that apply.

6738 Date your patient became markedly restricted: Year / Month

6740 The patient will be markedly restricted: 1. ☐ Permanently or Temporarily/Indefinitely ▶ Year — Please give the year the restriction ceased or should be reevaluated.

6742 Indicate how your patient is markedly restricted:

1. ☐ Vision 2. ☐ Walking 3. ☐ Speaking 4. ☐ Mental functions 6. ☐ Hearing 7. ☐ Feeding & Dressing 8. ☐ Elimination

6744 ☐ **DO NOT USE THIS AREA**

Continued on reverse ▶

T2201 E (97) (Ce formulaire existe aussi en français.) 1091 Canada

FIGURE 11–4
Disability Tax Credit Certificate. (Courtesy Revenue Canada.)

Illustration continued on following page

Part B — Continued (to be completed by a medical doctor, optometrist, or audiologist)

Indicate medical diagnosis relevant to the impairment and describe the restriction and aids used. Failure to complete this area might result in the claim being disallowed or the assessment of the income tax return being delayed.

Complete the boxes that apply. Note: If your patient requires an inordinate amount of time to perform one of these activities answer "no" to the applicable question.

1. **Vision**
   Is your patient able to see, using corrective lenses if necessary? (Your patient is considered blind if visual acuity in both eyes with proper refractive lenses is 20/200 (6/60) or less with Snellen Chart or equivalent, or when the greatest diameter of the field of vision in both eyes is less than 20 degrees.) — Yes ☐ No ☐

2. **Walking**
   Is your patient able to walk, using an aid if necessary? (For example, at least 50 metres on level ground.) — Yes ☐ No ☐

3. **Speaking**
   Is your patient able to speak so as to be understood in a quiet setting, using an aid if necessary? (Exclude language differences.) — Yes ☐ No ☐

4. **Mental functions**
   Is your patient able to think, perceive, and remember, using medication or therapy if necessary? (For example, can he or she manage personal affairs or do personal care without supervision?) — Yes ☐ No ☐

5. **Hearing**
   Is your patient able to hear (without speech reading) so as to understand a spoken conversation in a quiet setting, using an aid if necessary? (Exclude language differences.) — Yes ☐ No ☐

6. **Feeding & dressing**
   a) Is your patient able to feed himself or herself, using an aid if necessary? — Yes ☐ No ☐
   b) Is your patient able to dress himself or herself, using an aid if necessary? — Yes ☐ No ☐

7. **Elimination**
   Is your patient able to control and personally manage bowel and bladder functions, using an aid if necessary? (For example, has uncomplicated ostomy or uses a catheter.) — Yes ☐ No ☐

8. Has the impairment lasted, or is it expected to last, for a continuous period of at least 12 months? — Yes ☐ No ☐

9. Is the impairment severe enough to restrict the basic activity of daily living identified above all, or almost all, the time, even with therapy and the use of appropriate aids and medication? — Yes ☐ No ☐

Having read this form and the information sheet, I certify that, to the best of my knowledge, the foregoing information is true and complete.

Signature of medical doctor, optometrist, or audiologist

Name (please print)	Address	Date
		Telephone number

Printed in Canada

FIGURE 11–4 *Continued*

cost of living. To be eligible for the credit, a person must have a severe and prolonged physical or psychological impairment. More importantly, the person's ability to perform a basic activity of daily living must be markedly restricted because of the impairment. Generally, this occurs only when the individual is blind or is unable (or requires an inordinate amount of time) to perform such an activity, all or substantially all of the time, even with therapy and the use of appropriate devices and medication.[18] Basic activities of daily living include: walking; speaking; thinking, perceiving, and remembering; hearing; feeding and dressing; and eliminating. To apply for the credit, a disability tax credit certificate must be completed by the applicant and by his or her physician (Fig. 11–4). Optometrists, audiologists, psychologists, and occupational therapists also have the authority to certify (within their fields of expertise) the disability tax credit certificate. The completed certificate is filed as part of the applicant's income tax return.

Upon receipt of a new disability tax credit application, Revenue Canada reviews it to determine eligibility. In some cases, the department may ask a medical advisor for advice, who may in turn contact the claimant or health practitioner for more information to verify the claim.[17] If an individual is dissatisfied with Revenue Canada's ruling on a claim, he or she has the right to request a review of the case and, eventually, if still not satisfied, to appeal the decision. In 1998 the amount of the disability credit was $4233. If a disabled individual receives no tax advantage by claiming the entire credit, the remaining amount may, under certain conditions, be claimed by a spouse or supporting person.

CONCLUSION

This overview of the Canadian Disability System demonstrates a structure in flux. To provide the reader with up-to-date information, an appendix containing key government websites has been provided. In addition, provincial medical associations track changes that affect physicians in their provinces and periodically publish updates and third-party payment schedules for physicians doing medical evaluations not covered under the universal health-care system.

REFERENCES

1. American Medical Association: Guides to the Evaluation of Permanent Impairment, 4th ed. Chicago, American Medical Assocation, 1993.
2. Armitage A: Social Welfare in Canada Revisited: Facing Up to the Future, 3rd ed. Don Mills, Ontario, Oxford University Press Canada, 1996, p 76.
3. Bogyo TJ: Workers' compensation: Updating the historic compromise. In: Richards J, Watson WG (eds): Chronic Stress: Workers' Compensation in the 1990s. Toronto, CD Howe Institute, 1995, pp 92–135.
4. Op. cit. p 101.
5. Canada pension plan. Section 42(2). In: Canada Pension Plan, Old Age Security Act and Pension Benefits Standards Act & Regulations, 11th ed. North York, Ontario, CCH Canadian Limited, 1996, p 40.
6. Guest D: The Emergence of Social Security in Canada. Vancouver, University of British Columbia Press, 1980.
7. Op. cit. p 8.
8. Human Resources Development Canada: Disability Benefits. 1998a, Website: www.hrdc-drhc.gc.ca/isp, p 7.

9. Human Resources Development Canada: Facts About Reassessing Eligibility. 1998b, Website: www.hrdc-drhc.gc.ca/isp, p 1.
10. Human Resources Development Canada: (1998c). Annual Report of the Canada Pension Plan, 1996–1997. Ottawa, Minister of Public Works and Government Services Canada, 1998c, p 18.
11. Kumar P, Smith AMM: Pension Reform in Canada: A Review of the Issues and Options. Kingston, Ontario, Industrial Relations Centre, Queen's University, 1981.
12. Pals KC, Guidotti TL: Overview of the Canadian Disability System. In: Demeter SL, Andersson GBJ, Smith GM (eds): Disability Evaluation. St Louis, Mosby, 1996, p 31–35.
13. Op. cit. p 34.
14. Op. cit. p 32.
15. Personal communication with Veterans Affairs Canada staff.
16. Quebec Task Force on Spinal Disorders: A scientific approach to the assessment and management of activity-related spinal disorders: Spine 12(7 Suppl), S1–S59, 1987.
17. Revenue Canada: Disability Tax Credit and You. Website:www.rc.gc.ca/disability, 1996, p 3.
18. Revenue Canada: Medical Expense and Disability Tax Credits and Attendant Care Expense Deduction. Interpretation bulletin No. IT-519R2. Ottawa, Income Tax Rulings and Interpretations Directorate, 1998, p 4.
19. Smolkin S: What's happening to government benefits in Canada? In: The Law Society of Upper Canada: A Pension and Benefits Legislative Primer. Toronto, The Law Society of Upper Canada, 1996, p 4–3.
20. Stritch A: Homage to catatonia: Bipartite governance and workers' compensation in Ontario. In: Richards J, Watson WG (eds): Chronic Stress: Workers' Compensation in the 1990s. Toronto, CD Howe Institute, 1995, pp 136–172.
21. Op. cit. p 146.
22. Thomason T: The escalating costs of workers' compensation in Canada: Causes and cures. In: Richards J, Watson WG (eds): Chronic stress: Workers' Compensation in the 1990s. Toronto, CD Howe Institute, 1995, pp 23–65.
23. Op. cit. p 25.
24. Vaillancourt F: The Financing of Workers' Compensation Boards in Canada, 1960–1990. Toronto, Canadian Tax Foundation, 1994, p 82.
25. Veterans Affairs Canada: Disability Pensions (Cat. No. V44-5/1997). Ottawa, Minister of Public Works and Government Services Canada, 1997, p 4.
26. Veterans Affairs Canada: Benefits to Canadian Veterans Residing Outside of Canada. Website: www.vac-acc.gc.ca, 1998, p 1.
27. Williams Jr CA: An International Comparison of Workers' Compensation. Boston, Kluwer Academic Publishers, 1991.

APPENDIX 11-1

Web Site Addresses

FEDERAL PROGRAMS

REVENUE CANADA: Information for People with Disabilities Web Page
http://www.rc.gc.ca/disability

HUMAN RESOURCES DEVELOPMENT CANADA: Canada Pension Plan
http://www.hrdc-drhc.gc.ca/isp

VETERANS AFFAIRS CANADA (Home Page)
http://www.vac-acc.gc.ca

PROVINCIAL PROGRAMS

Information on provincial social assistance programs can be found via provincial government home pages listed below. Provincial Workers' Compensation Board websites are also listed.

NEWFOUNDLAND AND LABRADOR
Government Home Page: http://www.nfld.com
Workers' Compensation Commission: http://www.whscc.nf.ca

NOVA SCOTIA
Government Home Page: http://www.gov.ns.ca
Workers' Compensation Board: http://www.wcb.ns.ca

PRINCE EDWARD ISLAND
Government Home Page: http://www.gov.pe.ca
Workers' Compensation Board: http://www.wcb.pe.ca

NEW BRUNSWICK
Government Home Page: http://www.gov.nb.ca
Workplace Health, Safety and Compensation Commission:
http://www.gov.nb.ca/whscc

QUEBEC
Government Home Page: http://www.gouv.qc.ca

ONTARIO
Government Home Page: http://www.gov.on.ca
Workplace Safety and Insurance Board: http://www.wcb.on.ca

MANITOBA
Government Home Page: http://www.gov.mb.ca
Workers' Compensation Board: http://www.wcb.mb.ca

SASKATCHEWAN
Government Home Page: http://www.gov.sk.ca
Workers' Compensation Board: http://www.wcbsask.com

ALBERTA
Government Home Page: http://www.gov.ab.ca
Workers' Compensation Board: http://www.wcb.ab.ca

BRITISH COLUMBIA

Government Home Page: http://www.gov.bc.ca

Workers' Compensation Board: http://www.wcb.bc.ca

YUKON

Government Home Page: http://www.gov.yk.ca

SECTION IV

Physician Disability Practice Applications

CHAPTER 12

Independent Medical Evaluation

Steve R. Geiringer, MD

Performing disability evaluations encompasses providing an opinion; the more definite the opinion, the more valuable the evaluation, within the limits of medical knowledge. The opinion sought usually concerns "the severity of a medical problem, the appropriateness of a treatment plan, and an assessment of the degree of medical impairment in persons who claim they are entitled to disability benefits."[3] However, opinions may differ from one practitioner to another, and insurance companies or others may arrange for an independent (sometimes termed *impartial*) medical evaluation (IME). The requesting party is typically seeking "a medical opinion from a physician not involved in the care of the claimant and with no regular business ties to the insurance company."[3] The physician performing the IME does not develop a treating relationship with the examinee.

There are a number of potential confounders of recovery in litigated claims. For example, it has been well established that a person who is experiencing pain cannot objectively judge the severity of the condition. Injured workers using the legal system overestimate their health at baseline, and overstate the negative impact of injury.[6] Factors relating to a claimant's psychological makeup and current employment status may contribute to disability prolongation[2]; such factors may be only indirectly related to impairment.

Furthermore, a worker's treating physicians often contribute to prolonged disability status beyond that justified by objective information.[11] Work disability is also related to interpersonal conflicts on the job.[1] Or, an asymptomatic but deconditioned individual could be mistaken on examination for one with a lumbar impairment or for a "symptom magnifier."[7]

These are some of the reasons that an impartial opinion, based as much as possible on objective information, may be requested.[10] Although some work-simulating machines may be useful in that objective data are generated, the reasoned opinion of a physician skilled in disability evaluation is highly valued by referring sources.[4]

THE ETHICS OF PROVIDING INDEPENDENT MEDICAL EXAMINATIONS

The ethics of being an IME provider are the topic of extensive discussion, especially informally. Some practitioners insist that there is no such thing as an "impartial" opinion because the physician knows full well where the reimbursement is coming from for a given case. The reality is that payment has to originate from somewhere, and in these cases it is from the party requesting the IME. Most disability evaluators fall on the "defense" side of the equation (i.e., receiving IME referrals from employers, compensation insurance carriers, and case managers). A smaller number of IME physicians garner most of their referrals from attorneys for the "plaintiff," or injured worker. A physician's reputation (i.e., as "favoring" the plaintiff or defense viewpoint) often determines his or her referring sources.

Any clinician working in this arena can identify those physician outliers whose opinion can be counted on, regardless of the specifics of an individual case. This works both ways; some physicians will deem any claimant fully disabled for extended periods. The other extreme is the IME rater who feels that no one is disabled, even partially and/or temporarily, despite the objective findings of impairment that may exist. These examples are of course exaggerated to make the point.

The retort to these concerns is clear and simple: as a physician, treating or evaluating, one must always recommend what is in the best interest of the client. If an injured worker presents without any sign of impairment after careful search, it is clearly not in his or her best interest to remain off work indefinitely while receiving passive and inefficacious modalities and sliding further into the abyss of general deconditioning, occupational and social isolation, chronicity of suffering, and perhaps depression. Conversely, when an objective impairment does exist and could be made worse by working, it may be against everyone's best interest for the physician to allow a premature, unrestricted return to work. Finally, society, the ultimate consumer of goods and services provided by workers, benefits maximally when these considerations are followed to the best ability of an ethical physician.

There is clearly a place for the physician performing IMEs who is willing and able to make objective and fair determinations. However, when a referring source knows in advance what a physician's opinion will be because that opinion never varies among cases, the physician is doing a disservice to the field of disability evaluation. Referring sources also prefer physicians who diagnose and treat patients as the main component of their practices, to ensure that sufficient clinical experience supports the IME opinions.

REASONS FOR THE INDEPENDENT MEDICAL EVALUATION

There are myriad reasons for an IME to be performed, beyond the determination of whether the claimant actually has an impairment, although that is likely the most frequent reason. In that circumstance, the examining physician is asked to make or confirm a diagnosis, a question that translates in practical terms to whether an impairment is present to explain the symptoms and consequent disability. Additional reasons to request an IME include the following:

- Impairment
- Maximal medical improvement (MMI)
- Prognosis
- Diagnostic testing
- Treatment
- Causality
- Apportionment
- Work ability
- Follow-up

Impairment

An impairment is the objective physiological abnormality that can account for the examinee's symptoms. Impairment must be distinguished from the pain itself and from the disability arising from the pain. It generally is not fruitful to doubt whether someone is feeling pain; the IME physician's first task is to identify the underlying impairment that explains the pain. Function must also be differentiated from impairment, although as with pain, the two are usually related. Objective evidence of impairment in the realm of musculoskeletal medicine is typically documented on physical examination, radiographic studies, or electrodiagnostic testing.

Maximal Medical Improvement

The IME is often used to determine whether there is still potential for medical recovery from whatever impairment is found; if not, the worker has reached maximal medical improvement (MMI). A strict interpretation, applicable to the vast majority of occupational injury cases, is that MMI is considered to have been achieved *when further formal medical intervention (treatment) cannot be reasonably expected to improve the underlying impairment*. This concept is crucial for several reasons:

- MMI presupposes that in fact an impairment exists. When one has pain that cannot be correlated with an objective abnormality, it makes no sense to then discuss MMI.
- The timing of MMI must not be confused with the disappearance of symptoms. To illustrate, one may have ongoing pain in the injured area, but without identifiable impairment. If the residual pain can be expected to fade and eventually disappear simply with passage of time, MMI has been reached.
- Similarly, if the remaining symptoms can be ameliorated with palliative measures, for example cold or hot packs applied at home, MMI has already been achieved.
- This in turn should also highlight the fact that measures that are purely for the relief of symptoms, for example hot packs to the back, do not (in isolation) comprise a treatment that will favorably affect the underlying impairment. MMI has already been reached if the only interventions are for symptomatic relief only, and other measures will not improve the impairment.

Although the above definition of MMI is widely applicable, it is inadequate in at least two circumstances. The first, and least controversial, is when the impairment is stable, yet a new or previously untried treatment arises. To illustrate, a worker sustained an above-elbow amputation long ago and has been using a "standard" prosthesis with a shoulder girdle–driven terminal device. The switch to a myoelectric prosthesis might enable the worker to perform some job functions that were previously not feasible. Here, MMI had not been achieved initially even though the impairment (the amputation) was stable, because *a new or additional treatment allowed for reduction of disability.*

The second, more common occurrence in the disability evaluation realm is the client with disabling pain, to the point of not being able to work, but without demonstrable impairment. That combination presents more of a dilemma to the evaluator. It may be that further treatment would reduce the disability (i.e., improve the level of functioning) even though no impairment is present. It may also be that a restricted return-to-work schedule may be useful temporarily, as a transition to a status of full functioning. These possibilities should be considered in the IME opinion because it is not in anyone's best interest to adopt a punitive or pejorative attitude toward the examinee who has no impairment. Frank malingering seems rare, and often the lingering pain and disability are present through no "fault" of the person experiencing them.

In a subset of the "pain without physical impairment" group are those with chronic pain syndrome. The evaluator might then conclude that there is no impairment from the physical standpoint, but return to work should be deferred until evaluation by an expert in chronic pain, typically a psychologist, can be done. The greater the proportion of clients referred to a practice in the acute or subacute stages, the smaller will be this subset.

Prognosis

The determination of prognosis requires an educated medical guess but should take into account the objective information alluded to earlier. Prognosis is, of course, related to the impairment present. The most favorable prognosis predicts that the impairment will fully resolve, leaving no residual symptoms or loss of function. A less favorable prognosis typically means that some impairment will remain after MMI has been reached.

Diagnostic Testing

The IME physician might be asked whether tests done previously were in fact needed, and what further testing should be done. The answer to the inquiry about prior studies might be used to (retrospectively) deny payment for them. Most insuring bodies will not need to resort to that, as most studies must be authorized ahead of time.

An important point for clarification is that providing an opinion about diagnostic studies, and even ordering or performing them, does not violate the terms of an IME (i.e., it does not constitute treatment). Tests that are suggested should be necessary in the determination of objective impairment. An IME physician, for example, will sometimes perform electrodiagnostic studies before rendering a final report.

Treatment

Insurance companies providing workers' compensation or auto insurance benefits will often ask the IME physician if treatment rendered to date has been effective. This could be to deny payment, or to prevent future such treatment from being remunerated. It is wise to remember that it is easier to judge what was wrong after the fact, compared with prospectively anticipating which interventions will be useful.

The need for future treatment may also be addressed. The IME physician must be as specific as the circumstances allow when answering these questions. It is not helpful to state that "a 4-week course of physical therapy is warranted." Rather, the details of what that therapy should entail should be stated (i.e., the use of passive modalities only for the facilitation of an exercise program that has specific components). A prediction of MMI or prognosis might hinge on these treatment suggestions being followed, and the clinical response to them.

Causality

Simply put, one must determine as best as possible what led to the impairment that is identified. This is potentially an extremely difficult determination for the IME provider. An idealized history of work-related injury would find that the worker had no prior symptoms or impairment related to the newly diagnosed condition, no prior incidents involving those areas, and no underlying, preexisting problems such as degenerative arthritis affecting nearby regions. With that clean background, there should be no controversy about the origin of the current impairment.

Typically, though, the history is not so clear cut. There may be one or more of the following factors to consider:

- A similar impairment, now fully resolved, is known to have occurred previously
- A previous impairment has occurred and is not fully healed (i.e., MMI had not yet been achieved for a prior injury to the same structure)
- There is an underlying, preexisting condition that is clearly not work related, such as a significant leg-length discrepancy from a childhood fracture
- There is a preexisting condition that might or might not be work related, such as osteoarthritis in the lumbar spine, or carpal tunnel syndrome; in the most difficult of determinations, there has been no prior diagnostic testing to "establish the baseline" of the problem
- An underlying impairment is known to be present, but arose from employment elsewhere
- Myriad other situations and combinations of situations can and do arise routinely to complicate the determination of causality in an IME

One factor that simplifies the IME provider's task in this regard is the medicolegal definition of whether cause is present. In this setting, the term *medically probable* means that there is an equal to or less than 50% likelihood that the events are linked. *Medically possible* means that there is an equal to or less than 50% chance that the cause is linked to the impairment. Although that definition is much less rigorous than is used in typical medical logic, it describes an important distinction that the medicolegal system relies on, and on which award determinations might rest.

Apportionment

Apportionment is the assigning of the relative degrees to which various causes just identified have contributed to the impairment. This is a physician responsibility and is often a subjective determination. In some workers' compensation jurisdictions, the employer or its insurance company must assume responsibility only for that fraction of cause arising directly from the current work injury. In others, the responsibility falls fully on the employer even if there was only a minor aggravation of a severe, preexisting, unrelated impairment. Naturally, the IME rater must be familiar with local regulations because the meting out of apportioned responsibility for an impairment is critical in the former circumstance but irrelevant in the latter.

Work Ability

It is unusual for an IME to be requested when the claimant is still or again working full time and unrestricted, so most IMEs include a request to comment on the injured worker's ability to return to the job. The majority of costs related to workers' compensation arise from time off the job, not from medical expenses. The company's compensation specialists, therefore, are most eager to effect a rapid return to work, preferably without the limiting effects of physical or time restrictions.

The three broad categories for return to work include *unrestricted, with restrictions* (time or physical, or both), and *unable to work*. Unrestricted return to work is generally limited to situations in which the impairment has been healed or reversed, or no impairment was present initially. Some very minor impairments may still allow for heavy physical work, and some major impairments (e.g., a limb amputation) may allow for unrestricted work in a setting that does not include heavy labor, per NIOSH standards.[8] Restricted return to work can be allowed if the physical demands of the light-duty job will not worsen the impairment or impede healing. This is most often a temporary state, with the limitations to be reduced or removed when appropriate after clinical reevaluation. A related issue, but one that does not fall within the purview of the IME evaluator, is whether the stated restrictions are in fact met by the employer. Many clients maintain that on their return to work they are expected to perform physical tasks beyond those "allowed." Finally, keeping an examinee completely off work is necessary if even light duty could worsen the impairment, prevent or delay healing, or potentially put the worker or co-workers in peril.

The IME report may conclude that the worker is unable to return to work, typically for a time-limited period, although at times it may be on a permanent basis. The specific reasons for those opinions must be based on the nature of the objective impairment and its relationship to the job in question.

Follow-Up

A follow-up opinion may be needed once the recommended diagnostic tests have been performed, or results of prior testing have been forwarded for review. In those cases, the original IME report remains inconclusive regarding the questions posed.

Another circumstance is that the IME physician may recommend another examination after a specified amount of time has passed, a particular treatment has been rendered, a job change has been affected, or other events or conditions have occurred. A "serial" IME then occurs, with some cases involving numerous examinations over many months to a year or more.

ELEMENTS OF THE IME REPORT

The remainder of this chapter will detail the elements of the IME report, and as such will to some extent mirror the preceding sections. This portion will contain more detail about situations commonly encountered in practice, and should serve as a template for the performance and reporting of the IME for a physical medicine and rehabilitation practitioner.

It is wise to allow sufficient time in the daily clinic schedule for dictation of IME reports immediately after the appointment. The credibility of the report content will be greater if it is the physician's standard practice to dictate then instead of at the end of a busy day when numerous other evaluations could be commingled in memory. Elements of the report include the following:

- Introduction
- History of current condition
- Work history
- Diagnostic studies
- Prior treatment
- Review of systems
- Physical examination: musculoskeletal
- Physical examination: neurological
- Physical examination: nonphysiologic findings
- Diagnosis (impairment)
- Causality and apportionment
- MMI
- Prognosis
- Work ability
- Diagnostic testing
- Treatment
- Follow-up

Introduction

The referral source for the IME should be documented, as well as the specific questions that have been posed that the IME evaluator will attempt to answer. It is wise in the introductory paragraph to also include a statement acknowledging that, because this is an IME, no treating relationship will arise from the examination, and the examinee has been so informed. A signed disclaimer attesting to this fact may be useful.

The IME evaluator should summarize the medical records reviewed. Those files will be present in the chart should the case come to medicolegal testimony, so there is no need to record the source, date, and specific content of each medical narrative and/or diagnostic test result. Pertinent details from outside information can be dictated into the report as indicated, especially for objective test results. In the case of radiological reports, the IME evaluator should note whether the conclusions are his or hers alone from studying the films, or are taken from a radiologist's final report. In the former case, the IME evaluator's opinion will not be considered "expert" unless he or she is also board certified in radiology.

History of Current Condition

The history should be extracted as fully as possible from the client. If other records are used to supplement or provide the basic history, or a family member, friend, or case manager supplies information, that should be documented. There is no need for the dictated report to repeatedly read "The examinee states . . ." That is implied unless noted otherwise. With experience, the art of providing "just enough" detail of the history will evolve, particularly for reports on a chronic condition; once again, there is no need to detail the particulars of each physical therapy session ever attended, or of each radiograph ever taken. The reader should be left with a sufficient overview of the clinical course from start to finish, and fine points can always be retrieved later as needed. It is acceptable to refer to another medical narrative as a source of more detail, assuming the content of that report has been reviewed and appears consistent with the history obtained.

As with any aspect of a medical history, it is important to ask specific, rather than broad questions about prior, related problems. To illustrate, for a person with a herniated lumbar disc it is not useful to ask, "Have you had back pain before this?" Rather, the IME evaluator should inquire about prior diagnoses; any radiological examinations, scans, or EMGs that might have been performed; or any physical therapy received for a similar or related type of pain. He or she should also ask if any work was missed for those problems, or if light duty was needed, and for how long.

Work History

The IME physician should ask about the client's length of time with the current employer and about changes in job responsibilities while there. He or she should also determine if there is a temporal relationship between the pertinent symptoms and such a change. A general idea of "job satisfaction," including how favorably supervisors and management are viewed, may yield useful insight into a recurring problem. The IME physician should find out (from the employer if necessary) about prior physical or time restrictions the client may have had, and if he or she has had good or subpar attendance. He or she should also ask whether prior jobs were similar in physical demands, and why those positions were vacated. Finally, it can be very revealing to inquire about and gauge the sincerity of the response to the claimant's plans for the immediate and intermediate future. Some will be very forthcoming about having no intention whatsoever of returning to work, demonstrating a strong sense of entitlement after a work injury. Others will want nothing less than full return to work at the soonest possible time, and those feelings might need to be reflected in the report.

Diagnostic Studies

The IME physician should document what was available to him or her at the time of the IME:

1. Radiographic films (or EMG data) only
2. Films and formal report
3. Neither
4. Client's memory of prior results

Prior Treatment

For musculoskeletal conditions, the most important component of prior treatment is typically physical therapy. There might also be any of the following: surgical procedures; medications, either oral, locally injected, systemically injected, or applied topically, either by prescription or over the counter; manipulations; acupuncture; nutritional or home remedies; or other "alternative" interventions. Therapy efforts should be reviewed in detail regarding whether only modalities were used, or if in fact an active exercise program, monitored and advanced regularly and appropriate to the impairment present, was attempted. Was a home exercise program prescribed? Did the examinee follow it faithfully? How often were exercises actually performed, and how recently was it done? The IME evaluator should ask about further efforts such as back school, work hardening, or functional restoration programs.

Some patients have become accustomed to what can be called *palliative treatments,* those that could not be expected by themselves to improve an underlying impairment or reduce the level of disability. Passive modalities of hot packs, ultrasound, or massage are commonly applied for extended courses over months or even years. One must ascertain whether the examinee feels those are helpful, perhaps simply by asking, "Do you feel better after a treatment?" At some other time in the history, though, the IME evaluator should let the client estimate how much better his or her symptoms have become overall (e.g., "I'm only 5% better than right after my injury 7 months ago"). Those two lines of questioning often yield notably disparate answers, information that could be useful in the determination of whether current treatment is efficacious in reducing an impairment, ameliorating disability, or improving function.

Review of Systems

A general medical review of systems is not usually needed for the musculoskeletal IME. It is necessary, however, to record major medical problems (e.g., depression, diabetes mellitus, or cardiac disease). Some conditions that are not work related could affect the person's ability to undergo rehabilitation efforts that might otherwise be indicated.

Physical Examination: Musculoskeletal

All aspects of the physical examination must be performed and reported as objectively as possible.

- **Inspection and observation:** The IME physician should document asymmetries or deformities, posture characteristics, biomechanics of lumbar motion and of foot motions/gait if indicated, loss of contour of muscles (e.g., gastrocnemius on toe raise), obvious atrophy or swelling, distal trophic changes.
- **Measurements:** Shoulder heights, distances from thoracic spine to medial scapular borders, leg lengths, and arm, forearm, thigh, and calf circumferences should be measured.
- **Ranges of motion:** For axial joint contractures (e.g., at the elbow, hip, or knee), it might be helpful to use a goniometer for objective measurement of joint motion. Inclinometers for the spine are difficult to rely on and are often not necessary. It helps to develop an inherent sense of degrees of joint motion, and with practice it is usually possible to estimate within 5° motion at the ankle, knee, hip, wrist, elbow, and shoulder. For lumbar and cervical spine motion it is sufficient to estimate motion in 25% increments (e.g., "Neck rotation lacks about 50% to the right and left, whereas side bending lacks between 0 and 25% to the right, about 25% to the left.") More detail than that is unlikely to be clinically or legally useful. Any asymmetry and local, referred, or radiating pain with any motion should be reported.
- **Palpation:** Although the examinee's response to palpation (i.e., whether it is tender or not) is itself subjective, the evaluator can lend some objectivity by reporting whether tenderness was felt virtually everywhere, or if it was isolated to recognized points such as the superior medial scapular border, upper trapezius fibers, or posterior iliac crest. Similarly, the abnormal texture or consistency of a trigger point is not within the control of the client, and should be noted.

- **Provocative maneuvers:** Any inflamed tissue that is part of a contractile complex (e.g., muscle, musculotendinous junction, enthesis) will hurt when contraction is evoked. The IME evaluator should record what resisted motions hurt and where the pain was felt. For example, he or she should mention whether pain with resistance of supraspinatus function was felt in the typical rotator cuff area near the deltoid insertion or in the upper trapezius area. If the Spurling maneuver is performed, the provider should record where the pain was felt and if it was localized to the head or neck, or radiating down the limb. Joint examinations for laxity, instability, or pain should be carried out and reported as for any examinee.

Physical Examination: Neurological

Strength must be tested against body weight as needed, particularly for the lower limb groups (i.e., toe and heel walking, arising from a squat). Muscle stretch reflexes for lower limb or lumbar problems must be done not only at the knees and ankles, but always at the medial hamstring as well, to study L5 root integrity. This is most reliably accomplished with the person prone, with the IME physician tapping on his or her finger that overlies the tendon just distal to its origin from the ischial tuberosity.[5] In this position, the targeted muscle can be observed for the amplitude and briskness of the reflex response.

If straight leg raising causes pain, the quality and location of the pain should be recorded, as well as at what degree it occurs. Many times there will be a stretching sensation in the hamstring area, or low back pain without thigh or leg pain, not the characteristic radiating pain to the ankle or foot that sometimes accompanies L5 or S1 nerve-root irritation. The same guidelines hold for reverse straight leg raise testing while prone. Tinel's sign is useful for any nerve that has been injured and is currently in the process of regrowth, not just the median nerve.

Sensation testing always relies on the claimant's subjective responses, whether for pain, light touch, two-point discrimination, or proprioception. It is therefore impossible to objectify, and should be considered only adjunctive to other findings. If all other findings point to a C7 radiculopathy, for instance, it would not be justified to discount that impairment because of a "non-dermatomal" sensory loss. Conversely, if the only physical examination finding is a subjective decrease in light-touch sensation, the IME physician might consider that insufficient by itself to diagnose a nerve impairment.

Physical Examination: Nonphysiological Findings

Some nonphysiological findings were described by Waddell.[9] In general, the importance of these signs is to alert the examiner to findings that cannot be explained by known physiological mechanisms. One example is a straight leg raise test that yields severe pain at 0 or a few degrees while supine, but can be carried out to 80° or 90° later in the examination without complaint, and is observed while testing distal limb strength or sensation. Other nonphysiological findings include sensory loss that poorly matches dermatomes (but beware of typical individual variability from "textbook" dermatomes), remote spread of symptoms (e.g., neck pain while testing toe extensor strength), or discrepancies in manual versus functional strength (e.g., the claimant cannot extend the knee even with gravity removed, but is seen to ambulate normally in the parking lot).

Although these signs can provide useful insights, they must be considered in the larger picture before assigning significance to them. An injured worker who perhaps has been unjustly denied benefits by the employer or insurance company may feel the need to embellish certain aspects of the examination to "make sure" the IME physician notices the pain. The isolated finding of a discrepant supine versus seated straight leg raising test does not mean that impairment is absent.

Diagnosis: Impairment

From this point forward, the IME report will contain the provider's opinions and conclusions about the history and physical examination and will answer the questions put forth by the referring source. For some IMEs, the only question asked is whether there is any impairment to explain the symptoms or disability, and nearly every IME will include impairment as one of the items to be addressed. The most definitive positive response occurs when there is good correlation among the examination, diagnostic testing, and reported symptoms. It is then simple to state, for example, that the symptomatic numbness and weakness suggest a C7 radiculopathy, and the diminished triceps size, strength, and stretch reflex, combined with the MRI finding of a low cervical disc herniation, support that diagnosis. The IME physician's skills are tested more when the symptoms do not match with the impairment found, or when there is in fact no impairment found despite ongoing symptoms. When such a discrepancy exists, the report must highlight it and explain it in clear terms, or the conclusions will not be useful to the claimant, the referring source, and ultimately to the system within which the IME arose. In these cases, it is not useful to use terms such as *exaggeration, embellishment,* or *malingering.* A medicolegal report is not the place for judgmental statements that by definition cannot be supported by fact; if the IME physician is clear about the lack of impairment, the same result will occur without the need for unprofessional terminology.

One circumstance that may allow the IME physician to broach the issue of malingering is when a surveillance videotape is available showing the client doing heavy physical labor proximate in time to when any lumbar movement caused excruciating pain during the IME. The videotape, assuming the correct person has been identified, is useful and objective information. Even here it is best to summarize the discrepancy in a straightforward manner, without resorting to pejorative terms.

It may also be necessary to determine whether an impairment is expected to be temporary or permanent. If temporary, an expected time frame should be given, sometimes contingent on treatment recommended by the IME physician being carried out. The conclusion of permanent impairment naturally is an important decision for all concerned, and should be supported by careful reasoning.

Diagnosis: Disability

The step after specifying the impairment is to determine its relevance to work, daily functioning, or household activities. Work disability will be discussed later. In general, however, the physician must ascertain if and to what extent a given impairment diminishes the examinee's ability to carry out expected functions in various settings. Conclusions can then be made whether help is needed with activities of daily living such as light and/or heavy household chores.

Diagnosis: Prognosis

Only with considerable clinical experience can a physician attempt to foresee how an impairment will behave as time passes. Some conditions, such as the client having undergone a prior laminectomy, will of course never change. Most musculoskeletal conditions will change over time, for better or worse, and the expected prognosis might depend on subsequent treatment, job placement, or operative intervention. In those situations, it is most helpful if the report provides a prognosis for each of the variables of the case, so the referring source has a sense of cause and effect. To illustrate, the report might state that an injured worker could return to a restricted job 3 weeks after the recommended physical therapy regimen commences and to unrestricted work 6 weeks thereafter. If the examinee returns for a follow-up IME and no treatment has occurred, it is unlikely that return to work could take place; the reason for that delay will be obvious, however, and the system might then be prompted to respond.

Causality and Apportionment

A compensation insurance provider may have a strong interest in the opinion of the IME evaluator regarding the cause and effect relationship between a work injury, car accident, or personal health habits and the impairment. Additionally, if more than one cause is present, it is the physician's responsibility to assign the percentage of the impairment that arose from each cause. Perhaps a prior car accident resulted in the worker having a light-duty job over the past several years, and a recent work incident rendered him more limited yet. One may have underlying osteoarthritis and lumbar disc degeneration simply from having reached late middle age, and a work accident leads to substantially worsened symptoms. These and myriad other scenarios occur routinely, rather than as exceptions, in the setting of disability determination. Apportionment is the process of sorting out these factors.

Maximal Medical Improvement

It is critically important to understand the difference between ongoing symptoms (and even consequent disability) and an objective impairment that explains the symptoms. MMI is generally achieved when further formal medical intervention cannot be reasonably expected to improve or diminish the impairment (but consider again the additional aspects of MMI as discussed earlier in this chapter). Approached in another way, treatment after MMI is palliative, and the insurance carrier should not shoulder the burden of its provision. At MMI, the underlying condition might be totally resolved, partially resolved but not expected to further improve, or unchanged from when it occurred. Prognosis in most cases is linked to the medical condition at MMI.

Many soft-tissue injuries (e.g., rotator cuff tendinitis) can be successfully treated so that no impairment lingers; return to work could then occur without any restrictions. If a cuff tear occurs, the impairment remains indefinitely, even though there might be decreasing disability over time. Return to work might be successful only with restrictions against repeated overhead work, heavy pushing and pulling, and repetitive back and forth (wiping) motions of that shoulder. Once an operative cuff repair is performed, the employee will permanently retain the impairment of weakened tissue and consequent disabilities depending on the job demands.

The IME evaluator might be asked to ascertain retrospectively when MMI occurred, or when it would have occurred had proper treatment been undertaken originally. A review of the response to prior treatment efforts could be helpful. More useful, but rarely present in medical records, are objective measurements of motion, strength, and endurance that could have signalled MMI. These retrospective determinations are often requested for the purpose of after-the-fact denials of useless treatments. IME evaluators might also be asked to foresee when MMI will be reached. It is sensible to make those statements contingent on other factors, most importantly treatment, as illustrated earlier.

Work Ability

Work ability is the crux of many IMEs. The employer or the workers' compensation insurance carrier wants the IME physician's opinion about if and when the worker can return to the job. From the financial viewpoint, their interests would be served by an immediate return to work without restrictions and without any further diagnostic testing or treatment. That might indeed be the provider's recommendation, assuming an impairment is not present, or is clinically irrelevant if it does exist, and there is small likelihood of reinjury on return to work.

One must always keep foremost in mind the best interest of the claimant, and never more so than with the opinion about return to work. There are times when the only information available about the physical demands of the job is from the client interview, information that may not closely match reality. It can be helpful to have a detailed job analysis (JA) at the time of the IME. For controversial cases, such as when the worker argues that the JA does not reflect reality, a videotape of another worker on the job site is extremely helpful. If the IME physician's practice includes many referrals from a particular plant, a tour of that facility aids immensely in return-to-work decisions while simultaneously lending credibility to his or her opinions. Lacking such information, and keeping in mind the caveat against doing harm, it is wise to be conservative with return-to-work recommendations until the provider receives a detailed description of the specific physical demands of the job.

The three general categories of work recommendations include return to unrestricted work, return to work only with certain physical and/or time limitations, and complete disability from the job, either temporarily or permanently. The components of the IME report, as have been shown, are highly interrelated. It may not be possible to come to a firm conclusion about return to work until additional testing has occurred, or until specific treatment has been provided for a certain length of time. In those cases, a follow-up report or addendum is generated when the provider has reviewed the test results, physical therapy progress notes, and other pertinent items.

Return to work with temporary restrictions is a common recommendation. It is preferable to report specific physical limitations (e.g., no overhead work, no lifting over 15 lb, no heavy pushing or pulling with the right upper limb) than to try to foresee every job placement within a workplace, and judge yes or no to each. Job placement is the responsibility of the employer, not the physician, but should be done within the guidelines provided by the IME evaluator.

Many employers remain wary about restricted return to work, largely because of liability concerns. They want a worker to be 100% capable, or stay off the job. In those cases, it may still be feasible to suggest a return to work without physical restrictions but with time limits. For example, an IME evaluator might recommend 4-hour work days for the first 2 weeks, then 6 hours daily for the following 2 weeks, then 8 hours, and then full time (if overtime is an issue). Re-evaluation may be needed part way through this schedule (consider this several days after the 6-hour schedule has been in place, then again after the claimant is working full time) to ensure the impairment is not worsening. If neither physical nor time restrictions are allowed by the employer, formal, daily work hardening might be a solution.

A functional capacity evaluation (FCE) is sometimes used to more objectively determine a worker's capacity for lifting, carrying, reaching, overhead work, and other physical tasks. An FCE that is matched to a specific JA, when performed by a skilled clinician on a motivated client, can be helpful. When one or more of those factors is missing, however, the FCE results might appear objective and useful when in fact they are neither. A common quandary is for the FCE results to reflect the employee's lack of motivation, although the conclusions may seem to indicate a physical incapacity. The IME physician is then left with "objective" documentation of the worker's inability to match the prior job demands, when in reality other factors are more important. On the other hand, the FCE might prove useful to add objective credence to the concern of suboptimal claimant motivation. The physician, faced with this dilemma, can downplay the FCE conclusions in the final opinion, although that might appear punitive. A better strategy is to avoid ordering an FCE on workers for whom it will not be helpful for any of the reasons mentioned earlier.

If the IME physician's practice includes follow-up IMEs, the provider may have heard from workers, "I went back with your restrictions, but my supervisor ignored them, and I'm hurting again." IME providers should keep in mind that they cannot be there with the employee at the workplace, and it is not the provider's responsibility to contact the supervisor to ensure that return-to-work recommendations are being met. This complaint should be dealt with by the case manager, ergonomist, worker's compensation representative from the plant, or other such individual. Occasionally it is warranted to remove the claimant from work completely if the restrictions are indeed ignored, and particularly if the impairment is worsened as a result. Above all, the IME provider should not allow harm to be done.

Diagnostic Testing

Ideally, all pertinent diagnostic test results precede the client to the IME physician's office; often they do not. Final opinions may be delayed until the referring source is able to provide the test results (this is not the responsibility of the claimant). It is within the realm of an IME evaluator to recommend testing, either to establish the impairment more objectively, or to help with treatment or return-to-work decisions. An electromyogram (EMG), for example, might document that ongoing denervation is still present in the C7 distribution, therefore vigorous strengthening of that limb will be delayed. Ordering tests also falls within the purview of an IME evaluator, as does performing an EMG. None of those activities causes a doctor-patient (treating) relationship to be established. The final IME opinion about many of the other issues discussed might hinge on the results of such testing.

Most IME requests will authorize the examination only, or perhaps plain radiographs if needed, but not any further testing. The IME evaluator will then need to obtain approval before proceeding with scans, nerve conduction studies (NCS), EMG, or other studies.

Treatment

If the IME physician finds fault with prior treatment, it is best to record his or her opinion in a matter-of-fact, dispassionate manner. The IME report is not the place to cast aspersions on another practitioner. If the treatment has truly been useless, the examinee will have told the IME evaluator so directly or indirectly, depending on the skill of his or her line of questioning. The IME evaluator should ask about the effectiveness of each treatment session (e.g., whether the hot pack feels good when it is on, and for how long after it is removed). At another time in the interview, the IME physician should ask how the client's condition has changed in the big picture and what percent has he or she improved since the original incident. There is often a glaring discrepancy between these two responses, or the IME likely would not have been requested in the first place. It is then simple and honest to conclude that the best interest of the worker dictates that the palliative treatment be discontinued or supplanted with treatment that presumably will ameliorate or remove the impairment.

An IME determination might be that the first 2 to 3 weeks of a certain treatment were warranted as a trial, but when the claimant did not improve at all, further such treatment could not be justified. This reasoning can be extrapolated to initial efforts at physical therapy, soft-tissue or epidural injections, medications, use of a nerve or muscle stimulation unit, and so on.

For the initial IME report it is helpful to include details about the treatment regimen recommended, and the reasons for various aspects of the treatment. If that includes physical therapy, the IME evaluator should list the exercises that should be taught, monitored, and advanced over time. Guidelines should be given about frequency and duration of therapy; it may help to clarify that passive modalities should be used only to facilitate active treatment, such as stretching or strengthening, and not in isolation for temporary symptom relief. The IME evaluator should explain that after a certain point the client should be expected to continue the program independently. If the home program can only be successful with exercise equipment (not typically the case), the evaluator should consider recommending a finite trial (e.g., 6 months or less) subscription to a fitness facility, funded by the insurance company at many times less than the cost of ongoing physical therapy. That effectively shifts the responsibility for continuing exercise to the claimant.

Follow-Up

The IME report has potentially included numerous suggestions about what should happen from this point forward, addressing issues such as additional testing, treatment, return to work with or without restrictions, or a trial return to work. If so, it then makes sense to suggest follow-up or even serial examinations as those events occur. If diagnostic studies are the only intervention, another appointment is not needed. Intercurrent treatment or return to work, however, might cause a change in the underlying impairment, and could therefore warrant repeat examination (or NCS/EMG) some weeks or months after the initial visit. Neither the recommendation for nor the performance of additional visits constitutes a treatment relationship.

SUMMARY

The IME is an integral component of the system of disability evaluation, and is ideally performed by practitioners who can think logically and dispassionately about medical conditions. This chapter has outlined the many components of the IME, although they intertwine extensively and in fact are interdependent. When performed and reported carefully and as objectively as is feasible, the IME has the potential to do a great service to the disability system at large, but most importantly to the examinee, whose best interests should always be the primary concern of the physician.

REFERENCES

1. Appleberg K, Romanov K, Heikkila K, et al: Interpersonal conflict as a predictor of work disability: a follow-up study of 15,348 Finnish workers. J Psychosom Res 40(2):157–167, 1996.
2. Bonzani PJ, Millender L, Keelan B, et al: Factors prolonging disability in work-related cumulative trauma disorders. J Hand Surg [Am] 22(1):30–34, 1997.
3. Cumming GR: The independent medical examination: cardiology assessment. Can J Cardiol 12(12):1245–1252, 1996.
4. Dusik LA, Menard MR, Cooke C, et al: Concurrent validity of the ERGOS work simulator versus conventional functional capacity evaluation techniques in a workers' compensation population. J Occup Med 38(8):759–767, 1993.
5. Felsenthal G, Reischer MA: Asymmetric hamstring reflexes indicative of L5 radicular lesions. Arch Phys Med Rehabil 63:377–378, 1982.
6. Lees-Haley PR, Williams VW, English LT: Response bias in self-reported history of plaintiffs compared with nonlitigating patients. Psychol Rep 79(3 Pt 1):811–818, 1996.
7. Mandell PJ, Weitz E, Bernstein JI, et al: Isokinetic trunk strength and lifting strength measures: differences and similarities between low-back-injured and non-injured workers. Spine 18(16):2491–2501, 1993.
8. National Institute for Occupational Safety and Health: Work Practices Guide for Manual Lifting. Washington, DC, US Department of Health and Human Services, National Technical Information Service, 1981, PB82.
9. Waddell G, McCulloch JA, Kummel E, et al: Nonorganic physical signs in low-back pain. Spine 5:117–125, 1980.
10. White KP, Harth M, Teasell RW: Work disability evaluation and the fibromyalgia syndrome. Semin Arthritis Rheum 24(6):371–381, 1995.
11. Zinn W, Furutani N: Physician perspectives on the ethical aspects of disability determination. J Gen Intern Med 11(9):525–532, 1996.

CHAPTER 13

Disability Evaluation and Unexplained Pain

Richard T. Katz, MD   Raymond C. Tait, PhD

The basis of impairment rating in many contexts, including the AMA *Guides to the Evaluation of Permanent Impairment*, is to evaluate pain *in context to the underlying objectively defined impairment. Impairment* is defined as "the loss, loss of use, or derangement of any body part, system, or function."[1] In general the percentages awarded in the AMA *Guides* for various permanent impairments allow "for the pain that may occur with those impairments." Similarly, the Social Security Administration and the U.S. Department of Veterans Affairs view pain as significant only when it is associated with mental impairment.

Although the AMA *Guides* and other authorities consider pain to be of secondary importance relative to objectively defined impairment, many patients present for disability evaluation with subjective complaints and little or no objective findings. Among patients with low-back pain, for example, an estimated 85% cannot be given a definitive diagnosis because of weak associations among symptoms, pathological changes, and imaging results.[60, 70] Moreover, efforts to standardize guidelines for disability evaluation of these patients have met with little success.[13, 14, 58, 79, 83] Further complicating the picture is the one-time nature of a disability examination, a format that does not afford the examiner the opportunity to judge a chronic problem across time according to proposed sampling procedures.[42] Thus there are few benchmarks available to the disability examiner against which to assess this difficult patient group. This chapter will offer some guidelines that are hoped to be of value in assessing such patients more effectively.

THE EVALUATION OF PAIN IN THE AMA *GUIDES*

The International Association for the Study of Pain has defined pain as "an unpleasant sensory and emotional experience with actual or potential tissue damage or that is described in terms of such damage." This definition reflects the principal problem in evaluating pain: its subjectivity. Although a variety of psychological, physiological, and functional methods of quantifying pain have been proposed, there is no clearly accepted and validated method of objectively assessing this complex but commonplace problem. More specifically, no data are available to the examiner that facilitate determinations regarding a particular patient's future employability, despite investigations designed to develop such criteria.[69]

Recognizing the lack of a widely accepted template, the AMA *Guides* offers a classification system for the examiner to use in categorizing the nature of pain with which patients are likely to present (Table 13–1). Central to these classifications is assessment of objective impairment associated with a patient's

TABLE 13–1 Classifications/Models of Pain

Neuropsychiatric
- Nociceptive or somatic
- Neurogenic or central
- Psychogenic

Pathogenesis
- Primary
- Secondary

Biopsychosocial
- Acute
- Recurrent acute
- Cancer-related
- Chronic

From American Medical Association: Guides to the Evaluation of Permanent Impairment, ed 4. Chicago, American Medical Association, 1993.

complaint. Because it is known that pain and impairment do not correlate highly[89]—patients with clear evidence of impairment can experience no pain and vice versa—the classification system proposed by the AMA *Guides* clearly has shortcomings. Nonetheless, the AMA *Guides* do present a system that is useful in decision making, and the use of a system (even with flaws) is preferable to the lack of any workable system.

The *neuropsychiatric* construct divides pain into three principal types: (1) *nociceptive* or *somatic:* pain that is generated through established neuroanatomic/neurophysiologic pathways and that originates from actual or impending tissue damage, (2) *neurogenic* or *central:* pain arising from spontaneous excitation within the various parts of the nervous system without any specific noxious stimulus (e.g., deafferentation or neuropathic pain), and (3) *psychogenic pain:* a psychiatric disorder that may be part of various conditions such as somatization disorder, but for which there seems to be no nociceptive or neurogenic basis. A useful question to ask for psychogenic pain is, would the patient have pain if the mental disorder were absent? Although impairment is associated with nociceptive or neurogenic pain, there is no impairment associated with psychogenic pain.

Pathogenic classifications categorize pain as (1) *primary:* tissue damage or physiological disruption, or (2) *secondary:* the result of adverse pain behavior or ineffective medical treatment. Pain caused by the effects of chemotherapy for a neoplasm would be an example of secondary pain. Each of these conditions reflects a medical impairment.

The *biopsychosocial model* of pain recognizes the important interrelationships between nociception, pain, suffering, pain behavior, and how the pain patient fills the "sick role." Loeser's paradigm suggests that the initial noxious stimulus leading to nociception may be less important than the suffering the patient experiences and the illness behaviors that the patient exhibits.[47] This model is consistent with studies that have failed to find a direct relationship between tissue damage and the severity of pain.[6]

The biopsychosocial model classifies pain as *acute* (e.g., broken ankle), *recurrent acute* (e.g., trigeminal neuralgia), *cancer-related,* and *chronic* (benign or nonmalignant). Chronic pain is a state in which the pain becomes a destructive illness in its own right, rather than a symptom of underlying disease. This last category is likely the most difficult for the disability-evaluating physician.

Although these categorizations and models lend understanding to the treating physician, they do little to help the disability-rating physician give a fair and balanced assessment of a patient's functional decline (e.g., activities of daily living), which is one way that we can objectively measure loss of function caused by pain. Ford et al[27] have noted that pain, even severe and persistent, is widely found among the general population, especially as we age.[29] How is the disability-evaluating examiner to decide if pain impedes function in a significant way?

IS CHRONIC PAIN SYNDROME PRESENT?

The AMA *Guides* suggests that two or more positive characteristics from the eight "Ds" are considered to "establish a presumptive diagnosis of chronic pain syndrome"[1] (Table 13–2). These eight "Ds" are an expansion of a list of six described by Sternbach.[81] These criteria are superficially attractive, but careful examination reveals serious problems. Although some define chronic pain syndrome after a period of 6 months or more has elapsed, chronic pain behaviors may be noted very early after low back injury (within days!), and can accurately predict delay in return to work. For example, Hazard et al. developed the Vermont Disability Prediction Questionnaire and administered the tool to workers within 15 days of their initial injury.[38] Using a simple dichotomous scoring system, they were able to predict 3-month post-injury work status with 94% sensitivity and 84% specificity.

Patients with chronic pain may use dramatic terms to discuss their suffering, in a style similar to that exhibited by somatizing patients, who invariably have pain-related complaints. Chronic pain patients pose a "diagnostic dilemma" in that repeated work-ups fail to clearly define the etiology of their problem, another important feature shared with the somatizing patient. Substance abuse and dependency are problems common to the chronic pain patient, the somatizer, and the antisocial personality–disordered patient. Dependency is a

TABLE 13–2 The Eight "Ds" of Chronic Pain

Duration: >6 months?
Dramatization: emotionally charged, affective exaggerated, theatrical, etc.
Diagnostic dilemma: extensive work-up without clear diagnosis
Drugs: frequent substance dependence/abuse, large amounts of drugs
Dependence: dependent on physicians and demands excessive care, extensive passive physical therapy, dependent on family/spouse
Depression: hypochondriasis, hysteria, unhappiness, hostility, poor coping mechanisms
Disuse: immobilization causing secondary pain, overly cautious of further injury
Dysfunction: withdraw from the social milieu, disengage from social and work activities, feel rebuffed by the medical provider

From American Medical Association: Guides to the Evaluation of Permanent Impairment, ed 4. Chicago, American Medical Association, 1993.

feature shared with a variety of psychiatric disorders, including various personality disorders. Although depression is extremely common in those with chronic pain,[71] unfortunately it is also extremely common in the general population.[21] Finally, dysfunction within the social milieu is a frequent feature of a wide variety of psychiatric diagnoses and has no specificity for the patient with chronic pain. In summary, the eight Ds are so nonspecific as to be of questionable value in identifying, as well as differentiating, the chronic pain sufferer from a wide variety of psychiatric diagnoses that are well defined in the American Psychiatric Association's *Diagnostic and Statistical Manual of Mental Disorders, fourth edition* (DSM–IV).[2]

ESTIMATING PAIN IMPAIRMENT

Assessment of pain-related impairment by the disability-evaluating physician is a task complicated by two factors—poorly defined criteria for certain diagnoses, and questions that can arise regarding the validity of patient self-reports. Neuropathic and central pain are examples of diagnoses that reflect the first problem. Careful inspection reveals that 90% of those who clearly meet criteria for a diagnosis of central pain had a history of stroke or thalamic insult, whereas the remaining 10% had no such history.[34] The diagnosis of "neuropathic pain" is also used with less than rigorous criteria. Although neuropathic pain seems entirely reasonable when associated with a diagnosis such as diabetic polyneuropathy, other neuropathic pain syndromes are less clearly accepted (e.g., complex regional pain syndrome I and II).[63]

Evaluating the patient's experience of pain also can be problematic. As noted earlier, the disability-evaluating physician typically sees a patient on only one occasion, a protocol that makes difficult the task of evaluating a chronic problem. Consistent with prevailing literature that recommends sampling procedures to be used with patient pain ratings,[42] the AMA *Guides* suggests that patients construct a pain grid that documents the frequency and intensity of their pain. Unfortunately, such procedures are both unwieldy, making them subject to noncompliance, and sensitive to demand characteristics,[28] situational influences that can occasion symptom magnification,[53] especially in settings where disability status is at issue.

Other self-report procedures also can be used, including pain drawings, an assessment task that requires patients to shade in areas on an outline of a human figure that are consistent with their distribution of pain. Data indicate that such drawings can be scored reliably,[52] and that they have reasonable validity for both chronic[85] and subacute conditions.[64] Pain drawings have been used to guide the placement of electrodes in dorsal column stimulation protocols[62] and to assist in differential diagnosis of psychogenic and/or benign pain versus herniated discs.[51] Like visual analog scales, however, pain drawings also are subject to a variety of situational influences that can compromise their validity.

Because of validity questions associated with these and other self-report techniques, a number of procedures have been developed to address validity issues. For example, a functional capacity evaluation (FCE) can be requested to document systematically a patient's physical capacities and consistency of effort across a range of tasks, but the value of these expensive assessments is questionable when the patient is less than fully compliant.[37] Moreover, the administration of an FCE can be highly variable across facilities, further complicating the interpretations of these findings.

Another procedure has been proposed for those cases in which pain is associated with atypical sensory complaints such as numbness of an entire limb. This strategy for evaluating a patient with a "totally numb hand" has been described as the *forced choice paradigm.*[8] The patient, eyes closed, is forced to choose which of two totally "numb" fingers was scratched by the examiner's pin. Random guess would suggest a correct response approximately 50% of the time. The patient with conscious or subconscious need to demonstrate illness to the examiner may offer a markedly decreased rate of correct responses.

In 1984, Waddell noted several key signs for "non-organic" low-back pain sufferers who were not likely to respond to surgical intervention for their low back pain.[91] These "Waddell signs" have become an important part of every low-back evaluation today (Table 13–3).

Waddell attempted to find physical examination findings that discriminated the chronic low-back pain patient from patients with no low-back pain.[92] A constellation of changes within eight items on clinical examination—pelvic flexion, total flexion, total extension, lateral flexion, straight leg raising, spinal tenderness, bilateral straight leg raising, and sit-ups—were successful in distinguishing the normal and chronic back-pain groups. Contrary to common belief, patients with chronic low-back pain did not have decreased flexion. However, the author acknowledged that "all physical tests are open to conscious deception," and the value of these signs can be at best, only clues. Thomas et al. have reached similar observations.[87]

Nonclinical aids such as the Minnesota Multiphasic Personality Inventory (MMPI), Cornell Medical Index Health Questionnaire, McGill Pain Questionnaire, Beck and Zung Depression Indices, and the West Haven–Yale Multidimensional Pain Inventory have been used to assess the impact of pain on the patient, and are discussed elsewhere in this volume.[84] The MMPI has a long history in the detection of malingering, but the true incidence of malingering is simply unknown.[24] Unfortunately, none of these tests answers the key question for any pain patient: how has the physical impairment affected the person's ability to function in his or her normal milieu? Realistically, this may simply be beyond the capability of the honest clinician to assess.

Electrodiagnosis has little to add in the evaluation of most chronic-pain patients once radiculopathy, mononeuropathy, and peripheral neuropathy have been ruled out.[95] One does not need an electromyogram (EMG) to note "psychogenic recruitment pattern," which clinically is noted as ratchety or

TABLE 13–3 Waddell Signs

- Tenderness
  - Superficial
  - Nonanatomical
- Simulation
  - Axial loading
  - En bloc rotation
- Distraction
  - Straight leg raising discrepancy
- Regional
  - Weakness
  - Sensory
- Overreaction

give-way weakness.[88] Percutaneous twitch superimposition—demonstrating that an electrical nerve stimulus increases the torque generated by the patient for a given contraction that was supposedly maximal—has been advocated to document the presence of maximal or submaximal effort by the patient,[57, 72] but this is superfluous in the face of careful clinical evaluation. Surface electromygraphy has shown promise in experimental settings for performance evaluation of back muscles[17] but has not reached a level of clinical usefulness.[35]

Many have hoped that by objectively assessing strength, the examiner can determine whether pain has impaired function. For example, peak grip strength has been used in the hope of determining if a patient is giving maximum effort, and isokinetic machine torque curves have been used to determine whether the patient is malingering.[82] There is ample evidence to show that parameters other than simple peak strength and reproducibility are required to demonstrate patient compliance. Even more sophisticated means, such as the coefficient of variation (standard deviation divided by the mean multiplied by 100%), may not accurately assess compliance in functional capacity tests.[11, 20, 39, 40, 43, 76, 77]

Mayer et al. have collected a substantial body of data with hopes of quantifying the spinal physical capacity of normal and injured workers.[54, 56] However, Madsen has demonstrated considerable day-to-day variability in such testing[50] and Mooney et al.[59] have not found that preplacement strength testing data predicted workplace claims of injury. In an exhaustive review, Newton and Waddell noted that "there is inadequate scientific evidence to support isomachines in pre-employment screening, routine clinical assessment, or medicolegal evaluation."[61]

Some would argue that the disability-rating examination process is a futile exercise for which there is no solution.[36] Brodsky has noted "futile are attempts to find a single or simple factor that explains why some workers become and remain disabled while others, seemingly suffering no lesser injury, either do not enter into a disability status role or recover much earlier."[10] Loeser and Sullivan argue that adequate science is not available to rate disability in the chronic low-back pain patient, and that the disability becomes iatrogenic.[46]

PSYCHIATRIC CONDITIONS AS CONFOUNDERS OF PAIN COMPLAINTS

Because the argument has been made that we cannot find a good way to rate pain, what observations can we make in patients in whom pain is the principal complaint but we are unable to document underlying impairment? Although the role of psychological factors in chronic pain remain poorly defined,[31] clearly psychosocial factors have important effects on the relationship between pain and disability.[80] The studies at Boeing[7] demonstrated the importance of job satisfaction as a predictor of future disability in low-back pain patients. In a primary-care setting, psychiatric morbidity in a pain-free population predicted the development of back pain over a defined period.[16] Compensation seems to have an adverse effect on self-reported pain, depression, and disability before and after rehabilitation has been attempted.[68] Studies of Australian aboriginals highlighted how back pain is extremely ubiquitous, yet is "expressed" readily in western cultures while not so in others.[41] Although whiplash-related complaints seem to persist for extended periods in our litigious western society, a study of Lithuanian patients complaining of whiplash injuries—in whom there was no litigious recourse within their country—demonstrated that no patient had disabling or persisting symptoms 3 months after injury, and there was little awareness of the potentially disabling consequence of whiplash injuries.[74] Gallagher et al. demonstrated that although compensation is awarded on the basis of physical evaluation, the likelihood of receiving compensation is significantly determined by level of emotional distress exhibited by the patient.[30]

In addition to societal factors, it is important to recognize that many patients with persistent somatic/pain complaints may have unrecognized psychiatric diagnoses that either drive or complicate their symptoms or complaints. Polatin et al. found 98% of chronic low-back pain patients had one or more *DSM-IIIR* diagnoses—most commonly major depression, substance abuse, and anxiety disorder.[32, 66] Most diagnoses *preceded* the onset of low-back pain. Similarly, Long has noted that 75% of persons with chronic low-back pain had antecedent psychiatric disease.[48] Conversely, Wallis et al. found a significant reduction in emotional distress (to normal levels) among patients who derived significant pain reduction from a surgical procedure.[93] Thus psychological distress can also be a consequence of persistent pain.

Anxiety is the most common problem in acute pain states, whereas depression is most common in chronic pain conditions.[21] However, there are a wide variety of diagnoses that may complicate the ability of the patient with chronic pain to function, including somatization disorder, undifferentiated somatoform disorder, conversion disorder, pain disorder associated with psychiatric disorders, hypochondriasis, factitious disorder, malingering, and substance dependence and abuse.

A thorough review of these many psychiatric diagnoses can be found in standard textbooks, but the principal point to be made to the reader is how common many of these diagnoses are. For example, 77% of patients who meet criteria for psychiatric diagnoses in the United States are treated in the primary-care physician's office[75] and very commonly present with a somatic or physical complaint; less than 1 in 5 complain of psychosocial symptoms or distress.[33] Nonpsychiatric physicians need not have a detailed understanding of dozens of psychiatric diagnoses because only a special few deserve mention for the patient with enduring pain complaints.

Depression, anxiety, and *substance abuse disorders* are extremely common, and each can be associated with physical and pain complaints. Anxiety is a frequent symptom of depression and substance abuse, and should prompt the clinician in a search for these two disorders. Each patient should be screened for substance abuse with brief questionnaires such as the CAGE or PRIME-MD (see p. 268). Depression may be undetected in more than 50% of a primary-care population[15] because patients often present with physical complaints that mimic other conditions rather than the expected symptoms of sadness, hopelessness, or loss of pleasure in usual activities.[18] In a study of 500 adults presenting to a general medical clinic with a physical symptom, a depressive or anxiety disorder was present in 29% of those studied. Predictors of a mental disorder included recent stress, six or more physical symptoms, higher patient ratings of symptom severity, lower patient ratings of their overall health, physician perception of the encounter as difficult, and age less than 50.

Somatoform disorders are a spectrum of psychiatric disorders in which physical conditions are caused or aggravated by psychological factors.[4, 5] The "full blown" syndrome—somatization disorder[2]—requires a history of many physical complaints (four pain symptoms, two gastrointestinal, one sexual, one pseudoneurological) that begin before the age of 30 and markedly disrupt the patient's lifestyle (Table 13–4). Notice the commonality of pain complaints within the realm of somatization.

Somatization that meets *DSM-IV* criteria may be too restrictive; thus many patients present to a primary-care physician's office with forms of somatization that are underdiagnosed because they do not meet strict criteria.[67] A new diagnosis of "multisomatoform disorder" has been suggested that is defined as three or more medically unexplained, currently bothersome physical symptoms plus a long (≥2 years) history of somatization.[45] Undifferentiated somatoform disorder, defined within the *DSM-IV,* is even less restrictive (Table 13–5).

Leaving aside the details of each somatization diagnosis, it is important to note that somatizing patients have chronic problems (many pain related), with recurrent physical symptoms, often in different bodily systems, that wax and wane over time. Medical work-ups reveal little objective pathology. Problems often cluster in areas where complaints are subjective and difficult to verify by

TABLE 13–4 Somatization Disorder

A. A history of many physical complaints beginning before age 30 that occur over a period of several years and result in treatment being sought or significant impairment in social, occupational, or other important areas of functioning.
B. Each of the following criteria must have been met, with individual symptoms occurring at any time during the course of the disturbance:
   1. *Four pain symptoms*: a history of pain related to at least four different sites or functions (e.g., head, abdomen, back, joints, extremities, chest, rectum, during menstruation, during sexual intercourse, or during urination)
   2. *Two gastrointestinal symptoms:* a history of at least two gastrointestinal symptoms other than pain (e.g., nausea, bloating, vomiting other than during pregnancy, diarrhea, or intolerance of several different foods)
   3. *One sexual symptom:* a history of at least one sexual or reproductive symptom other than pain (e.g., sexual indifference, erectile or ejaculatory dysfunction, irregular menses, excessive menstrual bleeding, vomiting throughout pregnancy
   4. *One pseudoneurological symptom:* a history of at least one symptom or deficit suggesting a neurological condition not limited to pain (conversion symptoms such as impaired coordination or balance, paralysis or localized weakness, difficulty swallowing or lump in the throat, aphonia, urinary retention, hallucinations, loss of touch or pain sensation, double vision, blindness, deafness, seizures, dissociative symptoms such as amnesia, or loss of consciousness or other than fainting)
C. Either 1 or 2:
   1. After appropriate investigation, each of the symptoms in Criterion B cannot be fully explained by a known general medical condition or the direct effects of a substance (e.g., a drug of abuse, a medication)
   2. When there is a related general medical condition, the physical complaints or resulting social or occupational impairment are in excess of what would be expected from the history, physical examination, or laboratory findings
D. The symptoms are not intentionally produced or feigned (as in factitious disorder or malingering)

From American Psychiatric Association: Diagnostic and Statistical Manual of Mental Disorders, 4th ed. Washington, DC, American Psychiatric Association, 1994.

TABLE 13–5 Undifferentiated Somatoform Disorder

A. One or more physical complaints (e.g., fatigue, loss of appetite, gastrointestinal or urinary complaints)
B. Either 1 or 2:
   1. After appropriate investigation, the symptoms cannot be fully explained by a known general medical condition or the direct effects of a substance (e.g., a drug of abuse, a medication)
   2. When there is a related general medical condition, the physical complaints or resulting social or occupational impairment is in excess of what would be expected from the history, physical examination, or laboratory findings
C. The symptoms cause clinically significant distress or impairment in social, occupational, or other important areas of functioning
D. The duration of the disturbance is at least 6 months
E. The disturbance is not better accounted for by another mental disorder (e.g., another somatoform disorder, sexual dysfunction, mood disorder, anxiety disorder, sleep disorder, or psychotic disorder)
F. The symptom is not intentionally produced or feigned (as in factitious disorder or malingering)

From American Psychiatric Association: Diagnostic and Statistical Manual of Mental Disorders, 4th ed. Washington, DC, American Psychiatric Association, 1994.

objective laboratory or other types of studies. Many patients have a long list of past medical problems and a history of referral to specialists for investigation of these subjective complaints. Often the patient will say "they did a lot of tests but nothing was found." Often there is a similar pattern of enduring complaints in other body systems. Substantial differences in disability and medical visitation have been found in patients without significant difference in organic pathology. Differences in illness behavior may to some extent be reflective of degrees of somatization.[12] Results from the Primary Care Evaluation of Mental Disorders Study demonstrated that multisomatoform disorder is present in 8.2% of a primary care population—nearly one in twelve patients.[45] One can only speculate that the incidence may be higher in the disability-evaluating physician's office, where additional pressures from the worker's compensation arena are well known to prolong recovery from low-back pain.

The reporting of somatic symptoms that have no pathophysiological explanation appears to be increasing in primary care as well as specialty practice.[4] The average British neurologist fails to find adequate neurological explanation for symptoms of one in five outpatients.[49] Only 40 of 100 patients presenting to a neurological ward had an adequate organic explanation for their symptoms.[23] Although some of these patients may have organic disease that was yet to be diagnosed, there is adequate room to offer alternative explanation, that of somatoform illness.

Personality disorders are pervasive and persistent maladaptive patterns of behavior (including pain behaviors) that are deeply ingrained and are not attributable to other psychiatric disorders.[21, 65, 94] They require a history of long-term difficulties in a variety of spheres of life.[96] *DSM-IV* has divided personality disorders into three clusters: A, B, and C (Table 13–6).

Cluster B patients are often especially difficult to manage, and include antisocial, narcissistic, histrionic, and borderline personality disorders.[3] This group shares a tendency to the dramatic, intense moods that can rapidly shift,

TABLE 13–6 Personality Disorders

Cluster A: Odd/eccentric
- Paranoid
- Schizoid
- Schizotypal

Cluster B: Dramatic/emotional
- Antisocial
- Borderline
- Histrionic
- Narcissistic

Cluster C: Anxious/fearful
- Avoidant
- Dependent
- Obsessive-compulsive
- Passive-aggressive

From American Psychiatric Association: Diagnostic and Statistical Manual of Mental Disorders, 4th ed. Washington, DC, American Psychiatric Association, 1994.

impulsivity, and feelings of entitlement. They may be demanding and exhausting. The physician's own feelings of exasperation and anger with a patient may be important clues of personality traits or disorders in that patient.[19] Schafer and Nowlis evaluated the association between "difficult" patients and personality disorders in a family practice, and found that unrecognized personality disorders were significantly more prevalent in this population.[73] These patients are relatively common—a recent survey of non-selected primary-care outpatients demonstrated that 8% of men and 3.1% of women met *DSM-IV* criteria for antisocial personality disorder (Table 13–7). The frequency of childhood conduct disorder (the "bad boys" or "bad girls" that can grow up to become antisocial) was 13.4% for men and 4% for women.

These patients have high rates of substance abuse, which complicates matters further because chronic narcotic administration may be associated with substance abuse. Physicians need to be alert because patients with personality disorders may be superficially charming if they are getting their way; however, when limits are set with them they can quickly become irritable and demanding. Physicians should look for a chronic history of interpersonal and occupational difficulties as additional clues (frequent change of companion, frequent job loss, previous arrests or incarcerations, violent episodes). This quickly notifies the clinician of the potential in the patient for action on aggressive impulses.

Patients with characterologic traits or disorders may use physical complaints for secondary gain—monetary rewards, avoidance of arrest, solicitation of opioids or benzodiazepines. The concept of secondary gain is difficult, and perhaps at times misused, but certainly it carries great weight in certain cases seen by the disability-evaluating physician.[25] When these personality traits are found, one should be alert to the possibility of secondary gain issues.[90] Malingering—the deceptive creation of symptoms for secondary gain—is always in the differential diagnosis in this group and, to a lesser degree, for any diagnosis in which the symptoms are subjective (Table 13–8).[26]

Finally, pain may be a component of a "psychiatric pain disorder" (Table 13–9). Although this diagnosis has clinical value, it often is of little value to the

TABLE 13–7 Antisocial Personality

A. There is a pervasive pattern of disregard for and violation of the rights of others occurring since age 15; as indicated by three (or more) of the following:
   1. Failure to conform to social norms with respect to lawful behaviors as indicated by repeatedly performing acts that are grounds for arrest
   2. Deceitfulness, as indicated by repeatedly lying, use of aliases, or conning others for personal profit or pleasure
   3. Impulsivity or failure to plan ahead
   4. Irritability and aggressiveness, as indicated by repeated physical fights or assaults
   5. Reckless disregard for safety of self or others
   6. Consistent irresponsibility, as indicated by repeated failure to sustain consistent work behavior or honor financial obligations
   7. Lack of remorse as indicated by being indifferent to or rationalizing having hurt, mistreated, or stolen from another

B. The individual is at least 18 years of age

C. There is evidence of conduct disorder with onset before age 15

D. The occurrence of antisocial behavior is not exclusively during the course of schizophrenia or a manic episode

From American Psychiatric Association: Diagnostic and Statistical Manual of Mental Disorders, 4th ed. Washington, DC, American Psychiatric Association, 1994.

TABLE 13–8 Malingering

The essential feature of malingering is the intentional production of false or grossly exaggerated physical or psychological symptoms, motivated by external incentives such as avoiding military duty, avoiding work, obtaining financial compensation, evading criminal prosecution, or obtaining drugs. Under some circumstances, malingering may represent adaptive behavior (e.g., feigning illness while a captive of the enemy during wartime).

Malingering should be strongly suspected if any combination of the following is noted:
   1. Medicolegal context of presentation (e.g., the person is referred to the clinician by an attorney)
   2. Marked discrepancy between the person's claimed stress or disability and the objective findings
   3. Lack of cooperation during the diagnostic evaluation and in complying with the prescribed treatment regimen
   4. The presence of antisocial personality disorder

Malingering differs from factitious disorder in that the motivation for the symptom production in malingering is an external incentive, whereas in factitious disorder external incentives are absent. Evidence of an intrapsychic need to maintain the sick role suggests factitious disorder. Malingering is differentiated from conversion disorder and other somatoform disorders by the intentional production of symptoms and by the obvious, external incentives associated with it. In malingering (in contrast to conversion disorder), symptom relief is not often obtained by suggestion or hypnosis.

From American Psychiatric Association: Diagnostic and Statistical Manual of Mental Disorders, 4th ed. Washington, DC, American Psychiatric Association, 1994.

TABLE 13–9 Pain Disorder

A. Pain in one or more anatomical sites is the predominant focus of the clinical presentation and is of sufficient severity to warrant clinical attention
B. The pain causes clinically significant distress or impairment in social, occupational, or other important areas of functioning
C. Psychological factors are judged to have an important role in the onset, severity, exacerbation, or maintenance of the pain
D. The symptom or deficit is not intentionally produced or feigned (as in factitious disorder or malingering)
E. The pain is not better accounted for by a mood, anxiety, or psychotic disorder and does not meet criteria for dyspareunia

From American Psychiatric Association: Diagnostic and Statistical Manual of Mental Disorders, 4th ed. Washington, DC, American Psychiatric Association, 1994.

disability examiner because all other diagnoses must be "ruled out" before pain disorder is considered.

Screening for Psychiatric Disorders

Nonpsychiatric physicians may be inexperienced in their attempts to identify psychiatric diagnoses within their patient populations. Two newer, multiple-disorder psychiatric screening tools have been developed to assist physicians with this dilemma. The Primary Care Evaluation of Mental Disorders (PRIME-MD) and the Symptom-Driven Diagnostic System for Primary Care (SDDS-PC) are simple-to-use, two-part instruments consisting of a patient questionnaire and a guided interview for physicians to confirm or rule out disorders suggested by the questionnaire.[9, 78] A comparison of the two screening tools can be found in Table 13-10.

The PRIME-MD questionnaire requires the patient to complete 26 simple initial items before follow-up questions, and is extremely easy to use. The entire process is now available in a computerized format that does not require physician participation and has been validated in a phone-administered interview.[44] The PRIME-MD is relatively sensitive for anxiety disorders (69%), substance abuse/dependence (81%), and mood disorders (67% overall). The specificity is particularly high for mood disorders (92%), alcohol abuse (98%),

TABLE 13–10 Comparison of Screening Diagnoses for PRIME-MD and SDDS-PC

PRIME-MD: Mood disorders (major depressive disorder, dysthymia, partial remission or recurrence of major depressive disorder, minor depressive disorder, ruling out of bipolar disorder), anxiety disorder, somatoform disorder, alcohol-related disorder, eating disorder

SDDS-PC: Major depression, generalized anxiety disorder, panic disorder, obsessive-compulsive disorder, alcohol and drug abuse/dependence, suicidal ideation or attempts and eating disorders (99%), whereas the most false positives were found in the somatoform section. Patients tolerate the PRIME-MD very well.[78]

CONCLUSIONS

The subject of disability in the workplace caused by chronic pain is one of the thorniest problems the disability-evaluating physician can face. Contrarians suggest that reliable disability rating simply cannot be performed, so we should abandon the attempt.[36] This article has summarized some of the literature that suggests that psychosocial issues complicate pain assessment considerably. This subject has been recently probed and debated within *Pain Forum*, published by the American Pain Society. Two quotations summarize the situation well: "[while attempts to] label chronic pain disorders as solely psychosocial issues to the exclusion of biological issues appear to be misguided,"[86] we must also "explain to the patient the therapeutic benefit of work and the reality that giving disability to all 65 million or so Americans with chronic pain would bankrupt our society."[22] Thus the disability-examining physician has an ethical mandate to provide a rating that reflects but does not distort impairment, both for social and individual reasons.

Of course, a fair-minded disability evaluation may mean that some individuals will face the dilemma of managing pain while also coping with the demands of work and everyday living. Effective treatment of pain and its associated disability continues to be a significant problem for those individuals and others who live with intractable pain. Hopefully, recent approaches to treatment such as those that emphasize rehabilitation with integrated psychological and vocational counseling[55] will offer those who suffer from chronic pain an opportunity to improve their levels of function and comfort.

REFERENCES

1. American Medical Association: Guides to the Evaluation of Permanent Impairment, 4th ed. Chicago, American Medical Association, 1993.
2. American Psychiatric Association: Diagnostic and Statistical Manual of Mental Disorders, 4th ed. Washington, DC, American Psychiatric Association, 1994.
3. Barry KL, Fleming MF, Manwell LB, et al: Conduct disorder and antisocial personality in adult primary care patients. J Fam Pract 45:151–158, 1997.
4. Barsky AJ, Borus JF: Somatization and medicalization in the era of managed care. JAMA 274: 1931–1934, 1995.
5. Barsky AJ, Klerman GL: Overview: hypochondriasis, bodily complaints, and somatic styles. Am J Psychiatry 140:273–283, 1993.
6. Beecher HK: Relationship of significance of wound to the pain experienced. JAMA 161:1609–1613, 1956.
7. Bigos SJ, Battie M, Spengler DM, et al: Prospective study of work perceptions and psychosocial factors affecting the report of back injury. Spine 16:1–6, 1991.
8. Binder LM: Forced-choice testing provides evidence of malingering. Arch Phys Med Rehabil 73:377–380, 1992.
9. Broadhead WE, Leon AC, Weissman MM, et al: Development and validation of the SDDS-PC screen for multiple mental disorders in primary care. Arch Fam Med 4:211–219, 1995.
10. Brodsky CM: Factors influencing work-related disability. In: Meyerson AT, Fine T (eds): Psychiatric Disability: Clinical, Legal, and Administrative Dimensions. American Psychiatric Press, Washington DC, 1987.

11. Chengalur SN, Smith GA, Nelson RC, Sadoff AM: Assessing sincerity of effort in maximal grip strength tests. Am J Phys Med Rehabil 69:148–153, 1990.
12. Ciccone DS, Just N, Bandilla EB: Non-organic symptom reporting in patients with chronic non-malignant pain. Pain 68:329–341, 1996.
13. Clark W, Haldeman S: Development of guideline factors for the evaluation of disability in neck and back injuries. Spine 18:1736–1745, 1993.
14. Clark W, Haldeman S, Johnson J, et al: Back impairment and disability determination: another attempt at objective, reliable rating. Spine 13:332–341, 1988.
15. Coyne JC, Fechner-Bates S, Schwenk TL: Prevalence, nature and comorbidity of depressive disorders in primary care. Gen Hosp Psychiatry 16:267–276, 1994.
16. Croft PR, Papageorgious AC, Ferry S, et al: Psychological distress and low back pain: evidence from a prospective study in the general population. Spine 20:2731–2737, 1996.
17. De Luca CJ: Use of the surface EMG signal for performance evaluation of back muscles. Muscle Nerve 16:210–216, 1993.
18. De Wester JN: Recognizing and treating the patient with somatic manifestations of depression. J Fam Pract 43:S3–S15, 1996.
19. DeLong K, Smith G, Grange J: Does that "difficult" patient have a personality disorder? Emerg Med December 1996, pp 75–96.
20. Dvir Z, David G: Suboptimal muscular performance: measuring isokinetic strength of knee extensors with new testing protocol. Arch Phys Med Rehabil 77:578–781, 1996.
21. Eisendrath SJ: Psychiatric aspects of chronic pain. Neurology 45(suppl 9):S26–S34, 1995.
22. Evans RW: Concepts of disease, the physician and chronic pain in the workplace. Pain Forum 6:239–242, 1997.
23. Ewald H, Rogne T, Ewald K, et al: Somatization in patients newly admitted to a neurological department. Acta Psychiatr Scand 89:174–179, 1994.
24. Faust D: Detection of deception. Neurol Clin 13(2):255–265, 1995.
25. Fishbain DA: Secondary gain concept. Am Pain Soc J 3:264–273, 1994.
26. Folks DG: Munchausen's syndrome and other factitious disorders. Neurol Clin 13(2):267–281, 1995.
27. Ford CV: Dimensions of somatization and hypochondriasis. Neurol Clin 13(2):241–253, 1995.
28. Furnham A: Response bias, social desirability, and dissimulation. Personality and Individual Differences 7:385–400, 1986.
29. Gagliese L, Melzack R: Chronic pain in elderly people. Pain 70:3–14, 1997.
30. Gallagher RM, Williams RA, Skelly J, et al: Workers' compensation and return to work in low back pain. Pain 299–307, 1995.
31. Gamsa A: Role of psychological factors in chronic pain. I. Half century of study. II. Critical appraisal. Pain 57:5–15, 17–29, 1994.
32. Gatchel RJ, Polatin PB, Mayer TG, et al: Psychopathology and the rehabilitation of patients with chronic low back pain disability. Arch Phys Med Rehabil 75:666–670, 1994.
33. Goldberg D, Bridges K, Duncan-Jones P, et al: Detecting anxiety and depression in general medical settings. Br Med J 297:897–899, 1988.
34. Gonzales GR: Central pain: diagnosis and treatment strategies. Neurology 45(suppl 9):S11–S16, 1995.
35. Haig AJ, Gelblum JF, Rechtien JJ, et al: Technology assessment: use of surface EMG in the diagnosis and treatment of nerve and muscle disorders. Muscle Nerve 19:392–395, 1996.
36. Hadler NM: Point of view. Spine 19:1116, 1994.
37. Harten HA: Functional capacity evaluation. In: Malanga GA (ed): Low Back Pain: Occupational Medicine: State of the Art Reviews, vol 13, No. 1, January–March, Philadelphia, Hanley & Belfus, pp 209–212, 1998.
38. Hazard RG, Haugh LD, Reid S, et al: Early prediction of chronic disability after occupational low back injury. Spine 21:945–951, 1996.

39. Hildreth DH, Breidenbach WC, Lister GD, Hodges AD: Detection of submaximal effort by use of the rapid exchange grip. J Hand Surg 14A:742–745, 1989.
40. Hirsch G, Beach G, Cooke C, et al: Relationship between performance on lumbar dynamometry and Waddell score in a population with LBP. Spine 16:1039–1043, 1991.
41. Honeyman PT, Jacobs E: Effects of culture on back pain in Australian aboriginals. Spine 21:841–843, 1996.
42. Jensen MP, McFarland CA: Increasing the reliability and validity of pain intensity measurement in chronic pain patients. Pain 55:195–203, 1993.
43. Kilmer DD, McCrory MA, Wright NC, et al: Hand held dynamometry reliability in persons with neuropathic weakness. Arch Phys Med Rehabil 78:1364–1368, 1997.
44. Kobak KA, Taylor LV, Dotti SL, et al: Computer-administered telephone interview to identify mental disorders. JAMA 278:905–901, 1997.
45. Kroenke K, Spitzer RL, DeGruy FV, et al: Multisomatoform disorder: an alternative to undifferentiated somatoform disorder for the somatizing patient in primary care. Arch Gen Psychiatry 54:352–358, 1997.
46. Loeser JD, Sullivan M, Long DM, et al: Disability in the chronic low back pain patient may be iatrogenic. Pain Forum 4:114–133, 1995.
47. Loeser JD: Concepts of pain. In: Stanton-Hicks M, Boas R (eds): Chronic Low Back Pain. Raven Press, New York, 1982.
48. Long DM: Effectiveness of therapies currently employed for persistent low back and leg pain. Pain Forum 4(2):122–125, 1995.
49. Mace CJ, Trimble MR: Hysteria, functional or psychogenic? Survey of British neurologists' preferences. J R Soc Med 84:471–475, 1991.
50. Madsen OR: Trunk extensor and flexor strength measured by the Cybex 6000 dynamometer: assessment of short-tern and long-term reproducibility of several strength variables. Spine 21:2770–2776, 1996.
51. Mann NH, Brown MD, Hertz DB, et al: Initial impression diagnosis using low back pain patient pain drawings. Spine 18:41–53, 1993.
52. Margolis RB, Tait RC, Krause SJ: A rating system for use with patient pain drawings. Pain 24:57–65, 1986.
53. Matheson LN: Symptom magnification syndrome structured interview: rationale and procedure. J Occup Rehabil 1:43–56, 1991.
54. Mayer T, Gatchel RJ, Keeley J, et al: Male incumbent worker industrial database. Part I. Lumbar spinal physical capacity. Part II. Cervical spinal physical capacity. Part III. Lumbar-cervical functional testing. Spine 19:755–761, 762–764, 765–770, 1994.
55. Mayer T, Gatchel RJ, Mayer H, et al: Prospective two-year study of functional restoration in industrial low back injury. JAMA 258:1763–1767, 1987.
56. Mayer T, Tabor J, Bovasso E, et al: Physical progress and residual impairment quantification after functional restoration. Part I. Lumbar mobility. Part II. Isokinetic trunk strength. Part III. Isokinetic and isoinertial lifting capacity. Spine 19:389–394, 395–400, 401–405, 1994.
57. McComas AJ, Kereshi S, Quinlan J: Method for detecting functional weakness. J Neurol Neurosurg Psychiatry 46:280–282, 1983.
58. Michel A, Kohlmann T, Raspe H: Association between clinical findings on physical examination and self-reported severity in back pain. Spine 22:296–304, 1997.
59. Mooney V, Kenney K, Leggett S, et al: Relationship of lumbar strength in shipyard workers to workplace injury claims. Spine 21:2001–2005, 1996.
60. Nachemson AL: Advances in low back pain. Clin Orthop 200:266–278, 1985.
61. Newton M, Waddell G: Trunk strength testing with iso-machines. Part I. Review of a decade of scientific evidence. Spine 18:801–811, 1993.
62. North RB, Nigrin DJ, Fowler KR, et al: Automated "pain drawing" analysis by computer-controlled patient interactive neurological stimulation system. Pain 50:51–57, 1992.

63. Ochoa JL, Verdugo RJ: Reflex sympathetic dystrophy: common clinical avenue for somatoform expression. Neurol Clin 13:351–363, 1995.
64. Ohlund C, Eek C, Palmblad S, et al: Quantified pain drawing in subacute LBP. Spine 21:1021–1031, 1996.
65. Oldham J: Personality disorders: current perspectives. JAMA 272:1770–1776, 1994.
66. Polatin PB, Kinney RK, Gatchel RJ, et al: Psychiatric illness and chronic LBP. Spine 18:66–71, 1993.
67. Quill TE: Somatization disorder: one of medicine's blind spots. JAMA 254:3075–3079, 1985.
68. Rainville J, Sobel J, Hartigan S, et al: Effect of compensation involvement on the reporting of pain and disability by patients referred for rehabilitation of chronic low back pain. Spine 22:2016–2024, 1997.
69. Rucker KS, Metzler HM: Predicting subsequent employment status of SSA disability applicants with chronic pain. Clin J Pain 11:22–35, 1995.
70. Rudy TE, Turk DC, Brena SF: Differential utility of medical procedures in the assessment of chronic pain patients. Pain 34:53–60, 1998.
71. Ruoff GE: Depression in the patient with chronic pain. J Fam Pract 43:S25–S34, 1996.
72. Rutherford O, Jones D, Newham DJ: Clinical and experimental application of the percutaneous twitch superimposition technique for the study of human muscle activation. J Neurol Neurosurg Psychiatry 49:1288–1291, 1986.
73. Schafer S, Nowlis DP: Personality disorders among difficult patients. Arch Fam Med 7:126–129, 1998.
74. Schrader H, Obelienienne D, Bovim G, et al: Natural evolution of late whiplash syndrome outside the medicolegal context. Lancet 347:1207–1211, 1996.
75. Schurman RA, Kramer PD, Mitchell JB: The hidden mental health network: treatment of mental illness by nonpsychiatrist physicians. Arch Gen Psychiatry 42:89–94, 1985.
76. Simonsen JC: Coefficient of variation as a measure of subject effort. Arch Phys Med Rehabil 76:516–520, 1995.
77. Smith GA, Nelson RC, Sadoff SJ, Sadoff AM: Assessing sincerity of effort in maximal grip strength tests. Am J Phys Med Rehabil 68:73–80, 1989.
78. Spitzer RL, Williams JB, Kroenke K, et al: Utility of a new procedure for diagnosing mental disorders in primary care: PRIME-MD 1000 study. JAMA 272:1749–1756, 1994.
79. Spratt KF, Lehmann TR, Weinstein JN, et al: New approach to the low back physical examination: behavioral assessment of mechanical signs. Spine 96–102, 1990.
80. Steig RL: Futility of physical testing in the assessment of disability. Am Pain Soc J 3:187–190, 1994.
81. Sternbach RA: Pain Patients: Traits and Treatment. New York, Academic Press, 1974.
82. Stokes HM: The seriously uninjured hand: weakness of grip. J Occup Med 25: 683–684, 1983.
83. Strender LE, Sjoblom A, Sundell K, et al: Interexaminer reliability in physical examination of patients with low back pain. Spine 22:814–820, 1997.
84. Tait RC: Psychological factors in the assessment of disability among patients with chronic pain. J Back Musculoskel Rehab 3:20–47, 1993.
85. Tait RC, Chibnall JT, Margolis RB: Pain extent: relations with psychological state, pain severity, pain history, and disability. Pain 41:295–301, 1990.
86. Teasell RW, Merskey H: Chronic pain disability in the workplace. Pain Forum 6:228–238, 1997.
87. Thomas E, Silman A, Papageorgious AC, et al: Association between measures of spinal mobility and low back pain. Spine 23:343–347, 1998.
88. van der Ploeg RJO, Oosterhuis HJGH: Make/break test as a diagnostic tool in functional weakness. J Neurol Neurosurg Psychiatry 54:248–251, 1991.

89. Vasudevan SV: The relationship between pain and disability: an overview of the problem. J Disabil 2:44–53, 1991.
90. Voiss DV: Occupational injury: fact, fantasy, or fraud? Neurol Clin 431–446, 1995.
91. Waddell G, Bircher M, Finlayson D, et al: Symptoms and signs: physical disease or illness behavior? Br Med J 289:739–743, 1984.
92. Waddell G, Somerville D, Henderson I, et al: Objective clinical evaluation of physical impairment in chronic low back pain. Spine 17:617–628, 1992.
93. Wallis BJ, Lord SM, Bogduk N: Resolution of psychological distress of whiplash patients following treatment by radiofrequency neurotomy: a randomized, double-blind, placebo-controlled trial. Pain 73:15–22, 1997.
94. Weisberg JN, Keefe FJ: Personality disorders in the chronic pain population: basic concepts, empirical findings, and clinical implications. Pain Forum 6:1–9, 1997.
95. Wilbourn AJ: Electrodiagnostic examination with hysterical conversion reaction and malingering. Neurol Clin 13(2):385–404, 1995.
96. Zimmerman M: Diagnosing personality disorders: review of issues and research methods. Arch Gen Psychiatry 51:225–245, 1994.

CHAPTER 14

Life Care Planning: Using Childhood Developmental Disability as a Model

Richard T. Katz, MD

Physicians may be asked by attorneys or other patient advocates to help plan for the long-term needs of patients with catastrophic injury. Often for litigation purposes, attorneys or insurance companies want a detailed outline of future expenses with which to negotiate. The life care planning process is simple and straightforward, though it can be manipulated by some to fit the financial "goals" of the negotiating party. One of the keys to constructing successful life care plans (LCPs) is to be intimately familiar with the needs of the disabled person for whom one is planning. It is easy to make laundry lists of expenses, but it requires extensive experience and training to plan accurately for the needs of an injured child or adult.

Because there are certain routine constructs in the preparation of an LCP, it would seem most productive to use one diagnostic group as a model. I have selected childhood disability under the two loosely used rubrics of cerebral palsy (CP) and mental retardation (MR) because these categories are very broad and require extensive consideration of childhood developmental issues, physical disability, equipment needs, cognitive impairments, and consideration of future surgical and therapeutic interventions. Children with brain injury often fall into the loosely used rubric "cerebral palsy," although this term may be overused. Nonetheless, it is fruitful to examine life care planning needs in this particular diagnostic group, for which there is a substantial body of medical literature.

A recent consensus group[26] defined CP as an "umbrella term covering a group of nonprogressive, but often changing, motor impairment syndromes secondary to lesions or anomalies of the brain arising in the early stages of its development." Recent studies suggest that CP is a rather common cause of childhood disability, with significant associated disability. According to Newacheck and Taylor,[28] greater than 100,000 Americans less than 18 years of age are believed to have some neurological disability attributed to CP. Approximately 25% of children with CP in France and England cannot walk, and 30% are classified as mentally retarded.[13, 30] A simple examination of these statistics suggests that health-care practitioners and the social community need to plan for the survival and care of these children.[13]

LIFE CARE PLANNING

When planning the lifelong needs of a child (or adult), an LCP may be constructed. An LCP estimates what services likely will be needed to meet the

TABLE 14–1 Steps in the Formation of a Life Care Plan

1. Determine extent and sequelae of the child's physical and cognitive impairments
2. Estimate prognosis
3. Estimate the need for and benefit of further medical and habilitative interventions
4. Calculate the costs of future personal needs (e.g. wheelchairs, orthopedic equipment, home furnishings and modifications, medical supplies, and recreational equipment)

future needs of the child. When constructing an LCP, the physician first must determine the extent and sequelae of the child's physical and cognitive impairments during the course of several evaluations (Table 14–1).

A physician experienced with treating patients with CP can give increasingly accurate estimates of a child's prognosis for improvement during serial observations of the child's developmental areas: gross motor skills, fine motor and adaptive skills, personal/social skills, speech and language skills, and cognitive and emotional development. With this knowledge, one can develop a cogent plan to assess the needs and benefits of future medical treatments and habilitation interventions (e.g., physical, occupational, and speech therapies). In cases of alleged malpractice liability issues on the part of prenatal and perinatal caregivers, physicians may be asked to calculate the costs of these potential interventions and personal needs. This can be performed with an approach as outlined in Table 14–2.[3, 7, 10]

The initial step in formulating these costs is to estimate the life expectancy of the child, which has been a source of considerable debate and a topic that will be dealt with extensively in this review.

Second, the physician must estimate the need, duration of need, and costs for a wide variety of hardware items and services. Examples of such devices include wheelchairs, seating systems, orthopedic aids, orthotics, home furnishings, architectural modifications, aids for independent function, drugs, supplies, and leisure-time equipment. The costs of the child's future home or facility care can similarly be approximated by planning for the appropriate level of daily care (e.g., home aid, skilled care within the home, or children's home occupant). The life care costs must include services rendered by physical, occupational, and speech therapists, and other educational and psychological services if they are not readily available. Finally, costs for future medical and surgical care, and the

TABLE 14–2 Estimating Future Costs in a Life Care Plan

1. Estimate life expectancy
2. Estimate costs of yearly services: evaluations by caregivers, therapy services, hardware needs (e.g., wheelchairs, orthopedic devices/equipment, maintenance, independence devices), home modification and furnishings, architectural changes, drugs and supplies, home or facility care, transportation, leisure time and/or recreational equipment, future medical/surgical care, costs of potential complications
3. Financial adjustment of estimated costs for future interest rates and inflation (generally within the expertise of an economist)

costs of potential future medical complications and procedures must be appraised.

After the total cost of an LCP is calculated in present dollars, a financial adjustment must be made to account for future interest rates and inflation. Such calculations need to account for the increasing costs of health care versus the consumer price index, return on investments, estimations of the present value of goods versus future costs (the discount rate), and taxes on investments. Economic modeling of these items is considered within the purview of an economist and is generally not carried out by a physician unless he or she has special expertise in financial matters.

SERVICES GENERALLY AVAILABLE FROM THE PUBLIC SECTOR

Planning for children with CP often involves a variety of social services because children with physical and mental handicaps have a variety of psychosocial challenges. A discussion of these challenges is beyond the scope of this review, but interested readers are referred to other sources for further inquiry.[5, 18, 22, 36] It is useful, however, to examine what types of social support services are available within the locality of the disabled child.

In the St. Louis metropolitan area, for example, there are a number of financial and funding resources that serve individuals with CP. The first is the Missouri Department of Mental Health (DMH) through the Division of Mental Retardation and Developmental Disabilities (DMDD). The St. Louis and St. Charles Regional Centers for Developmental Disabilities are the major case management and referral services funded through the DMH. Another important agency is the Productive Living Board (PLB) for St. Louis County Citizens with Developmental Disabilities. The PLB provides funding for a variety of services and programs, including employment, residential resources, respite care, recreational services, and family support. St. Louis city residents can receive funding through the St. Louis Office for Mental Retardation and Developmental Disability Resources. Programs and services funded are similar to those funded by the PLB. More specialized services, such as employment and attendant services, are funded through Vocational Rehabilitation, Division of Aging, and Division of Medical Services. In addition to the aforementioned funding sources, agencies such as the St. Louis Variety Club and United Way also provide additional funding to service providers and programs that serve adults and children with developmental disabilities.

There are a multitude of provider agencies throughout the greater St. Louis area that serve individuals with CP and who receive funding from one or all of the aforementioned funding sources. Residential services both in the natural home and in community placement models are primarily designed around the concept of "supported living." This concept dictates that the supports provided to the individual are specifically tailored to the needs and desires of the individual and family. Services are customized to each individual—the individual is not expected to fit into or adjust to preexisting service capabilities. Rather, the service provider must develop a specific and individually tailored approach and environment to best meet the needs and desires of the individual served. Some of the agencies in St. Louis that provide this type of service include the United Cerebral Palsy Association of Greater St. Louis (UCPA), Specialized Transitional Activities and Rehabilitation Training (START), Creative Concepts, Lifestyle Options and Opportunities, Gateways, Lifeskills, Council for Extended Care (CEC), and St. Louis Association for Retarded Citizens

(SLARC). Agencies in St. Charles that provide this service include Emmaus House, Willows Way, and Community Living Incorporated. In addition to supported living models, there are group-home settings and specialized residential facilities available, such as those operated by the Magdala Foundation and the Children's Home Society of Missouri.

Employment and vocational services include supported employment (which mirrors the concept of supported living outlined earlier) and sheltered workshops. Among the providers of supported employment services for people with CP are UCPA, Lifeskills, SLARC, and START. Sheltered workshop services are also provided by UCPA, SLARC, ITE Inc., Worth Industries, Universal Workshop, Lafayette Industries, and others. Respite services are provided in two different models (in-home and facility). Providers of facility-based respite services include UCPA, Children's Home Society, SLARC, Ranken Jordan, and New Horizon Center. In-home respite services are provided by SLARC, Olsten, Kimberly, Quality Care, and New Horizon Center. In addition, there are camping models provided by CEC and SLARC.

Generally, the Regional Center, under the auspices of the DMH, serves as the main case-management and referral source for the majority of the services outlined above. In most cases, an individual must have an active file with the Regional Center before funding will be approved. An individual is assigned a case manager who serves as the primary link between the individual and service provider.

ESTIMATING LIFE EXPECTANCY

As discussed earlier, one of the key issues in creating a robust LCP is to provide an estimate of life expectancy. There is a considerable amount of epidemiological literature to provide guidance in this regard. It is surprising that such literature is often left unconsulted by parties in negotiation. This literature will be reviewed here as it applies to both children with CP, as well as those with MR in general, because both parts of the literature add considerable insight. In many cases epidemiologists mix the two populations together. The following review selects some of the more methodologically useful studies conducted over the last 25 years.

As a preface to this analysis, the interface between scientific and legal thought should briefly be addressed. One of the important issues in bridging the gap between physicians and attorneys in this regard relates to the issue of what constitutes a fact. Taylor[35] has described it as follows:

> Health-care providers tend to view facts as being those observations which are based upon empirical evaluation. For a fact to be accepted as *true* it usually must be confirmed with *certainty.* On the other hand, for lawyers involved in civil litigation, facts are established by the legal construct of *probability.* Thus, even in the absence of complete scientific certainty, a legal fact is deemed to be true, if the observation is more likely than not found to be correct.

Herein lies a key point of miscommunication between lawyer and physician. The physician needs to understand that litigation situations hold to a standard of "more likely than not" or "less likely than not." Another often-used phrase is something like "within the realm of medical certainty." All of this simply means the probability is greater than 50%. With this construct in mind, the following epidemiological studies have been summarized (when possible) to address the important question, "when is it more likely than not that a child with CP or MR will no longer be alive?"

Studies in Children With Cerebral Palsy

Before the epidemiological examination, some additional definitions may be helpful to the reader less briefed in medical terminology. CP generally is grouped into four main categories: *spastic* (approximately 70%), *athetoid* (approximately 20%), *ataxic* (approximately 10%), and *mixed* forms. Spastic syndromes are most common, and are characterized by muscular hypertonicity and loss of motor control. Spastic syndromes may affect predominantly one side (hemiplegia), both legs (paraplegia), legs greater than arms (diplegia), or all four limbs (quadriplegia or tetraplegia). Athetoid or dyskinetic syndromes are characterized by slow, writhing, involuntary movements, and sometimes abrupt, distal, jerky movements. Ataxic syndromes are uncommon (~10%) and may be marked by weakness, incoordination, wide-based gait, and tremor. Many patients have mixed features.

Through the Mayo Clinic patient data bank, Kudrjavcev et al.[24] identified 60 cases of CP between 1950 and 1976. They stratified patients with CP into four groups: (1) *mild:* functions without marked difficulty and without mechanical aids; (2) *moderate:* functions with marked difficulty but without mechanical aids; (3) *severe:* functions only with the assistance of mechanical aids; and (4) *very severe:* does not function even with the assistance of mechanical aids. Seventy-three percent were spastic, 16% ataxic, and 6% were dyskinetic CP. Survival was calculated for the first 10 years of life. Intelligence was characterized as normal (IQ >80), mild to moderate MR (IQ 36–80), and severe/profound MR (IQ <35). For severely or profoundly mentally retarded children, survival was 68% at 5 years and 54% at 10 years. A life-table analysis showed 68% survival at 5 years for normal/mild mentally retarded children and 54% survival at 10 years for severe and profound mentally retarded children.

Emond et al.[11] studied the prevalence of children with CP in two cohorts, from the 1958 and 1970 British Births Survey. The prevalence of CP remained constant at 2.5/1000 births. The prevalence at 10 years after birth was higher in the second cohort. All children with CP born in 1970 survived until age 10, whereas 9 of 40 children born in 1958 were dead before 10 years of age. This study suggests that survival may have improved in children with CP, but more importantly it demonstrates that although obstetrical practices have changed, there was no decrease in the occurrence of CP.

Evans et al.[12] have presented two of the more important recent studies dealing with survival in patients with CP. First, they investigated death certificates from 732 children with CP in South East Thames born from 1970 to 1979. They found that death certificates did not offer accurate data in ascertaining the mortality of children with CP. Evans et al.[13] also prospectively followed children with CP in South East Thames born from 1970 to 1979, with an average follow-up of 15 years. Immobility (defined as being confined to bed or unable to propel a wheelchair) and severe mental subnormality were the strongest predictors of mortality. Spastic quadriplegia, dyskinesia, and mixed CP were most severely affected. Nearly all ataxic, 90% of dyskinetic, and 72% of quadriplegic patients reached 18 years of age. Seizures covaried with mental subnormality and were negatively correlated with survival. Hydrocephalus may

TABLE 14–3 Survival in Three Groups of Developmentally Disabled Children

Age interval	Subgroup I (% surviving to beginning of age interval)	Subgroup I (No. of years remaining if child survives to beginning of age interval)	Subgroup 2 (% surviving to beginning of age interval)	Subgroup 2 (No. of years remaining if child survives to beginning of age interval)	Subgroup 3 (% surviving to beginning of age interval)	Subgroup 3 (No. of years remaining if child survives to beginning of age interval)
1–4	58.6	4.1	92.9	8.1	97.5	23.4
5–9	21	4.8	57.1	8.3	89.3	21.4
10–14	7.2	4.8	30.1	8.7	66.6	22.9
15–19	2.5	4.5	17.1	8.5	57.8	21.5
20–24	0.79	4.4	9.0	9.1	48.3	19.8
25–29	0.21	5.4	4.5	10.8	39.2	18.8
30–34	0.07	7.0	2.7	11.6	32.3	17.4
35–39	0.029	8.9	2.1	9.5	32.3	12.4
40–44	0.020	6.4	1.5	7.3	28.0	8.7
45–49	0.008	8.1	0.78	6.7	13.1	11.0
50–54	0.004	9.2	0.42	5.3	—	—
55–59	0.004	4.2	0.18	4.6	—	—
>60	0.001	2.6	0.062	3.9	—	—
>65	—	—	0.0015	4.0	—	—

Modified from Eyman RK, Grossman HJ, Chaney RH, Call TL: Life expectancy of profoundly handicapped people with mental retardation. N Engl J Med 323:584–589, 1990.

also be a negative risk factor. Ninety percent of children survived between 10 and 20 years.

Four studies by Eyman et al.[14–16, 32] have added significantly greater insight into the survival of children with CP as well as other developmental disabilities. In 1990, they reported on 99,543 persons with developmental disability from the California Department of Developmental Services between 1984 and 1987.[14] The best predictors of mortality were (1) deficits in cognitive function, (2) limitations on mobility, (3) incontinence, and (4) inability to eat without assistance. They provided a life-table analysis of survival, which is shown in Table 14–3.

Analysis was based on defining three subgroups of children:

Subgroup 1: Immobile, not toilet trained, required tube feeding
Subgroup 2: Immobile, not toilet trained, but could eat with assistance
Subgroup 3: Mobile but not ambulatory and could eat with assistance

According to this life-table analysis, most children in subgroup 1 would not survive their eighth birthday; most in subgroup 2 would not reach age 12, and most in subgroup 3 would not reach age 23.

Eyman et al. extended these observations in three more recent papers. In the first,[15] they examined the relationship between mortality and the acquisition of basic skills by children and adults with severe disabilities. There were several very important conclusions:

1. Subjects who were tube fed and immobile showed very little likelihood of becoming mobile or feeding themselves and had a high probability of death

2. Individuals who had some mobility had a better outcome
3. Self-help skills generally should be achieved by around 5 years of age if they are likely to occur; after age 6, the most likely outcome for those who were immobile and could not feed themselves was death, or no improvement in self-help skills
4. There was a very high mortality associated with tube feeding
5. There was no evidence that these severely involved subjects could be helped by special training
6. Low IQ was the major deterrent to the acquisition of skills

In the third study, Eyman et al.[16] once again directly assessed the survival of profoundly disabled people with severe MR. A refinement of the earlier 1990 work, this paper demonstrated that voluntary arm-hand movement and the ability to roll over were associated with improved survival. They again divided their observations into functional categories, including mobility (ability to walk, crawl, creep, scoot), rolling (any type), hand use (e.g., grasp), arm use (functional use), toileting skills (trained), eating skills (help with their feeding), and need for tube feeding. Many of the children were also diagnosed with CP. In this study, six subgroups were defined:

Subgroup 1: Immobile, could not roll, required tube feeding, no arm-hand use

Subgroup 2: Immobile, could not roll, required tube feeding, some arm-hand use

Subgroup 3: Immobile, could not roll, could take food if fed by others, no arm-hand use

Subgroup 4: Immobile, could not roll, could take food if fed by others, some arm-hand use

Subgroup 5: Immobile, could roll over, could take food if fed by others, some arm-hand use

Subgroup 6: Immobile, could roll over, tube fed, some arm-hand use

Several survival charts (which plot additional years children would be expected to live) are presented for children of different ages in each of the different groups. Table 14–4 summarizes the median expected additional years

TABLE 14–4 Median Survival in Six Groups of Developmentally Disabled Children

Subgroup	1 year of age	1–15 years of age	16–49 years of age
1	0.9 years	4.8 years	10.4 years
2	1.4 years	5.3 years	Not available
3	1.2 years	5.7 years	10.4 years
4	3.2 years	10.0 years	Not available
5	Not available*	Not available*	Not available*
6	8.4	10.9	10.9

* Children in subgroup 5 had a comparatively good life expectancy. Over 70% of those <1, 70% of those 1–15, and 80% of those 16–49 were alive after 11 years.

of survival for three different age groups (<1, 1–15, and 16–49 years), according to the six subgroups defined above.

Note in the table that median survival could not be calculated for all subgroups and all ages. The survival in subgroup 5, for example, was comparatively good. None of the age groups in subgroup 5 evidenced a 50% cumulative death rate in the 11-year follow-up period. Another important finding in this study was that "improved medical care has not altered significantly the poor prognosis for those with the most severe impairments."

Finally, in 1996 Strauss, Eyman, and Grossman[32] set out once again to assess predictors of mortality, but also to carefully compare risk-adjusted mortality rates for those children living in institutions with those in the community. The population was once again from the California Department of Developmental Services, and data comprised over 7000 severely disabled children over a 12-year period. Variables included age, measures of mobility, tube feeding, level of retardation, and certain adaptive skills. Confirming their previous studies, reduced mobility and use of tube feeding were the strongest predictors of increased mortality. In addition, newly discovered negative predictors included the following:

1. Lack of hand use
2. Inability to creep/crawl/scoot
3. Inability to speak intelligible words
4. Inability to recognize voices
5. Inability to interact with peers

The most surprising result was that children cared for within their home residence or within community care facilities had an estimated 25% *higher* risk-adjusted odds of mortality than those in institutions or health-care facilities. This increased relative risk of mortality in community placement has been confirmed in further work by Strauss.[33] More recently Strauss et al. have further refined their understanding of the increased mortality associated with tube feeding. The risk was greater in children with less severe rather than those with very severe disabilities, and there was a trend toward reduction in relative risk when the child had a tracheostomy.[34]

Hutton et al.[20] reported the survival of a large cohort of patients with CP. All children with CP born between 1966 and 1984 to mothers in the Mersey Regional Health Authority were identified, including 1258 subjects with idiopathic CP. The 25-year survival rate was 89.3% for females and 86.9% for males overall. They studied three types of disability in the population: (1) ambulation (assistance needed for propulsion), (2) manual dexterity (unable to feed and dress), and (3) mental ability (IQ <50). For subjects with no severe functional disabilities, 20-year survival was 99%. Children who were severely disabled in all three functional groups had a 20-year survival of 50%. Functional disability was the strongest predictor of survival, whereas gestational age and birth weight predicted little. Girls had slightly greater survival. The percentage surviving to 27 years of age was 90%, 80%, and 44% for children with one, two, and three severe disabilities, respectively. This data is summarized in Table 14–5.

Median term survival rates have been calculated for 3189 children born with CP in British Columbia between 1952 and 1989. Investigators noted four categories of CP (quadriplegia/diplegia, hemiplegia/monoplegia, athetosis, other), seizure type (generalized, partial with/without secondary generalization, infantile spasms, unclassified), and presence of MR (nonexistent/mild, moder-

TABLE 14–5 Survival in CP Children According to Three Key Disabilities

Age	No disability (% survival)	One disability (% survival)	Two disabilities (% survival)	Three disabilities (% survival)
5	99.9	100	95.2	85.1
10	99.7	96.8	92.1	70.0
15	99.0	95.5	90.4	54.5
20	98.8	93.5	84.7	50.3
25	98.8	90.6	80.5	44.2
27	98.8	90.6	80.5	44.2

Modified from Hutton JL, Cooke T, Pharaoah H: Life expectancy in children with cerebral palsy. Br Med J 309:431–435, 1994.

ate, severe, profound). The data clearly support the adverse effects of mental retardation, epilepsy, and type of CP on survival. The spastic quadriplegia group had the worst prognosis. Overall survival rate at 30 years was at least 87%.[6]

Studies in Children Primarily With Mental Retardation

Several studies have also examined the life expectancy of children with MR, distinct from those with developmental disability with mental retardation. Using present nomenclature,[1] MR is categorized according to intellectual impairment into mild (IQ level 50–55 to 70), moderate (IQ level 35–40 to 50–55), severe (IQ level 20–25 to 35–40), and profound MR (IQ level below 20 or 25). These terms have for many years supplanted the following outdated designations: (1) feeblemindedness (former name for MR), (2) moron (IQ 50–69), (3) imbecile (IQ 25–49), and (4) idiot (IQ <25).[8] These antiquated terms are defined only because they are found in some of the older literature, such as Table 14–6.

Heaton-Ward[19] studied the life expectancy of hospitalized mentally retarded patients, including 108 females and 105 males. The age at death was strongly correlated to IQ. The average age of death for "non-Mongoloid" persons (i.e., MR not associated with the genetic defect trisomy 21 or Down syndrome) was 29 years for males and 32 for females with an IQ <25, and 39.5 years for males and 45.2 for females with an IQ of 26–50.

TABLE 14–6 Average Age at Death in Three Older Studies of Mentally Retarded Adults

Survey	Feeble-minded male*	Feeble-minded female*	Imbecile male	Imbecile female	Idiot male	Idiot female
Primrose 1966	45.1	47.5	45.1	46.2	25.2	25.0
Heaton Ward 1968	—	—	40.0	49.8	28.8	29.3
McCurley 1972	58.1	49.8	37.1	40.8	17.3	14.0

*As used by these authors, feeble-minded designates the "moron" (outdated term) or "mildly retarded" group of mentally handicapped individuals.

Modified from McCurley R, MacKay DN, Scally BG: Life expectation of the mentally subnormal under community and hospital care. J Mental Def Res 16:57–67, 1972.

McCurley et al.[25] examined the average age at death in mentally retarded persons and compared his data to earlier studies (summarized in Table 14–6). All individuals with MR had a significantly decreased life expectancy, which decreased dramatically with the severity of the mental deficit. They included patients cared for in a hospital, as well as a community setting. In this study, patients in a community care program had a better prognosis. Specific data for patients with CP showed the mean age of death was 8.3 years for males and 10.5 for females.

The life expectancy of mentally retarded persons in Canadian institutions from 1966 to 1968 was published by Balakrishnan and Wolf.[2] This study primarily involved more severely retarded individuals. For the profoundly retarded, the average age of death was approximately 23.5 years for males and 23.7 for females. For the severely and moderately retarded, average age of death was 37.9 years and 42.5 for males and females, respectively. These results were more recently replicated in a facility within the southwestern United States.[29]

Kaveggia[21] performed a survival analysis of 1915 severely and profoundly mentally retarded individuals who were institutionalized at the Central Wisconsin Center. CP survivors comprised 442 of the total studied, which included a wide gamut of etiologies for mental retardation. On admission, the median remaining lifetime was 8.81 ± 4.16 years for residents with inborn errors of metabolism, 18.56 ± 4.26 years for residents with primary central nervous system (CNS) malformations, and 24.66 ± 4.05 years for residents with unknown syndromes.

Chaney et al.[4] reviewed 1146 patients who had died and were autopsied from 1944 to 1983 from Lanterman State Hospital, a South Carolina hospital for mentally retarded persons. They evaluated survival by reported CNS "insult." Of those with perinatal insult, 34.6% survived beyond age 21. Similarly, 29.6% of prenatal, 16.7% of postnatal, and 47.4% of those in whom time of insult was uncertain survived beyond age 21. When considering all groups, 34.1% survived beyond age 21. This study is limited by the wide variety of etiologies causing MR. Furthermore, even in those cases with the diagnosis of "perinatal asphyxia," recent literature suggests that the ability of an investigator or caregiver to accurately determine the time of CNS insult is highly limited, suggesting the information in this study must be cautiously interpreted.[11, 27] As stated by one author, "epidemiologic studies . . . have not provided any reasons to change the impression that our ability to identify modifiable, presumed causes of cerebral palsy is limited."[23]

Simila et al.[31] prospectively followed 12,058 children from Finland, Oulu, and Lapland born in 1966 (96% of all children born) until they reached the age of 17. One hundred and sixty-five children had MR; 97 were classified as severe (IQ <50) and 68 as mild (IQ 50–70). The death rate was 158 per 1000 for those with MR as compared with 22 per 1000 for those with normal intelligence.

In one of the most methodologically sound and clinically important studies to date on the survival of those with MR, Dupont et al.[9] studied the mortality, life expectancy, and causes of death of individuals in Denmark with mild mental retardation. A total of 7314 persons were included. Even in the mildly mentally retarded population, the 50% survival for men and women was approximately 65 and 75 years of age, respectively, significantly less than a "normal" population. When examining those who had already survived to 10 years of age, only 50% survived to be 68 to 70 years. When comparing those who were and were not institutionalized, the type of residence had no effect on life expectancy.

Wolf and Wright[37] examined changes in life expectancy of mentally retarded

TABLE 14–7 Key Disabilities Diminishing Life Expectancy in CP and MR Children

Presence and severity of mental retardation
- Inability to speak intelligible words
- Inability to recognize voices
- Inability to interact with peers

Physical disability
- Limitations on mobility
  - Inability to propel wheelchair
  - Inability to roll over
  - Inability to creep/crawl/scoot
- Lack of upper extremity function
- Inability to eat without assistance

Tube feeding
Incontinence
Presence and severity of seizures

persons in Canadian institutions by using life-table analysis. Less than 50% of the profoundly mentally retarded population lived beyond 41 years, and only 50% of moderate to severely mentally retarded lived beyond 58 years. Even in the borderline to mild group, only 50% lived beyond age 67. Wolf calculated that the life expectancies for institutionalized mentally retarded Canadian children (who had reached 5 years of age from 1976 to 1978) was 39.6 for those who were profoundly retarded, 48.2 for moderately and severely retarded, and 58.0 years for borderline and mildly retarded. There had been a mild increase in life expectancy between an earlier cohort (1966–1968) and the most recent cohort (1976–1978) studied.

Forsgren et al.[17] studied a cohort of all children with mental retardation living in a noninstitutionalized setting within a single Swedish province for a span of 7 years. The standardized mortality ratio was 1.6 times the general population in those with MR only, 5 times greater in those with MR and epilepsy, and 5.8 times greater in those with MR, epilepsy, and CP. The mortality increase was seen in both those with partial seizures that generalized and those that did not. The highest mortality, 8.1, was seen in those who always generalized from the onset. Pneumonia was the most common cause of death.

In summary, there are a large list of factors that in many well-designed studies have been shown to decrease survival in early childhood brain injury. These are summarized in Table 14–7.

A SAMPLE LIFE CARE PLAN

For the novice life care planner, it may be helpful to see an actual life care plan to serve as a template. The following is an actual case prepared several years ago. The prices included are meant to be illustrative only. Every life care planner needs to explore actual list and discounted prices in their geographic region. Life care planning reports also have stylistic differences, and this represents only one such style.

I have added some running commentary for the reader in italicized print. These comments are, again, for illustrative purpose only.

I: COVER PAGE

LIFE CARE PLAN FOR R. K. Date of Birth: 8/27/91

Richard T. Katz, MD
4660 Maryland Ave.
#250
St. Louis, MO 63108

II: BRIEF OVERVIEW

R. K. is a nearly 5-year-old boy with severe developmental delay subsequent to an anoxic/hypoxic encephalopathy that occurred subsequent to a cardiopulmonary arrest on 10/3/91, when he was approximately 6 months of age. He was transferred from his community hospital to St. Mary's Hospital of Anytown, Missouri. He was diagnosed with streptococcal meningitis, and suffered sepsis, shock, severe metabolic acidosis, adrenal insufficiency, respiratory failure, disseminated intravascular coagulation, anemia, hematuria, leukopenia, and thrombocytopenia. His deficits include a severe uncontrolled seizure disorder, severe mental retardation and global developmental delays, oculomotor dysfunction resulting in bilateral medial rectus recessions, and spastic tetraparesis (worse on the left). His medications as of 5/6/96 were Depakote (125 mg) ii + iii + ii capsules per day, Klonopin (0.5 mg) 1.5 tablets per day, and phenobarbital (15 mg) iii tablets at qhs. His medical history is summarized in my report of May 6, 1996.

His most recent Individualized Educational Program of February 1996 from the County Special Education Cooperative was not available at the time of my initial report, and so shall be summarized here.

In the Physical Therapy Evaluation it was noted that he demonstrated frequent self-stimulatory behaviors. Movement patterns were dominated by extensor tone. Ankle-foot orthoses (AFOs) were present bilaterally. He would roll about the room, primarily with leftward rotation. He had functional head control. Sitting control was poor. He showed reasonable sitting in the booster chair. He propelled himself 5' in a gait trainer. He had emerging trunk control. His left side was more involved than the right. The physical therapist recommended 50 minutes of physical therapy per week in two sessions. In the June 10, 1996 update, the physical therapist was able to apply techniques to decrease self-stimulatory behaviors. He was able to sit with minimal-to-standby assistance for 20–30 seconds. A Freedom stander was used daily to increase tolerance of standing and to allow for better hip socket development. A *Body Vibes by Conair* was used to decrease self-stimulatory behaviors. He received a manual wheelchair in April. He propelled himself in the gait trainer for 100'.

Psychological evaluation on 1/4/96 revealed he functioned at the 7-month level, which did not include motor skills. He was able to ring a bell and rattle a spoon on a cup. His adaptive behavior was in the moderate-to-severe deficit range. Moderate deficits were reported in communication, daily living skills, and socialization.

Additional reports indicated his communication delays hinder his ability to effectively communicate with others. He communicates using an eye point and on occasion by reaching for objects or pictures presented. He does some babbling and makes signs (to eat or drink) with hand over head assistance. He understands most concepts and one-step commands. He is not toilet trained, and requires diapering. It is at times difficult to persuade R. K. to eat. He drinks from an open-ended cup with handles and some assistance. He is dependent in all other self-help skills. He displays little interest in his peers, and does not engage in any parallel play.

This life care plan is also constructed with the concept that physical therapy is especially important in preschool and early school years for children with cerebral palsy and similar static encephalopathies, but wanes in importance thereafter. In early adolescence and adulthood, cerebral palsy children essentially plateau in function. "Therapeutic exercise" should be carried out in "recreational" rather than "therapeutic" settings, especially for children with mild-to-moderate physical impairment. Finally, while R. K.'s essential needs are fully outlined in the following report, it is acknowledged that some of these services may be available within the public sector.

In terms of life expectancy, this plan is based on an estimated mortality at 36 years of age. Factors that mitigate R. K.'s life expectancy are his physical disability, inability to propel a wheelchair, incontinence, and presence of a severe seizure disorder. However, he is able to roll over, is able to assist in some aspects of feeding, has some useful upper extremity function, and he is not tube fed. Although children with this profile certainly have a marked limitation of life expectancy, as noted in the estimated additional lifespan of 31 years, he is in a group that is not as severely limited as those with tube feeding and complete lack of mobility.

Comments: After a succinct summary of the case outlining the major challenges for which to plan, the life expectancy is clearly stated. Note that in terms of expenses, the three most important factors for any life care plan are: (1) the amount of years surviving; (2) the amount, duration, and intensity of long-term care; and (3) the amount, frequency, and duration of therapy services. Thus there should be reasonable justification for each. The life expectancy in this case was based on the review of literature cited earlier. Although it is not possible to foresee the future, the process of litigation asks the "expert witness" to make a best estimate of future life expectancy. As there is no "crystal ball," the best estimate can be made by a systematic review of the literature.

III: ESTIMATE OF FUTURE COSTS

An estimate of future costs can be created by looking at the various aspects of needs outlined in Table 14–2. It should be emphasized at this point that although one would hope a life care planning process would be "objective" and "attending to the needs of the child," it unfortunately follows the adversarial process of polarization of plaintiff and defense views. What follows is hopefully an example of a plan that is down the middle. Although it may be difficult for the novice to envision an appropriate life care plan for a child's lifetime, it should be pointed out that the planner generally has but one "bite at the apple" (i.e., if provisions are not included in the original life care plan, they likely will never be addressed again). Finally, for what level of care should the life care planner provide: the standard within the community, the best possible care, barely adequate care? There are no simple answers to these questions, but plaintiff attorneys will argue that the child deserves "every opportunity available" to have a successful and productive life, whereas the defense attorney will argue that certain expenses are abusive and excessive. Note that costs are annualized both for one-time and recurrent expenses, so that a simple spreadsheet of future costs can be constructed.

Projected Evaluations

Evaluation	Age/Year at Which Initiated	Age/Year at Which Suspended	Frequency	Base Cost Per Year
Psychological rehabilitation	5/1996	1 time only	1 time only	Evaluation ($750–$800)
Vocational rehabilitation	21/2112	1 time only	1 time only	$950–$1250 at age 21
Physical therapy	5/1996	21/2112	1 time/year	$75
Occupational therapy	5/1996	21/2112	1 time/year	$75
Speech therapy	5/1996	21/2112	1 time/year	$150
Rehabilitation engineer	14/2005	21/2012	1 time/year at ages 14 and 21	$450

Comments: Many areas of life care planning are controversial, and some controversies exist here under evaluation. Although it is true that the child was evaluated as part of the Individualized Educational Plan as required by federal law, some schools may have suboptimal programs for children with developmental disability, and the life care planner may request adjuvant evaluations. Also, it was highly unlikely that this child would ever be competitively employable. However, a vocational rehabilitation specialist assessment at the age of graduation (remember disabled children are able to continue school until age 21) might be indicated to determine if schools for supervised workshop were existent.

Projected Therapeutic Modalities

Evaluation	Age/Year at Which Initiated	Age/Year at Which Suspended	Frequency	Base Cost Per Year
Family counseling/ family education	5/1996	21/2112	Weekly sessions for a block of 3 months three times over his childhood	$1020 on three occasions during his childhood (based on $85/hr)
Physical therapy	5/1996	15/2006	3 times/week to supplement school program	$11,700 based on sessions of $75/hr
Occupational therapy	5/1996	15/2006	1 time/week to supplement school program	$3900 based on sessions of $75/hr
Speech therapy	5/1996	21/2012	3 times/week to supplement school program	$11,700 based on sessions of $75/hr
Sheltered workshop guidance	21/2012	1 time only	2 times/week for 2–4 months at age 21	$2000 at age 21

Comments: Obviously not all patients and their families need counseling, and the lack of clear guidelines and endpoints makes this an area for potential "abuse" within the LCP.

However, there are times when this may be appropriate. The life care planner should have familiarity with the literature concerning supportive counseling, because most therapeutic relationships are by no means open-ended and interminable. To those unfamiliar with the needs of developmentally disabled children, one would assume that therapy services are well-provided for in the school environment. This varies greatly between school districts, and in some the therapy contact hours are sorely lacking because of budgetary restraints. For example, this child was not receiving any *occupational therapy services in the school setting. The life care planner thus needs to assess the "supplementary services" appropriate for each child.*

Diagnostic Testing/Educational Assessment/Schooling				
Diagnostic Recommendation	**Age/Year at Which Initiated**	**Age/Year at Which Suspended**	**Treatment Frequency**	**Base Cost Per Year**
Educational testing	5/1996	5/1996	1 time/year	$250–$300
Special education: Option 1	5/1996	21/2012	Throughout the year, 175 school days/year	Anytown School District reimburses Another School District $76.18/day or $13,331.50/year; in addition, an aide is paid approximately $9000/year, totaling $22,351.50/year; transportation is covered below
Special education: Option 2	5/1996	21/2012	The Stookey School is the only private option in the geographic area; the cost is $78/day; there are 217 program days per year	The yearly cost would be $16,926, plus the cost of an aid at approximately $9000/year

Comments: In this case the Anytown School District had no provisions for developmentally disabled children. They paid Another School District a daily fee to educate R. K. so that they did not have to provide this service. The family hired a woman to transport R. K. to and from school, which was a 45-minute drive. The family wished to stay in the public school setting, because the private setting was less desirable. Again, plaintiff and defense attorneys would have opposing views as to the inclusion of such educational costs within the LCP because they are provided for by public funds.

Wheelchair Needs/Maintenance/Accessories				
Wheelchair Type	**Age/Year at Which Purchased**	**Replacement Schedule**	**Base Cost**	**Base Cost Per Year**
Manual wheelchair including lap tray	5/1996	Every 5 years	$2000	$400
Manual wheelchair maintenance	5/1996	1 time/year	$175/year	$175
Shower/commode chair	5/1996	Every 5 years	$500	$100
Shower/commode chair maintenance	5/1996	1 time/year	$50/year	$50
Electric wheelchair	5/1996	Every 5 years	$8200	$1640
Electric wheelchair maintenance	5/1996	1 time/year	$400/year	$400
Back pack	5/1996	1 time/year	$35–$40	$35–$40

Comments: Although it was by no means clear when evaluating this 5-year-old child, he might be a candidate for an electric wheelchair in the future. Again, settlements are generally structured on a one-time basis, and the life care planner does not have the option of revisiting the issue in the future should the situation change. It is assumed that the generic wheelchairs available in a nursing home would not be appropriate for such a child, if that were his post-21 years of age placement (see below).

Orthopedic and Orthotic Equipment Needs				
Equipment Description	**Age/Year Purchased**	**Replacement Schedule**	**Base Cost**	**Base Cost Per Year**
Tumble form feeder seat	5/1996	1 time only	$240	$240
Platform walker	7/1998	1 time only	$60	$60
Prone stander	5/1996	1 time only	$680	$680
Helmet	5/1996	1 time/year to age 18	$35	$35
AFOs	5/1996	1 time/year	$400	$400
Wrist-hand splints	5/1996	1 time/year	$100	$100

Comments: An interesting debate that will arise between plaintiff and defense attorney is who is responsible for what expenses. For example, should a defendant found responsible for a child's cerebral palsy be responsible for equipment already purchased through Medicare/Medicaid? The plaintiff will argue that the "public sector" should not have to pay for the defendant's negligence. The defense will argue that the items were "already paid for."

Home Furnishings and Accessories				
Equipment Description	**Age/Year at Which Purchased**	**Replacement Schedule**	**Base Cost**	**Base Cost Per Year**
Exercise mat	5/1996	1 time/10 years	$200	$20
Electric bed with side rails	10/2001	1 time/10 years	$1800	$180
Hoyer lift	10/2001	1 time/10 years	$1250	$125
Maintenance on lift and replacement slings	12/2003	1 time/2 years	$100 every 2 years	$50

Aids For Independent Function				
Equipment	**Age/Year at Which Purchased**	**Replacement Schedule**	**Base Cost**	**Base Cost Per Year**
Environmental control unit	11/2002	Every 5 years	$2400	$480
Basic home computer	8/1999	1 time/4 years	$2400	$600
Upgrade and maintain computer; purchase software	8/1999	Every 2 years	$500 each time	$250

Comments: Again, the child was not able to use any computerized device or environmental control unit (ECU) at present, but therapists believed there was strong potential for both devices in the future.

Drug/Supply Needs				
Supply Description	**Age/Year Initiated**	**Age/Year Discontinued**	**Unit Cost Per Month**	**Yearly Cost**
Depakote 125 mg iii in am and pm ii at noon	5/1996	36/2127	$41/100 or $98	$984
Klonopin 0.5 mg 1.5 tabs qd	5/1996	36/2127	$88/100 or $40	$475
Phenobarbital 15 mg iii tabs qhs	5/1996	36/2127	$6.5/100 or $1.63	$20

Comments: Obviously there is no way to assess what drugs will be used in the future. Also, needs for medication dosage will increase as R. K. ages. It is also likely that he will try new medications as they are introduced on the market.

Home/Facility Care					
Facility Recommended	**Home Care/ Service**	**Age/Year Initiated**	**Age/Year Suspended**	**Hours/Shifts/ Days of Attendance of Care**	**Base Cost Per Year**
Before age 21	Weekday attendant care to help with wakening in AM, after-school care, feeding, bowel routine, bathing, etc.	5/1996	21/2012	6 hours/day, 5 days/week, 41 weeks/year (1320 hours) @ 12.50/hour	$15,375
	Weekend attendant care	5/1996	21/2012	6 hours/day, 2 days/week, 52 weeks/year (624 hours)	$7800
	Summer (8 weeks) and school (2 weeks) vacations, miscellaneous holidays (1 week) attendant care	5/1996	21/2012	12 hours/day, 5 days/week, 11 weeks/year (660 hours)	$8250
	Respite care	5/1996	21/2012	Additional 6 hours/day, 2 days/week, 12 weeks/year (144 hours)	$1800

Home/Facility Care After 21, Option 1					
Facility Recommended	**Home Care/ Service**	**Age/Year Initiated**	**Age/Year Suspended**	**Hours/Shifts/ Days of Attendance or Care**	**Base Cost Per Year**
After age 21	Live-in attendant	21/2012	36/2027	Live-in attendant services	$47,450 (based on $130/day)
	Additional costs of a live-in for food and utilities	21/2012	36/2027		$2700
	Sheltered workshop or supported workshop	21/2012	36/2027	Daily for 5 days/week; 50 weeks/ year	$12,500 (based on $50/day)
	Interior/exterior home repairs (assumes own home)	21/2012	36/2027	Regular services	$2100 (based on $40/ week)

Home/Facility Care After 21, Options 2 And 3				
Facility Recommended	**Age/Year Initiated**	**Age/Year Suspended**	**Hours/Shifts/ Days of Attendance or Care**	**Base Cost Per Year**
Option 2				
Group home residential living	21/2012	36/2027	Residential care	$43,800 (based on $120/day)
Day activity/ sheltered workshop	21/2012	36/2027	Day program	$12,500
Option 3				
Long-term residence in nursing facility	21/2012	36/2027	24-hour residential care	$61,000

Comments: A quick glance will point out that this section is "where the money is." Once life expectancy has been calculated, the decisions regarding type and intensity of long-term care are the major variances in the cost of an LCP. Again, controversies abound in this section. How much care does a developmentally disabled child need while at home? Should the parents provide the care? Plaintiffs would argue that if the child were not "injured," he or she would have a much higher level of independence after the first few years of life, and thus the defendant should have extraordinary responsibility to provide for home care. The stresses on any family with a developmentally disabled child are large. How much respite care is reasonable? How many hours after school should be provided for? Secondly, the type of long-term care is an extremely sensitive issue. The option of putting someone in a long-term skilled facility seems less expensive, but advocates for the disabled argue that this is an unsatisfactory setting to care for this population, and that they should be reintegrated into the community. The purpose here is not to settle this controversy, but to emphasize these issues for the reader.

Future Medical Care: Routine

Routine Medical Care Description	Frequency of Visits	Purpose	Cost Per Visit	Cost Per Year
General medicine	2 times/year	Routine care	$60	$120
Physiatrist or orthopedist	1 time/year	Routine care	$60	$60
Neurologist or psychiatrist	4 times/year	Routine care	$60	$240
Dentist	2 times/year	Routine care	$100	$200

Potential Complications

Complication	Estimated Costs	Comments
Contractures	$6600	There is a strong likelihood he may need surgical release of certain lower extremity contractures
Scoliosis	$15,000	He has not developed a significant scoliosis, but there is a distinct possibility in a patient with severe CNS injury
Additional ophthalmological surgery to correct disturbances of extraocular movement	$2000	He has already required two such procedures, and additional difficulties may be anticipated

Comments: Potential complications such as scoliosis surgery or contracture release seem like large expenses. However, because they are one-time costs, they are small in comparison to the cumulative long-term care costs. Surgical and hospitalization costs can be found in a hospital's accounting department or in textbooks. See for example, 1997 Physicians Fee and Coding Guide: A Comprehensive Fee & Coding Reference. *Healthcare Consultants of America, Inc., 609 15 St., Augusta, GA 30901.*

Transportation				
Equipment Description	**Age/Year Purchased**	**Replacement Schedule**	**Base Cost**	**Comment**
Van with wheelchair lift and tie downs	5/1996	1 time/6 years through age 36	$20,000 above the cost of the usual family vehicle	$3333; ends at age 21 if facility option is chosen
Transportation to school	5/1996	175–217 days/year depending on school option	$37.50/trip, totaling $6562–$8137	Paid for by the Livingston School District

Comments: Should the entire wheelchair-accessible van be scheduled, or merely the portion above the usual family car? Note that the costs end at age 21, if the option is to place R. K. in a setting where a van is provided.

Architectural Renovations		
Accessibility Needs	**Costs**	**Total Cost**
Ramping	$500	Anticipated $2000
Fire alarms	$200	
Smoke detectors	$100	
Pavement of rear patio and driveway	$1200	

Leisure Time and/or Recreational Equipment				
Equipment Description	**Special Camps or Programs**	**Age/Year of Purchase or Attendance**	**Replacement or Attendance Schedule**	**Base Cost**
Camping experience: 4 days and 3 nights	Cerebral Palsy of Southwestern Illinois	5/1996	2 times/year (to age 21)	$55/experience plus cost of personal attendant care hours; cost for attendant ~$392, totaling $447/experience and $864/year

Comments: Note that if camp is utilized, the attendant care must be eliminated for that period. This gives the life care planner a variety of combinations that must be considered.

Summary Of Expenses			
Category	**Expense**	**Frequency**	**Lifetime Cost**
Projected Evaluations			
Rehabilitation psychology	$800	Once	$800
Vocational rehabilitation	$1250	Once	$1250
Physical therapy	$75	16	$1200
Occupational therapy	$75	16	$1200
Speech therapy	$150	16	$2400
Rehabilitation engineer	$450	Two occasions	$900
		Subtotal	**$7750**
Projected Therapeutic Modalities			
Family counseling	$1020	3	$3060
Physical therapy	$11,700	10	$117,000
Occupational therapy	$3900	10	$39,000
Speech therapy	$11,700	10	$117,000
Sheltered workshop	$2000	1	$2000
		Subtotal	**$278,060**
Diagnostic Testing and Educational Assessment			
Educational testing	$300	Once	$300
Option 1 vs. Option 2	$22,351.50–$25,926	16	$357,624–$414,816
		Subtotal	**$300–$415,116**
Wheelchair and Maintenance			
Manual wheelchair	$400	31	$12,400
Wheelchair maintenance	$175	31	$5425
Shower chair	$100	31	$3100
Shower chair maintenance	$50	31	$1550
Electric wheelchair	$1640	31	$50,840
Electric wheelchair maintenance	$400	31	$12,400
Backpack	$40	31	$1240
		Subtotal	**$86,955**
Orthopedic and Orthotic			
Tumble form	$240	1	$240
Platform walker	$60	1	$60
Prone stander	$680	1	$680
Helmet	$35	13	$455
AFOs	$400	31	$12,400
Wrist-hand splints	$100	31	$3100
		Subtotal	**$16,935**

Summary Of Expenses *Continued*			
Category	**Expense**	**Frequency**	**Lifetime Cost**
Home Furnishings			
Exercise mat	$20	21	$620
Electric bed	$180	31	$5580
Hoyer lift	$125	31	$3875
Hoyer lift maintenance	$50	31	$1550
		Subtotal	**$11,625**
Aids for Independence			
Environmental control unit	$480	16	$7680
Computer	$600	31	$18,600
Software	$250	31	$7750
		Subtotal	**$34,030**
Drugs and Supplies			
Depakote	$984	31	$30,504
Klonopin	$475	31	$14,725
Phenobarbital	$20	31	$620
		Subtotal	**$45,849**
Home/Facility Care			
Weekday before 21	$15,375	16	$246,000
Weekend before 21	$7800	16	$124,800
Summer	$1800	16	$28,800
		Subtotal	**$399,600**
After 21, Option 1			
Attendant	$40,000	15	$600,000
Additional attendant expenses	$2700	15	$40,500
Sheltered workshop	$12,500	15	$187,500
Home repairs	$2100	15	$31,500
Option 2: Group Home			
Residential setting	$43,800	15	$657,000
Sheltered workshop	$12,500	15	$187,500
Option 3: Long-term center	$61,000	15	$915,000
		Subtotal	**$844,500–915,000**
Future Medical Care			
General	$120	31	$3720
Physiatrist	$60	31	$1860
Neurologist	$240	31	$7440
Dentist	$200	31	$6200
		Subtotal	**$19,220**

Table continued on following page

Summary Of Expenses *Continued*			
Category	**Expense**	**Frequency**	**Lifetime Cost**
Complications			
Contractures	$6600	1	$6600
Scoliosis	$25,000	1	$25,000
Ophthalmological	$2000	1	$2000
		Subtotal	**$33,600**
Transportation			
Van (Option 1)	$3333	31	$103,323
Van (Option 2 or 3)	$3333	15	$49,995
		Subtotal	**$49,995–103,323**
Architectural Renovations	$2000	Once	**$2000**
Camping	$864	15	**$12,960**

As can be seen, the life care budget can be enormous. In this particular plan, the costs vary between $1,828,619 and $2,367,263, depending on the options chosen and assumptions made (e.g., does one include the cost Anytown makes to Another Town School District for educational needs for a developmentally disabled child?).

IV: ADUSTMENT FOR FUTURE COSTS

As mentioned in Table 14–2, the final step in construction of a life care plan is to adjust costs for inflation, cost of living, etc. Generally, unless a physician has a specific credential in business or finance, this is left to a qualified economist or financial planner.

CONCLUSIONS

The construction of an LCP is a simple process; the difficulty is understanding the long-term needs of the patient and predicting future costs with accuracy. An economist or social worker can collect data as to the costs of each of the items cited above and construct an LCP as polished as a physician. Many do just that. The unsettled question is whether a physician who is experienced in life care planning needs for persons with chronic disability can provide a more accurate projection. There is no data available to answer this question, and the opportunity for "abuse" is large. For example, in a recent LCP for a child with cerebral palsy, a plaintiff expert testified that a severely disabled child would have a normal life expectancy, and offered a care plan totaling greater than $13 million. His opinion seems to conflict with the literature reviewed above, and he stated in his deposition that he did not hold the epidemiological data in high regard. Within the civil law arena, however, he is certainly entitled to his opinion. It remains within the arena of the discovery deposition and courtroom testimony for each expert to make a solid case as to the credibility of his or her opinion. If two expert witnesses can offer LCPs on the same patient with totals of $2 million versus $13 million, it would suggest that life care planning has the potential for abuse based on "personal opinion." Although these facts may be discomforting, they should be understood by persons wishing to enter the arena of life care planning.

In summary, this review has attempted to synthesize a large amount of information concerning LCP, and uses CP and MR as a model because they are some of the most complicated LCPs to perform. Several key points summarizing this review include the following:

- An LCP may be a useful construct to plan for and manage the needs of the disabled child with CP or brain injury
- A cost analysis for an LCP depends on the life expectancy of the child, and a careful review of the equipment, psychosocial, therapeutic, medical, nursing, and domiciliary needs of the child
- An LCP must be adjusted for future interest rates and inflation
- A wide variety of support services are available in the public sector, and must be accounted for in the LCP
- Lifespan of the child is curtailed by the presence of certain key disabilities, which are summarized in Table 14–7
- Decreased cognitive abilities are associated with diminished lifespan, even in the absence of physical impairment
- Life expectancy for physically and mentally disabled persons has increased slightly with time
- There was no clear evidence suggesting that institutionalized children had shorter lifespans than those cared for in a noninstitutionalized setting
- Improvements in medical care have not clearly altered the poor prognosis for the most severely disabled children

ACKNOWLEDGEMENTS

Thanks to Mr. Gary Strange for his assistance in the section on services available within the public sector.

REFERENCES

1. American Psychiatric Association: Diagnostic and Statistical Manual of Mental Disorders, 4th ed. Washington, DC, American Psychiatric Association, 1994.
2. Balakrishnan TR, Wolf LC: Life expectancy of mentally retarded persons in Canadian institutions. Am J Mental Deficiency 80:650–662, 1976.
3. Bush GW: Calculating the cost of long-term living: a four-step process. J Head Trauma Rehabil 5:47–56, 1990.
4. Chaney RH, Givens C, Watkins GP, Eyman RK: Birth injury as the cause of mental retardation. Obstet Gynecol 67:771–775, 1986.
5. Cox AD, Lambrenos K: Childhood physical disability and attachment. Dev Med Child Neurol 34:1037–1046, 1992.
6. Crichton JU, Mackinnon M, White CP: Life-expectancy of persons with cerebral palsy. Dev Med Child Neurol 37:567–576, 1995.
7. Deutsch PM: Discharge planning: structuring the home environment. In: Deutsch PM, Fralish KB (eds): Innovations in Head Injury Rehabilitation. Matthew Bender & Co, New York, 1989.
8. Dorland's Illustrated Medical Dictionary, 26th ed. W.B. Saunders Co, Philadelphia, 1981.
9. Dupont A, Vaeth M, Videbach P: Mortality, life expectancy, and causes of death of mildly mentally retarded in Denmark. Upsala J Med Sci (suppl) 44:76–82, 1987.

10. Dussault W: How to keep settlement funds and maintain government benefits. In: The Head Injury Case: What the Trial Lawyer Needs to Know. Southboro, Mass. National Head Injury Foundation, 1989, pp 688–726.
11. Emond A, Golding J, Peckham R: Cerebral palsy in two national cohort studies. Arch Dis Child 64:848–852, 1989.
12. Evans PM, Alberman E: Certified cause of death in children and young adults with cerebral palsy. Arch Dis Child 65:325–329, 1990.
13. Evans PM, Evans SJW, Alberman E: Cerebral palsy: why we must plan for survival. Arch Dis Child 65:1329–1333, 1990.
14. Eyman RK, Grossman H, Chaney R, Call TL: Life expectancy of profoundly handicapped people with mental retardation. New Engl J Med 323:584–589, 1990.
15. Eyman RK, Grossman HJ, Chaney R, et al: Survival of profoundly disabled people with severe mental retardation. Am J Dis Child 147:329–336, 1993.
16. Eyman RK, Olmstead CE, Grossman HJ, Call TL: Mortality and the acquisition of basic skills by children and adults with severe disabilities. Am J Dis Child 147: 216–222, 1993.
17. Forsgren L, Edvinsson SO, Nystrom L, Blomquist HK: Influence of epilepsy on mortality in mental retardation: an epidemiologic study. Epilepsia 87:960–963, 1996.
18. Hallum A, Krumboltz JD: Parents caring for young adults with severe physical disabilities: psychological issues. Dev Med Child Neurol 35:24–32, 1993.
19. Heaton-Ward W: Life expectation of mentally subnormal patients in hospital. Br J Psychiatry 114:1591–1592, 1968.
20. Hutton JL, Cooke T, Pharaoah H: Life expectancy in children with cerebral palsy. Br Med J 309:431–435, 1994.
21. Kaveggia FF: Survival analysis of the severely and profoundly mentally retarded. Am J Med Genetics 21:213–223, 1985.
22. Kokkonen J, Saukkonen AL, Timoenen E, et al: Social outcome of handicapped children as adults. Dev Med Child Neurol 33:1095–1100, 1991.
23. Kuban KCK, Leviton A: Cerebral palsy. New Engl J Med 330:188–195, 1994.
24. Kudrjavcev T, Schoenberg BS, Kurland LT, Groover RV: Cerebral palsy: survival rates, associated handicaps, and distribution by clinical subtype (Rochester, MN 1950-1976). Neurology 35:900–903, 1985.
25. McCurley R, MacKay DN, Scally BG: Life expectation of the mentally subnormal under community and hospital care. J Mental Def Res 16:57–67, 1972.
26. Mutch L, Alberman E, Hagberg B, et al: Cerebral palsy epidemiology: where are we now and where are we going? Dev Med Child Neurol 34:547–551, 1992.
27. Nelson KB, Ellenberg JH: Antecedents of cerebral palsy. New Engl J Med 315: 81–86, 1986.
28. Newacheck PW, Taylor WR: Childhood chronic illness: prevalence, severity and impact. Am J Public Health 82:364–371, 1992.
29. O'Brien KF, Tate K, Zaharia ES: Mortality in a large southeastern facility for persons with mental retardation. Am J Mental Retardation 95:397–403, 1991.
30. Rumeau-Rouquette C, du Mazaubrun C, Mlika A, Dequae L: Motor disability in children in three birth cohorts. Int J Epidemiol 21:359–366, 1992.
31. Simila S, von Wendt L, Rantakallio P: Mortality of mentally retarded children to 17 years of age assessed in a prospective one-year birth cohort. J Mental Def Res 30:401–405, 1986.
32. Strauss D, Eyman RK, Grossman HJ: Predictors of mortality in children with severe mental retardation: effect of placement. Am J Public Health 86:1422–1429, 1996.
33. Strauss D, Kastner K: Comparative mortality of people with mental retardation in institutions and the community. Am J Mental Retardation 101(1):26–40, 1996.
34. Strauss D, Kastner T, Ashwal S, White J: Tubefeeding and mortality in children with severe disability and mental retardation. Pediatrics 99:358–362, 1997.

35. Taylor JS: Neurolaw: towards a new medical jurisprudence. Brain Injury 9:745–751, 1995.
36. Thomas A, Bax M, Coombes K, et al: The health and social needs of physical handicapped young adults: are they being met by statutory services? Dev Med Child Neurol (suppl 50):153–158, 1985.
37. Wolf LC, Wright RE: Changes in life expectancy of mentally retarded persons in Canadian institutions. J Mental Def Res 31:41–59, 1987.

CHAPTER 15

Medicolegal Testimony and the Expert Witness

Richard T. Katz, MD *Richard Z. Freemann, Jr., BS, JD*
Richard P. Bonfiglio, MD

PHYSICIAN AND THE LAW

Physicians may not wish to take part in legal proceedings, but eventually most physicians will do so. Every time a patient is treated and becomes injured or incapacitated, there is the potential that the circumstances giving rise to the injury or the consequences of the injury may lead to litigation. Litigation may be criminal, civil, or administrative, but only civil litigation will be discussed in this chapter. "The Law" is a term referring to the rules controlling litigation.

Physicians may be asked to testify subsequent to the treatment of an injured patient; in this role they normally serve as a *medical fact witness*. Physicians who perform independent medical evaluations (IMEs) are frequently deposed so the findings of an evaluation can be entered into the legal record. Lastly, physicians may be asked to serve in the capacity of an *expert witness*, a setting in which they provide expert testimony (see p. 305). Therefore it behooves most physicians to learn enough about the world of lawyers, depositions, trials, and civil litigation to feel comfortable in the "lawyer's world." Table 15–1 includes a few Latin legal phrases in common usage.

The physician uninitiated as to lawyers and legal proceedings may initially be puzzled by a discipline of thought somewhat foreign to medical training. Physicians are taught to practice medicine within a scientific model. Such a model is generally *collaborative;* involved parties share their data and insight through scientific meetings and publications to develop a cogent understanding of clinical science that is held up as "truth."

The legal model is different, and a brief overview might be helpful. The legal system within the United States is based on precedents from British common law that date back for centuries. The theory of the *adversarial system* is that truth is best ascertained by witnessing the combat of minds, rather than the wisdom of a single Solomon-like judge. Opposing attorneys initially assume antipodal positions, each viewing the client's position as correct. To ferret out the truth, each side of the adversarial process must be able to attack the other as vigorously as possible, a scenario sometimes uncomfortable for the uninitiated physician.

To understand legal concepts more clearly, it would be helpful to provide a clinical scenario to which the physician can relate. Consider a construction worker who was employed by a moderate-sized construction company as a professional carpenter and who was assigned to use a nail gun to join lumber in the process of hanging drywall. Suppose that the nail gun had a safety switch

TABLE 15–1 Commonly Used Latin Phrases Within the Law

Res ipsa loquitur The thing speaks for itself. For example, a negligent act so obvious that an expert witness is not necessary to establish a relationship.

Voir dire Say true. The initial stage of testimony in which the attorney examines the expert witness' qualifications to testify.

In limine motions Motions made before trial seeking the court's ruling on the admissibility of a particular piece of evidence.

Subpoena duces tecum A subpoena requiring the witness to produce documents.

provided to avoid accidental firing of nails, and that the safety feature allegedly malfunctioned. Horribly, a nail was misfired into the carpenter's left leg just below the knee, severing the popliteal artery. The man underwent emergency surgery to repair the vessel and save the limb, but after several attempts, the man underwent a below-knee amputation. The stump healed well, and he was fitted with a below-knee prosthesis with excellent cosmesis and function.

First Steps on the Litigation Trail

The carpenter may decide to sue the manufacturer of the nail gun, and procures the services of a *plaintiff attorney.* Plaintiff attorneys generally work on a contingency basis, with the expectation that they will collect a percentage (perhaps one third) of any judgment or settlement. The plaintiff attorney files a personal injury suit in *civil court* in the proper jurisdiction, and once notified of the suit, a *defense attorney* is procured by the defendant (i.e., the nail gun manufacturer) to defend the case. Defense attorneys, often paid by insurance companies, generally work for an hourly fee.

Civil litigation involves a lawsuit brought by one party seeking monetary damages against another. Physicians most often will be involved in *tort,* or personal injury law suits. A tort is a breech of duty that gives rise to an action for damages. In contrast to a contractual suit, where there is a prior agreement between parties, there is no prior agreement between parties in a tort liability case. There are four critical components in tort liability:

1. A legal duty must exist between the two parties involved
2. There must be a breach of that duty by one party onto the injured party
3. There must be proximate or direct cause
4. There must be harm or damage inflicted onto the injured party

Each lawyer attempts to build a cogent argument to support his view of the case, based on factual data available from witnesses and documentation. Attorneys begin the *discovery* process through a series of elaborate procedural rules to find out about the opposing party's case. Paper discovery involves *interrogatories,* or written questions to which the other party is required to respond in writing and under oath, as well as *requests for production of documents.* For example, the plaintiff attorney may ask the physician to state the substantive facts and opinions about which the physician will be testifying. The attorney may request copies of the incident report of the accident, all medical records and imaging studies, plans for manufacturing the nail gun, instructions for assembly of the tool by the distributor, and safety regulations for worksites regulated by the federal government. Equipment maintenance logs from the employer may be solicited, as well as safety protocols on the work site. Witnesses are interviewed by the plaintiff's attorney to examine the material facts of the case. In addition, it is common in such matters that the technical nature of these circumstances may exceed a lay person's knowledge, and *expert witnesses* may be brought in to offer insight or explanation.

Serving as an Expert Witness

A witness who is qualified as an expert by knowledge, skill, experience, training, or education has the scientific, technical, or specialized knowledge to assist the trier of fact in understanding the evidence or determining a fact in issue. Although treating physicians may be brought in to testify about the care rendered to the patient, physicians may also be asked to serve in an *expert* capacity to discuss prognosis, limitations in work and non-work activities, and also the future costs of medical and prosthetic care (see Chapter 14). Non-physician expert witnesses may also be recruited to discuss the design of the nail gun, workplace safety procedures, prosthetic design, or vocational rehabilitation potential. Attorneys generally seek expert witnesses who will reach a valid conclusion favorable to their case, convey their opinion within the deposition and courtroom setting in an effective manner, and have the necessary credentials and experience to impress the judge and jury.

Expert witness opinions are admissible into courtroom testimony if they are based on *scientific validity*, a controversial concept under constant scrutiny and evolution. The Supreme Court has set a standard for "scientific validity" in the case of *Daubert v. Merrell Dow Pharmaceuticals, Inc.,* 113 S. Ct. 2786 (1993), in which prenatal use of the drug Bendectin was purported to have caused birth defects in newborns. When assessing what is scientifically valid, trial judges generally must determine whether the scientific theory or technique:

1. Has been tested
2. Has been subjected to peer review and publication
3. Has potential for error and what that error rate is
4. Has a standard controlling its operation
5. Has achieved widespread acceptance within the scientific community

Although the concept of scientific validity is complex and left for legal texts to review,[10] the reader should be aware that this volatile subject may be important in his or her own medicolegal testimony. There has been extensive lay and professional press concerning the recent class-action settlement by breast implant manufacturers, which some feel was based on a questionable standard of scientific validity.[3] The American Academy of Neurology and the American College of Physicians (among others) have questioned the quality of medical testimony by expert witnesses and have offered guidelines and suggestions for reform.[1, 2, 8, 9, 11]

When physicians perform an IME as an expert witness, their evaluations should generally meet the following goals:

- Offer a diagnosis and qualify the severity of the condition (e.g., below-knee amputee with excellent fit, appearance, and function)
- Establish *causality* (did "A" cause "B?" Did the nail gun cause the loss of limb?)

- Ensure that necessary tests and treatment have been completed (Are more tests needed to study the vascular supply? Has an optimal prosthesis been formulated?)
- Perform additional tests or treatment if necessary
- State whether the patient has reached maximal medical improvement
- Provide an impairment rating according to the rules of the appropriate jurisdiction (in Missouri, 100% loss of the lower extremity at the level of the knee)
- Assign apportionment (100% caused by the accident with the nail gun)
- Offer permanent restrictions for the patient to return to work (e.g., no climbing ladders, no walking on markedly uneven surfaces, no underwater labor). Generally a physician cannot be sued for negligence if a worker returns to work and is reinjured when following the physician's restrictions, unless the physician made false statements and statements were made recklessly. A second opinion that corroborates the physician's goes a long way toward establishing the credibility of his or her opinion in controversial cases.

Causality

Lawyers are keenly interested in the physician's comment on causality because it is one of the key components of tort liability (see p. 304). To establish causality, the claimant must have a condition or impairment that is a direct result of the event that caused the condition. Although this is quite clear cut when a nail gun severs the popliteal artery, causality is far less obvious with impairments such as soft-tissue pain or low-back pain. U. S. worker's compensation statutes generally require that there be a discrete work-related episode that precipitated the problem before an employee can receive worker's compensation benefits. Yet pain in general, as well as low-back pain, in particular, is widely found in the general population.[4, 5, 7] The implications for physicians who serve as expert witnesses are powerful to consider.

When a physician is asked whether "A" caused "B," he or she must understand that the question has different implications in the lawyer's world than in the physician's. In medicine, cause and effect are viewed in statistical terms, based on analyses of correlation or regression. For example, epidemiologic and interventional studies have shown that smoking and diabetes are major causes or risk factors for coronary artery disease. That is, people who possess these traits have significantly higher risks (both statistically and clinically) for the disease.

The situation is a bit different in civil litigation. When the attorney asks a physician whether "A" caused "B" within a "reasonable degree of medical certainty" (or some very similar language, depending on statutes within that jurisdiction), he or she means, is there a greater than 50% probability that "A" caused "B?" If so, the legal standard for civil proceeding is met, which means that "A" did indeed cause "B." Thus if a physician states a lifting episode *probably* was the cause of the low-back pain (greater than 50% chance), the employer may be fiscally responsible, and worker's compensation benefits will be paid. When the physician states that the episode *possibly* was the precipitant, this would not meet the standard within civil litigation, and the employer would not be responsible. Note also the contrast between civil and criminal proceedings, where the standard of proof is "beyond a reasonable doubt."

The plaintiff's attorney would argue that there was a *legal duty* on the part of the nail gun manufacturer to provide a functioning safety switch that would comply with certain standards within the industry. The malfunction of the safety switch and failure to comply with industry standards was the alleged *breach* of that legal duty. The faulty switch allegedly resulted in the inadvertent expulsion of the nail into the man's leg, which was the *direct or proximate cause* of the popliteal artery tear and eventual amputation. The damages that might be collected for the tort could include *special damages* (medical bills, lost wages, compensation for loss of limb, loss of future earnings because he could no longer climb a ladder to work in construction, future costs of medical and prosthetic care) and *general damages* (commonly referred to as *pain and suffering*).

Tort liability cases may be filed as a result of an intentional act by one party against another (e.g., assault and battery, false imprisonment, malicious prosecution), but most often medicolegal expert testimony will focus on acts of *negligence*. In our example above, the plaintiff attorney would claim that the nail gun manufacturer was negligent for not adhering to industry standards in the design or manufacture of the nail gun's safety switch. Depending on the jurisdiction, the concept of *contributory negligence* or *comparative negligence* may come to bear. The concept of contributory negligence refers to which parties contributed to the negligence for which tort liability has been sought. For example, did the nail gun company manufacture the gun properly? Did the tool supply house forget to assemble the safety switch properly when sold to the contractor? Did the owner of the tool maintain it properly? Did the worker knowingly use the tool other than in the manner for which it was intended? Did the worker read the instruction and safety manual? Were proper safety warnings placed on the tool? In some claims, if the plaintiff was contributorily negligent there will be no recovery.

Comparative negligence refers to the relative contribution of each allegedly negligent party for the damage done. For example, was the manufacturer 100% responsible, or did the worker bear the major share of the responsibility because of misuse of the tool? Was the distributor 0% negligent because the tool was assembled properly prior to sale? The degree of compensatory negligence may reduce the plaintiff's recovery.

INDEPENDENT MEDICAL EXAMINATION AND PHYSICIAN COMMUNICATION

There are unique aspects to IMEs that relate both to patients and attorneys. The physician should be explicitly clear to the patient that this appointment is for evaluation only, and that no ongoing care or treatment will be offered. That is, no physician-patient relationship is to be established. Most health-care attorneys advise the physician to have the patient sign a disclosure explaining the purpose of the IME, and that the patient understands the proceeding is for evaluation purposes only.

When communicating with attorneys about IMEs, physicians should realize that some attorneys may wish to discuss the findings before the physician has committed them to paper. In this way, if the findings do not support the argument of the lawyer who solicited the IME, the physician's opinion may not be discoverable by an opposing attorney. Most physicians believe that there is no ethical dilemma in leaving an IME undictated as long as they are truthful in their opinion, that no physician-patient relationship has been established, and because the physicians are paid for their time and not for their opinion.

Disability-evaluating physicians also should remember that opposing attorneys have the right to request all of your materials related to a particular case, including but not limited to dictations, notes, computer files, pictures, old medical records, bills, and letters between the physician and the attorney who requested the evaluation. Physicians may need to decide if they want to keep preparatory examination notes after they have completed the final dictation, and should be aware that during a deposition they may be questioned by the attorney as to the contents of any notations contained within.

Physicians should also be careful about with which attorney they are communicating. Generally, if a physician was retained as an expert witness, opposing counsel is not permitted to speak with him or her other than in the deposition setting.

ENTERING THE MEDICOLEGAL ARENA

The physician's first entrée into the lion's den may be in the form of a deposition subsequent to the IME. The physician, or any other person who is to be deposed, is summoned to give a deposition through an official legal document called a *subpoena.* A subpoena gives the date, time, and location of the deposition and cannot be ignored without risking sanctions from the court. Subpoenas may also be issued to obtain medical records only. Generally the attorney who subpoenas the physician is responsible for the charges associated with the deposition. Legally, the attorney must pay the physician a minimal witness and mileage fee; however, reasonable hourly fees are customarily paid.

A *discovery deposition* is attended by one or more attorneys representing each of the parties involved in a suit. In the example of the amputee, lawyers representing the nail gun manufacturer, the distributor of the tool, the employer, and the plaintiff all may be present, as well as a court stenographer, who captures each word uttered "on the record" using a shorthand typewriter, and/or a tape recorder. Often, before the deposition, the plaintiff's attorney may discuss the pending deposition with the physician to prepare him or her for the questions and strategies he or she will face. The physician may later be asked to disclose the content of this conversation with the attorney, as well as any previous communications that transpired.

At the onset of the deposition, the court reporter will generally ask the physician to raise his or her right hand and give an oath pledging that the testimony given will be complete and truthful. The opposing attorneys will have decided among themselves an order in which to question (examine) the physician, and this will generally commence with a review of the physician's credentials and experience to determine whether he or she has the right qualifications to be an expert witness in this area. The discovery deposition is how each of the represented parties gains insight into the witnesses' qualifications, views, and knowledge. There is no judge, and the "rules of evidence" do not apply. (Rules 702 through 706 of the Federal Rules of Evidence deal with the admissibility of expert testimony). Evidence (in this case, the physician's opinions) from the discovery deposition can normally be entered into courtroom testimony only if the physician's courtroom and deposition testimony conflict. In other words, the testimony should be consistent. Sometimes, in lieu of appearing in court, an *evidentiary deposition* may be held at the physician's office, where testimony may be videotaped and later shown to the jury. Formal rules of evidence do apply in the evidentiary deposition. After each attorney has had an opportunity to ask questions, the attorney who solicited the opinion may do likewise, after which additional turns may be taken.

At the end of the deposition, the physician will be asked whether he or she wishes to *waive signature,* to which the reply should always be "no." Waiving signature implies that the physician does not wish to read the transcript of the deposition for errors, after which he or she signs his or her name, witnessed by a notary public. Physicians should always ensure that omissions or errors are not present in the deposition transcript that might complicate testimony should a case proceed to trial. An agreement should be made with the attorney that review of court transcripts is billable time for the physician's involvement with the case.

If a case is not settled by the parties, they may proceed with *alternative dispute resolution,* in which an arbitrator (often a retired judge) is given authority by the parties to adjudicate the case, or it may proceed to trial. As an expert witness, a physician may be asked to come to the state or federal court building to offer testimony in the presence of judge and jury.

Preparation for Deposition

Most emphatically, disability-evaluating physicians should make sure each and every IME they perform is thorough, inclusive, and well documented. Physicians should always request that the attorney supply all relevant documents, medical records, and clinical tests. Events that have transpired to date in the case should be accurately summarized, and physicians should precisely note the positive as well as negative features of the history and physical. Conclusions should be clearly delineated at the end of the evaluation report. Dictations should be read carefully before giving testimony, although physicians are normally free to consult any written documentation during testimony. A picture of each patient should be kept in the medical record so a clear and vivid recollection of the patient can be made even though years may have passed since the IME. This can be inexpensively achieved by photocopying a picture identification or driver's license. A well-organized curriculum vitae, which summarizes all of your training, experience, research, publications, organizations, and lectures, should be prepared. Attorneys will be especially interested in those that are pertinent to the present case.

Deposition Testimony

On entering the room where the deposition is held, the physician should introduce himself and find out the name and firm of each attorney present, as well as which party they represent. This may help him or her to understand why certain questions are asked or why they are framed in a certain way. The physician should comport himself or herself with professionalism but not be overly friendly. After the physician is sworn in, the attorneys will begin their questioning. Time should be taken to carefully consider each question an attorney poses. There is a specific reason for each question, and the physician should be comfortable with the answer he or she gives and that the answer is consistent with any testimony that could be given in the future. The physician should wait for the entire question to be asked and to see if his or her attorney wishes to object to the question.

Generally, initial questions will refer to the physician's experience and training, and each attorney will have a copy of the curriculum vitae. The physician should emphasize his or her diversity of experience, which indicates that he or she is neither the cloistered academic within the ivory tower nor the private practice entrepreneur who hasn't followed the literature carefully enough.

Often, physicians will be asked how a patient was referred to them, and how often they have worked for a particular insurance company or attorney in the past. The attorney is attempting to lay groundwork here that the physician's opinion is for hire, and that he or she is dependent on a particular referral source for the success of his or her practice, thereby compromising the physician's objectivity as an expert witness. The physician should emphasize (if true!) that he or she works both for plaintiff and defense attorneys, as well as insurance companies and health maintenance organizations, and that his or her professional skills are offered to any ethical person or firm that requests the services.

When asked just how many cases a physician has worked for each side, he or she might wish to indicate that no such records are kept, if that is the case. Note that attorneys do have access to previous testimony given by a physician through legal search services, so they will know whether a specific physician testifies consistently on certain issues in similar cases. The physician will also be asked how much of his or her income is derived from medicolegal testimony; he or she should answer honestly, but the "golden answer" seems to be around 10%. Physicians who advertise their expert witness services or actively solicit attorneys may have their objectivity undermined for such activities.[6]

The attorneys will ask what the physician's hourly charges are, as well as the fees earned in this particular case. The physician should note to the attorney that he or she is paid for his or her time, not the testimony, and that he or she charges the same fee for all legal services. These legal charges may be somewhat higher than the physician's customary charges, which do not require the level of pressure and expertise needed within the medicolegal arena.

Physicians should keep their answers to the point. The goal of deposition testimony is to avoid damaging admissions. Physicians should not unnecessarily educate opposing counsel in the deposition and should squelch any impulse to be the professor on ward rounds. Although honesty is required, answers should be kept short. It is not the physician's role to point out material that the interrogator has not covered. "Yes" or "no" is an appropriate response to many questions, but the physician should avoid being forced to answer in such a manner when it is inappropriate. For example, in response to "did you stop beating your spouse?" neither response is the correct one.

Physicians should avoid quoting medical literature. Although this may impress colleagues or disciples during ward rounds, it generally is a losing proposition in deposition testimony. By quoting papers, physicians are providing a complementary literature search for opposing counsel. Although a physician may have read thousands of articles in his or her career, these are part of ongoing self-education as a physician, and these papers were not read specifically for today's deposition. Attorneys may ask whether there is a "definitive" source of information within a physician's field of expertise. However, in medicine there is no definitive source of information because all scientific knowledge is in a state of flux and changes with time. The caveat of identifying a certain textbook as definitive is that the physician will then be responsible for defending himself when any page of that work has a statement that may differ from his or her opinion. The physician's knowledge as an expert witness is a distillation of residency and fellowship training, clinical experience, and the large volume of textbooks and articles reviewed during a career.

Particular articles should also not be quoted during courtroom testimony that have not been previously mentioned during deposition. Opposing attorneys may object that such materials had not been previously presented during discovery and thus should be inadmissible as evidence at time of court.

Courtroom Testimony

In the small percentage of cases that do not settle, the physician may be asked to appear before the judge and jury. Scheduling a court appearance has far less flexibility than a deposition, and the physician's charges may reflect the need to block significant periods of time from his or her schedule.

The deposition transcript should be reviewed before trial. The physician should also dress neatly and conservatively. Professionals should look as if they dress for success, but not give the appearance of the avaricious physician who decorates himself or herself with expensive suits and lavish cars. On entering the witness box and after being sworn in, the physician should face the jury and make eye contact, appear confident and sincere, and direct his or her verbal responses to the jury. Delivery should be informational, but not preachy, and the physician may wish to use audiovisual materials. The physician should listen carefully to the questions posed, even if the interchange becomes increasingly heated or impolite. Responses should demonstrate self-control and expertise, but the physician should avoid jargon and information overkill. Facts should be separated from inferences. Physicians should remember that despite all the changes in health care, people still have a great deal of respect for physicians.

Strategies During Interrogation

In contrast to the deposition setting, the physician's courtroom appearance begins with questions from the attorney who requested his or her services. Generally, the physician and attorney have discussed what areas will be covered, and this part of the examination is quite straightforward. Subsequently, some or all of the attorneys who represent other interests in the case may cross-examine the physician, and this part of the proceeding may be more antagonistic. Simply put, the opposing attorney's goal is to minimize the impact or credence of the physician's testimony by attacking his or her credentials, independence, thoroughness, and analysis. Several strategies that may help the physician through a difficult cross-examination include the following:

- *You are the batter. Hit only what is in the strike zone.* Although questions are generally straightforward, it is the attorney's responsibility to pose the question. If the question is grammatically incomprehensible, or contains certain misinformation, it is perfectly permissible for the physician to state that he or she does not understand the question and it should be reframed. Questions may become exceedingly long, to a point it seems that the cross-examining attorney is presenting the expert testimony. The physician should make sure he or she understands the question asked, but should not feel pressured to affirm the diatribe that was just delivered. The physician might state, "if the question was . . . then my response would be . . ."
- *Explain limitations in current knowledge but don't apologize for them.* Medicine does not have the answer for every question that can be posed. For example, "doctor, isn't it true that you cannot make a precise diagnosis of the cause of low back pain in 85% of cases?" The answer could be "Yes,

but the overwhelming number of these are benign musculoskeletal back pain cases and will resolve within days to weeks. With or without adequate medical care, the vast majority of these cases will improve dramatically." However, an expert witness is not an omniscient physician. "I don't know," is a perfectly acceptable response when the answer is unknown.

- *Stick to your guns when you are right.* The physician should not be intimidated or bullied from an opinion when he or she is correct, provided he or she has the knowledge and experience to support it. The physician should be polite but firm; he or she should not get into a fencing match with the attorney, but answer in an objective and straightforward manner. He or she should also know the medical literature that supports the opinion because an experienced attorney may have thoroughly researched the area in which testimony is being given.
- *Beware of certain types of questions.* Constructs that include the words "always" and "never" are dangerous, and physicians should think twice before answering and beware of leading questions that suggest the answer to the question. Hypothetical questions should be carefully evaluated because the physician might not be able to answer a supposition such as the following: "Doctor, if a new leg could be grafted onto this man's lower extremity in the future, what would his disability be?" The answer would depend on whether science progresses to that point in any of our lifetimes, if the graft is successful, and if laws regulating disability evaluation do not change. No one has the knowledge to answer this question adequately. The physician should also beware of summary questions in which the attorney attempts to condense the physician's opinion into a sound bite that may not accurately convey the meaning of his or her testimony.
- *Keep control of your responses.* The physician should explain the entire opinion, even if he or she is interrupted. The physician has the right to answer completely, although at times it might not seem so. Yes or no questions should be answered only when they are appropriate. The physician should know his or her limitations. If the attorney asks, "Doctor, if this gentleman who suffered a below-knee amputation were trained as a sales clerk, is it likely he could return to work?" most physicians would feel comfortable responding in the affirmative. However, if the question is, "Doctor, from what percentage of the work force is this amputee now excluded?" and the physician is not a vocational rehabilitation specialist or does not have the experience to answer within an expert capacity, the question should be deferred as "outside my field of expertise." Physicians should take care if the attorney twists a previous response and uses that distortion as a basis for a succeeding question. The physicians should respond firmly if his or her opinion was misstated.
- *Maintain your credibility.* In an effort to diminish the weight of the physician's testimony, attorneys may utilize several strategies. Physicians may be asked how long they spent in each aspect of their chart review, history, and physical examination or the attorney might say "Doctor, can you really develop any kind of valid opinion as to this man's future employability based on the 1-hour contact you had with my client?" Physicians should explain that they are not able to accompany each patient for a week-long period of observation, and that generally a 1- to 2-hour evaluation does permit them to make reliable and valid observations about a patient and to draw conclusions from such observations. Physicians may be painted as a "hired gun" whose opinions are for sale. They should answer such ques-

tions as they did in the deposition testimony (discussed earlier). Most importantly, physicians should remember that they are serving as expert witnesses and it is their job to testify; it is the lawyer's job to win the case. If a question undermines the argument for the physician's side, it should be answered simply and honestly. A jury will recognize when a physician makes extraordinary contortions in response to a straightforward question.

- *Wait for objections before answering questions.* As in deposition testimony, attorneys have an opportunity to object before the physician answers the question posed. Rules of evidence generally preclude *hearsay,* in which a person's testimony includes the statements of others, rather than his or her own opinion. *Badgering the witness* refers to the "roughing up" of witnesses in the witness box by the attorney, and may prompt an objection from the adversary. An objection of *asked and answered* refers to an interrogation strategy in which the cross-examining attorney will attempt to ask witnesses the same question many times in subtly different ways in the hope that they might contradict themselves. Within limits, physicians should not have to answer the same question repeatedly. An objection of *irrelevant* refers to questions that do not pertain to the case, and the judge decides whether such questions are irrelevant or not. Questions concerning the income of the expert witness may fall into a gray area as to their relevance to the case. *Leading the witness* is another strategy ripe for objection, in which the attorney feeds questions to the witness to obtain responses favorable to his or her argument. Again, the judge decides whether such objections are approved (sustained) or disapproved (overruled).

SUMMARY

Most physicians will at some time need to offer testimony in a deposition as fact witnesses for patients they have treated. Some physicians will also choose to offer their services as expert witnesses to attorneys and insurers. Physicians who wish to make IME a significant part of their medical practice need a familiarity with the rules of law to serve as a successful consultant. Expert witnesses must have experience and training that serve as a foundation for their opinion. They must perform evaluations that are comprehensive and authoritative and support their conclusions. Expert witnesses must convey their opinions effectively and must exhibit confidence and professionalism within the deposition and courtroom settings. Physicians who serve as witnesses for both plaintiff and defense attorneys are better able to maintain a balanced perspective, as well as credibility within the medicolegal community.

REFERENCES

1. American Academy of Neurology: Qualifications and guidelines for the expert witness. Neurology 39:9A, 1989.
2. American College of Physicians: Guidelines for the physician expert witness. Ann Intern Med 113(10):789, 1990.
3. Angell M: Shattuck lecture: evaluating the health risks of breast implants: the interplay of medical science, the law, and public opinion. N Engl J Med 334(23): 1513–1518, 1996.
4. Ford CV: Dimensions of somatization and hypochondriasis. Neurol Clin 13(2): 241–253, 1995.

5. Gureje O, von Korff M, Simon GE, et al: Persistent pain and well-being: WHO study in primary care. JAMA 280:147–151, 1998.
6. Kunin CM: Expert witness in medical malpractice litigation. Ann Intern Med 100: 139–143, 1984.
7. Linton SJ, Hellsing AL, Hallden K: Population based study of spinal pain among 35–45 year old individuals: prevalence, sick leave, and health care use. Spine 23: 1457–1463, 1998.
8. Martensen RL, Jones DS: Expert medical testimony: opinions, conflicts of interest and the court's quest for the 'truth.' JAMA 273(20):1707, 1997.
9. Omenn GS: Enhancing the role of the scientific expert witness. Environ Health Persp 102:674–675, 1994.
10. Piorkowski JD: Medical testimony and the expert witness. In: Sanbar SS, Gibofsky A, Firestone M, LeBlang TR (eds): Legal Medicine, 3rd ed. Mosby, St. Louis, 1995.
11. Weintraub MI: Expert witness testimony: time for self-regulation? Neurology 45: 855–858, 1995.

ADDITIONAL READINGS

American College of Legal Medicine Foundation: Medicolegal Primer. 1200 Centre Avenue, Pittsburgh, PA 15219, 1992.

Baldwin S: Art of Advocacy: Direct Examination. Matthew Bender, New York, 1985.

Besford HR: Physician as expert witness. In: Sanbar SS, Gibofsky A, Firestone M, LeBlang TR (eds): Legal Medicine, 3rd ed. Mosby, St. Louis, 1995.

Demeter SL, Andersson GBJ, Smith GM: Disability evaluation. Mosby, St. Louis, 1996.

Gordon EJ: Independent medical evaluations. Ortho Review 14:109–114, 1985.

Poynter D: What to tell your expert about cross-examination. Missouri Lawyer's Weekly 10/22/90.

Quinn NK: How to give a deposition. Orthop Review 15:94–96, 1986.

INDEX

Page numbers in italics indicate illustrations; *t* indicates tables.

C

D

E

R

S

T

U

V

W